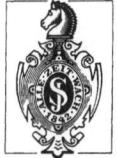

K. Hirohata · K. Mizuno
T. Matsubara (Eds.)

Trends in Research and Treatment of Joint Diseases

With 112 Figures, Including 4 in Color

Springer-Verlag
Tokyo Berlin Heidelberg
New York London Paris
Hong Kong Barcelona

KAZUSHI HIROHATA, M.D.
KOSAKU MIZUNO, M.D.
TSUKASA MATSUBARA, M.D.
Department of Orthopedic Surgery
Kobe University School of Medicine
Chuo-ku, Kobe, 650 Japan

ISBN 978-4-431-68194-6   ISBN 978-4-431-68192-2 (eBook)
DOI 10.1007/978-4-431-68192-2

On the front cover: Electron micrograph of shadow-cast of lesion in tendon, see Fig. 4/p. 54, and Fixation of the osteotomized site, see Fig. 2/p. 87.

Typesetting: Best-set Typesetter Ltd., Hong Kong

Preface

A half century ago, orthopedic surgeons needed to specialize in only the pathophysiology and treatment of the neuromuscular and skeletal systems in order to treat patients. However, since then, surprising progress has been made in medicine, and through the limitless avenues for research orthopedics is now divided into many subspecialities, with terms such as orthopedic pathology, orthopedic oncology, orthopedic rheumatology, and orthopedic traumatology becoming commonplace. Interdisciplinary studies in this and other related fields are now indispensible. As a result, the half-life of the information accumulating yearly has been estimated at five years. In times such as these, if one stubbornly adheres to treatment alone, progress comparable to that in other fields will not be made. If one opens an orthopedic textbook, it is easy to see that there are still many diseases of undetermined etiology; in the last quarter of a century, there has been no evidence of even of these diseases' etiology having been resolved internationally. This is a direct result of the ineptitude of basic orthopedic research. Therefore, recently in the United States, Japan and Canada, orthopedic research institutes and associations have been established, and SIROT has been organized internationally.

This book contains the manuscripts presented by international and Japanese speakers at the 5th Annual Meeting of the Orthopedic Research Society of the Japanese Orthopedic Association, and the Second International Cherry Blossom Conference of Rheumatology. The speakers included not only orthopedic surgeons also but rheumatologists, bio-engineers, chemists, anatomists, and immunologists of international reknown. The gathering of speakers of this calibre, the level of interdisciplinary approach, and a book such as this presenting their findings is surely a first. I recommend this book highly to the new generation of orthopedic surgeons, for the reason that orthopedic basic research should not be the sole domain of Ph.Ds (chemists, immunologists, and bioengineers). Basic research is an essential part of becoming of a leading orthopedic surgeon; it is a basic aspect. On the occasion of the publication of this book, I would like to thank the staff members of Springer-Verlag for their dedication and support.

KAZUSHI HIROHATA
Chairman of Orthopedic Surgery
Kobe University School of Medicine
Kobe, Japan

Contributors

Contents

Part III: Miscellaneous Conditions in Orthopaedics

Part I. Pathogenesis of Joint Diseases

Changes in the Extracellular Matrix of Articular Cartilage in Human Osteoarthritis

A. Robin Poole, G. Rizkalla, A. Reiner, M. Ionescu[1], and E. Bogoch[2]

Summary. Articular cartilage is carefully organized to provide an articulating surface that provides almost frictionless movement and the ability to absorb and dissipate compressive load and resist tensile forces. The cartilage is organized into zones, the structures of which reflect the mechanical forces acting upon the cartilage. Type II collagen, together with type IX and type XI collagens, forms a fibrillar network throughout the matrix which is secreted by the chondrocytes. The large aggregating proteoglycans and the smaller proteoglycans interact directly or indirectly with this fibrillar network. The collagen and the proteoglycans can be degraded by metalloproteinases produced by the chondrocytes. In osteoarthritis, early damage to the collagen fibrillar network is seen at the articular surface and in the upper mid-zone. It is accompanied by a local loss of the large aggregating proteoglycan and small proteoglycans. Large proteoglycans exhibit degradative changes at this stage. With further progression of disease, fibrillation of cartilage occurs and proteoglycans are lost and replaced by larger more intact molecules with different glycosaminoglycan chains. Collagen damage now extends throughout the cartilage. There are also significant changes in the organization of the small proteoglycans, decorin and biglycan, in the osteoarthritic cartilage. Overall, a major reorganization of proteoglycans occurs with net collagen damage. We now know which proteases degrade both the collagen and the proteoglycan and how their synthesis, secretion and activity may be stimulated. The arthritis probably results from a mechanical stimulation of protease activity with impaired collagen fibril assembly although proteoglycan synthesis continues actively. Thus, the key to the survival of the cartilage is the protection and preservation from damage of the inact type II collagen fibrillar network. Clearly, there is no evidence of impaired proteoglycan synthesis, but retention of proteoglycans is prevented when collagen is damaged.

Key words. Cartilage — Osteoarthritis — Proteoglycans — Collagen — Proteinases

Introduction

General Organization of the Collagen Fibrillar Network and Cartilage Proteoglycans

Articular cartilage, lubricated by synovial fluid, provides almost frictionless articulation in a diarthrodial joint. The collagen fibrillar network (Fig. 1), composed of type II collagen, to which type IX and type XI collagens are bound, [1,2] endows cartilage with its strength and hence its tensile properties. Its organization reflects the mechanical forces which act upon the cartilage: ranging from predominantly shear forces at the articular surface, where fibrils are thin and are aligned parallel to the articular surface, to compressive forces within the cartilage in the mid and deep zones (Fig. 2). Here, the fibrils are thicker and arranged in a more random manner although there is evidence for the arcading of fibrils, originally described by Benninghoff [3] and confirmed by others [4]. The calcified cartilage (Fig. 2) acts as an intermediate zone,

[1] Joint Diseases Laboratory, Shriners Hospital for Crippled Children, Division of Surgical Research, Department of Surgery, McGill University, Toronto, Ontario, Canada
[2] Division of Orthopaedics, Department of Surgery, Wellesley Hospital, Toronto, Ontario, Canada

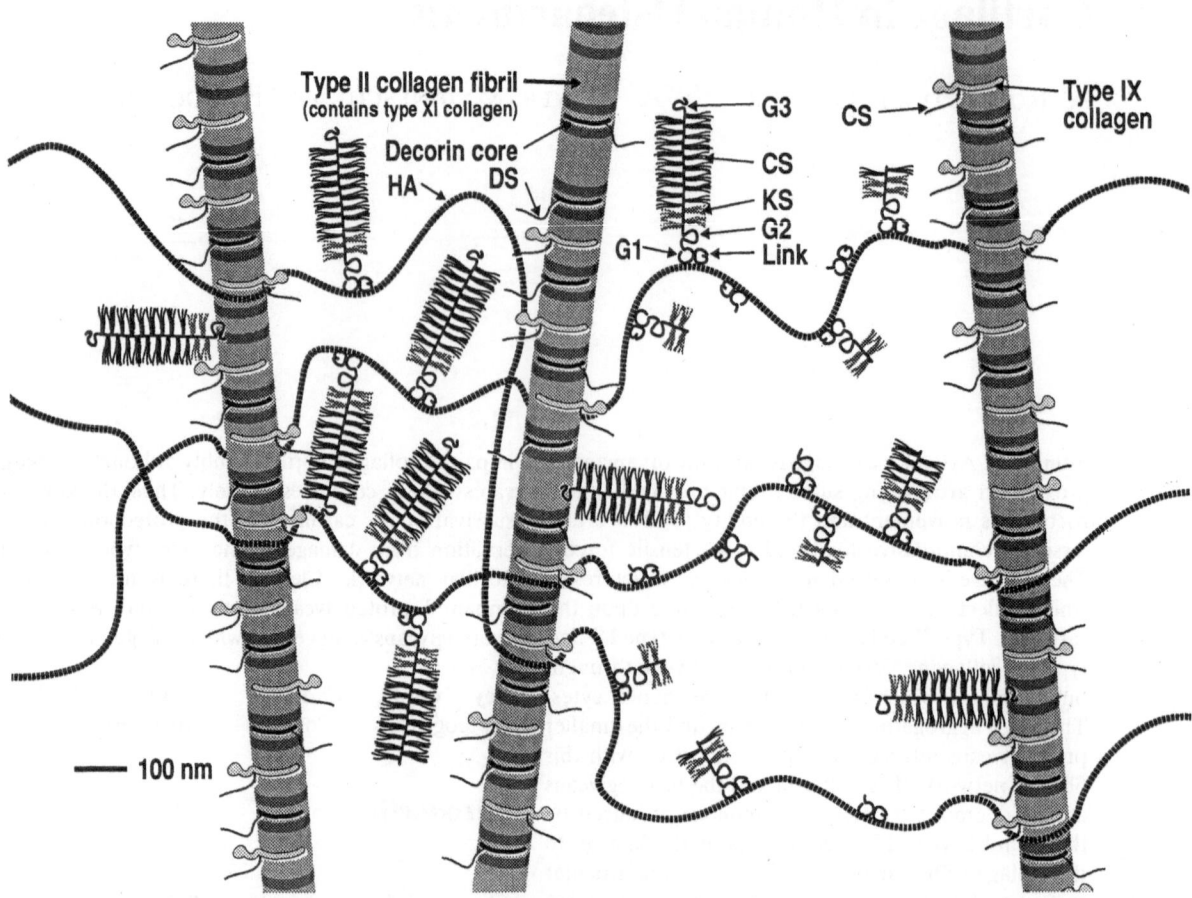

Fig. 1. Organization of type II collagen fibrils, containing type IX and type XI collagen, and aggregating proteoglycans that bind to hyaluronic acid in the extracellular matrix of adult articular cartilage. Hyaluronic acid (*HA*) interacts directly or indirectly with collagen fibrils in a periodic manner as shown by Poole et al. [32]. It may bind to the basic NC4 domain of type IX collagen (shown as a globular terminal component). This collagen is covalently bound to and has a periodic distribution on type II collagen. Decorin also binds to type II collagen though its core protein [33] in a periodic manner. Its single dermatan sulfate chain (*DS*) is shown. Biglycan, which is co-distributed with decorin, (AR Poole, A Reiner, M. Ionescu and PJ Roughley, manuscript in preparation, see Fig. 3) is not shown but it may also be bound to type II collagen. Intact aggrecan molecules contain a G3 globular domain at the C-terminus. They are attached to HA via a globular N-terminal domain called G1. The G2 and G3 globular domain have no known function. Keratan sulfate (*KS*) and chondroitin sulfate (*CS*) are bound to core protein as shown. Link protein stabilizes the interaction of G1 with HA. Degradation products of aggrecan are shown that remain bound to HA via the functional G1 domain. These proteoglycans can bind 50 times their weight of water, leading to hydration of the extracellular matrix. In reality this hydration is limited by the collagen fibrillar network. As a result these molecules exhibit a swelling pressure which endows cartilage with its compressive stiffness. The figure is drawn approximately to scale. (From [32], with permission).

sitting between the uncalcified articular cartilage of the deep zone (bounded by the tidemark) and the subchondral bone. It appears to be formed by a process of endochondral ossification but normally remains uninvaded by capillaries. In osteoarthritis capillary invasion of the calcified zone and of the tidemark occurs in more advanced disease.

The cellular organization of adult articular cartilage also reflects the differences in biomechanical properties, structure, and metabolism. At the articular surface, the cells are

Fig. 2. Organization of articular cartilage into different zones and regions. (Modified from [32])

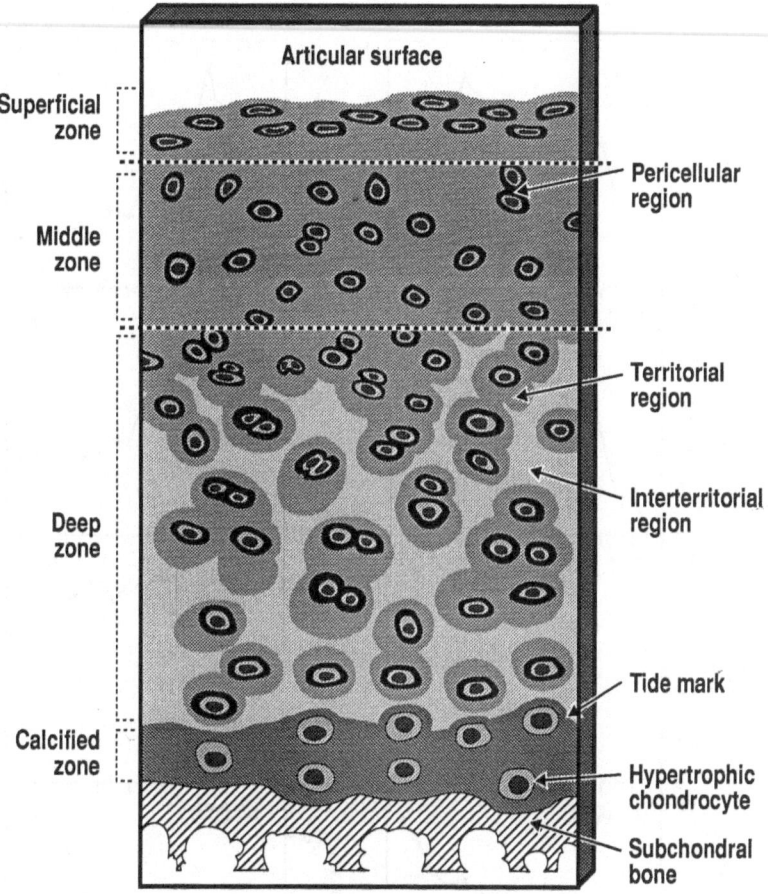

flattened as a result of the shear and compressive forces acting upon them. Here the content of the large aggregating proteoglycan (called aggrecan) is at its minimum (Fig. 3). But attached to these more superficial fibrils is a small proteoglycan called decorin [5] which is most concentrated at and just under the articular surface (Fig. 3). Another small proteoglycan called bigylcan or PG I [5] is also concentrated here (Fig. 3) and may also be attached to collagen fibrils.

In the mid-zone, the cells are rounded and cell density is higher than in the deep zone. The matrix is richly endowed with aggregating proteoglycans, which are distributed throughout the matrix.

In the deep zone of cartilage, cell density is at its lowest [6]. The aggregating proteoglycans are mainly concentrated in the narrow pericellular and the broad territorial domains that surround these cells (Fig. 2). Comparatively little proteoglycan is detectable in the interterritorial matrix of the deep zone in adult human articular cartilage. Surprisingly, however, the concentration of these proteoglycans is at its greatest in the deep zone (Fig. 3). This means that the majority of these molecules are highly concentrated in the deep zone of the cartilage in the pericellular and territorial domains. In contrast, the content of the small proteoglycans, biglycan and decorin, is low in the deep zone (Fig. 3), where collagen fibril diameters are largest and where interfibrillar space is very limited in adult human articular cartilage.

The structure of the large aggregating proteoglycan (aggrecan) is shown in Fig. 1. These proteoglycans endow cartilage with its compressive stiffness and ability to dissipate load. Their presence also protects collagen fibrils from mechanical damage. When they are normally present in low concentration, as at the articular surface (Fig. 3), the small proteoglycans, decorin and biglycan, replace them. These large proteoglycans undergo progressive damage within the extracellular matrix. Consequently,

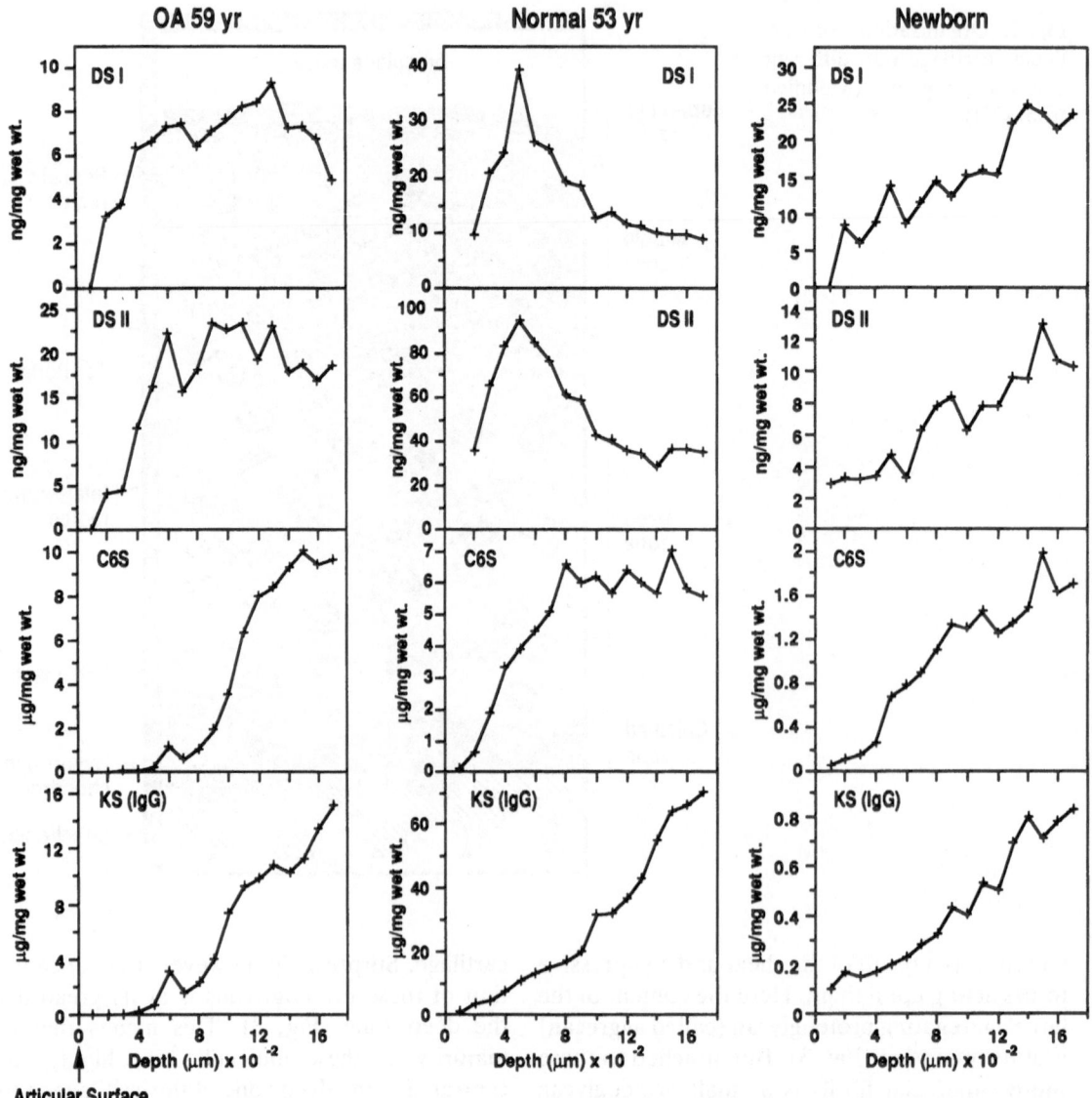

Fig. 3. Distribution of aggregating proteoglycans containing chondroitin 6-sulfate (*C6S*) and keratan sulfate (*KS*) and the proteoglycans decorin (*DSII*) and biglycan (*DSI*) in healthy newborn, adult and osteoarthritic human articular cartilage. In normal cartilage aggrecan is concentrated in the deep zone. In contrast, decorin and biglycan are most concentrated close to the articular surface (*AS*). There is an altered distribution of biglycan and decorin in osteoarthritic cartilage compared with that seen in normal cartilage. This altered distribution resembles move that seen in newborn cartilage. The distribution of aggrecan is unchanged and is the same in all cartilages. Concentrations of biglycan and decorin are expressed as equivalents of synthetic peptides used in the radioimmunoassays. Each peptide, which is approximately 1/20th the size of the intact secreted core protein, is approximately 20 residues long. Contents of aggrecan (C6S and KS) are based on equivalents of intact adult human aggrecan. (A.R. Poole, A. Reiner, M. Ionescu, E. Bogoch, L.C. Rosenberg, and P.J. Roughely, unpublished work). (From [34], with permission)

various degradation products can be identified which are mainly represented by a keratan sulfate-rich fragment and a free hyaluronic acid-binding region. These are retained in the extra-

cellular matrix, in part because they retain their ability to bind to hyaluronic acid through their G1 domain (Fig. 1). Fragments of these proteoglycans are released into synovial fluid.

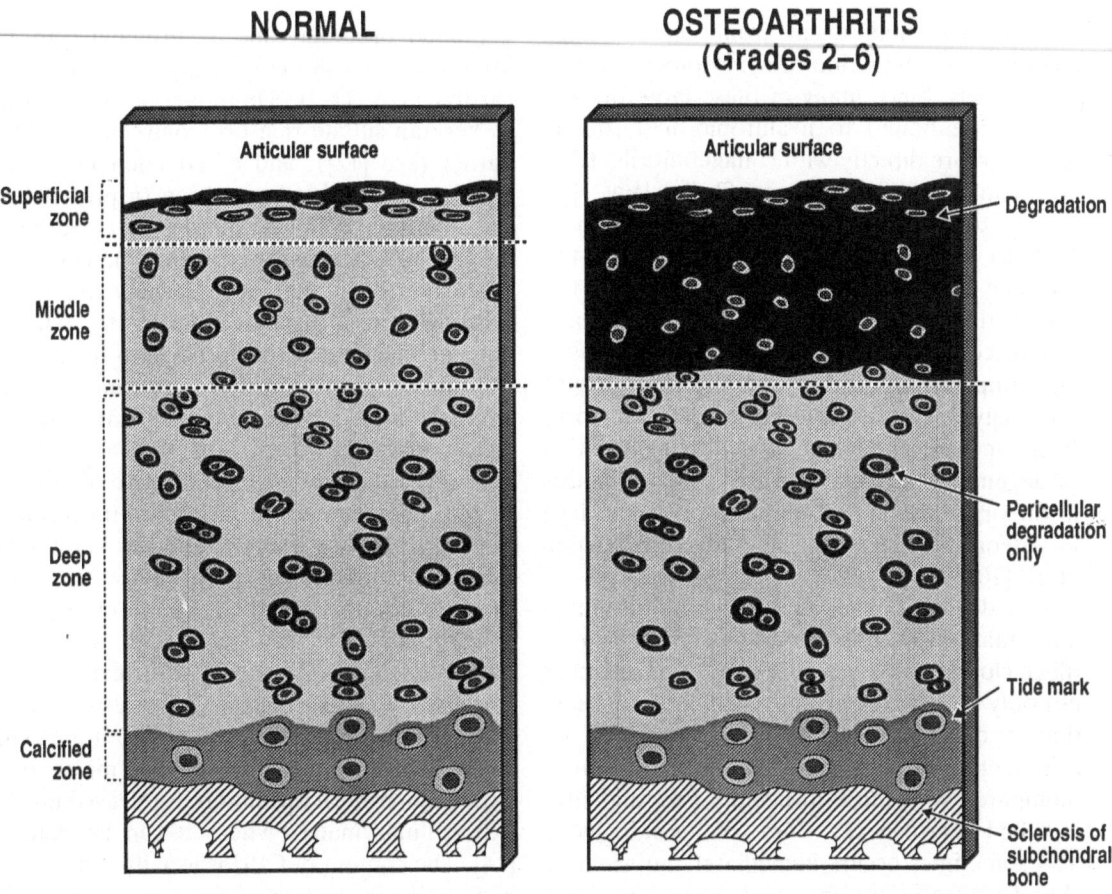

Fig. 4. Sites of degradation (in black) of type II collagen in normal and early (grades 2–6) osteoarthritic cartilages, to reveal pathological damage to collagen in the superficial and mid zones. Pericellular degradation is normally seen in healthy cartilage. Results are a summary of those of Dodge and Poole [8]. (From [34], with permission)

These fragments consist of different molecular species derived from the chondroitin sulfate and keratan sulfate-rich regions, in addition to the G1 domain [7].

Molecular Changes in the Extracellular Matrix in Osteoarthritis: Evidence for Increased Degradation of Collagen and Proteoglycan and Changes in Synthesis and Reorganization of These Molecules in the Extracellular Matrix

Early osteoarthritis is recognizable as a roughening and degeneration of the articular surface, characterized by fibrillation of superficial cartilage. Splits appear which subsequently extend into the mid and the deep zones. This fissuring and fibrillation occurs as a result of damage to the network of collagen fibrils in the superficial

and upper mid zones early in the disease process (Fig. 4). This was demonstrated recently using antibodies that react only with collagen in which the triple helix has unwound as a result of damage caused by mechanical and/or enzymatic forces [8]. As a result of this damage, the integrity of the network is violated and its strength is lost. It becomes susceptible to mechanical rupture; matrix splitting and degeneration develop. Associated with this damage to the fibrillar network is a loss from the upper zones of cartilage of the small proteoglycans, decorin and biglycan (Fig. 3) which may both interact with collagen fibrils. With damage to the fibrils, it is likely that these proteoglycans lose their ability to bind to collagen, at least in the case of decorin. Moreover, some aggrecan may be lost from the upper parts of the cartilage, but it becomes concentrated in the deep zone (Fig.

3). This loss may result from fibril damage reducing the interaction of hyaluronic acid with those fibrils. Since many of these large proteoglycans are bound to hyaluronic acid (others interact more directly with collagen fibrils, (Fig. 1]), damage to the collagen fibrils, [Fig. 1]), damage to the collagen fibrillar network not only leads to a loss of the tensile properties of the cartilage [9], but also leads to a loss of the aggregating proteoglycans that provide cartilage with its compressive stiffness and ability to resist the compressive forces within the joint. These proteoglycans also protect the collagen fibrils from mechanical damage caused by articulation of degenerate articular surfaces. These changes in the organization and composition of cartilage in osteoarthritis have been graded by Mankin et al. [10].

This degradation of proteoglycans, although most marked in those regions of articular cartilage closest to the articular surface, is reflected not only by a loss of proteoglycan in these sites, that is detected histochemically, but also by a reduction in the sizes of these molecules (compared with those in healthy age- and site-matched cartilages). Loss of proteoglycan also sometimes occurs immediately adjacent to chondrocytes in the mid and deep zones and is indicative of an active degradative process which, in this case, is probably enzymatic in nature. This occurs in cartilages of Mankin grades 2–6.

As the disease progresses to greater than Mankin grade 6, so the damage to the type II collagen network and the fissuring of the cartilage extends deeper and are more pronounced. In advanced disease, there is a net loss of proteoglycan from the cartilage, not only locally, but also in other areas, such as at the surface. Earlier in the disease there is no evidence for a net loss of proteoglycan from all the cartilage: the loss is mainly local, restricted to regions at and close to the articular surface. The content of these molecules increases in the lower, mid and deep zones to compensate for this local loss. In advanced disease (grades 9–13), however, there is a net loss of proteoglycan throughout the cartilage; this is accompanied by a loss of hyaluronic acid [11]. Examination of the molecular sizes of these molecules in more advanced disease (greater than grade 6) reveals, however, that there is extensive replacement of

degraded proteoglycans by proteoglycans that are larger than those normally found in healthy cartilage (see [12]). There is a reduced content of keratan sulfate-rich proteoglycans, as shown earlier (see [12]), and a reduction in the free hyaluronic acid-binding region (a proteoglycan degradation product which is retained by its binding to hyaluronic acid) (Fig. 1). The loss of hyaluronic acid that accompanies the loss of proteoglycan is probably due to the extensive damage throughout the cartilage to the collagen fibrillar network to which hyaluronic acid and aggrecan are directly and/or indirectly attached.

The larger proteoglycans that are retained have a changed chemistry indicative of new synthesis. They contain less chondroitin 6-sulfate, more chondroitin 4-sulfate and less keratan sulfate, as in fetal cartilage [12]. They exhibit structural differences in their chondroitin sulfate chains which are detectable with monoclonal antibodies [13]. There is also evidence for increased type II collagen synthesis. The C-propeptide of the type II procollagen molecule, which is used to align procollagen molecules in extracellular fibril formation, is released into the extracellular matrix where it can be detected [14]. The content of CPII is usually considerably increased in osteoarthritis, indicating that type II collagen synthesis is increased [14]. This increase is seen mainly in the mid and deep zones where most of the aggregating proteoglycans are found.

The small proteoglycans, decorin and biglycan, both decrease in content at the articular surface and in the upper zone, but increase in content in the deeper layers (Fig. 3). Their distribution is the reverse of that found in adult normal cartilage and resembles that found in the fetus. Thus in osteoarthritis, before overt degeneration sets in with deep fibrillation, most synthesis appears to be concentrated in the deeper half of the cartilage matrix, while degradation is concentrated in the superficial half of the matrix. This degradation then spreads to and involves collagen in the deeper half.

How is Cartilage Degraded in Osteoarthritis?

Damage to the type II collagen fibrils is a pivotal event in cartilage degradation. This is because

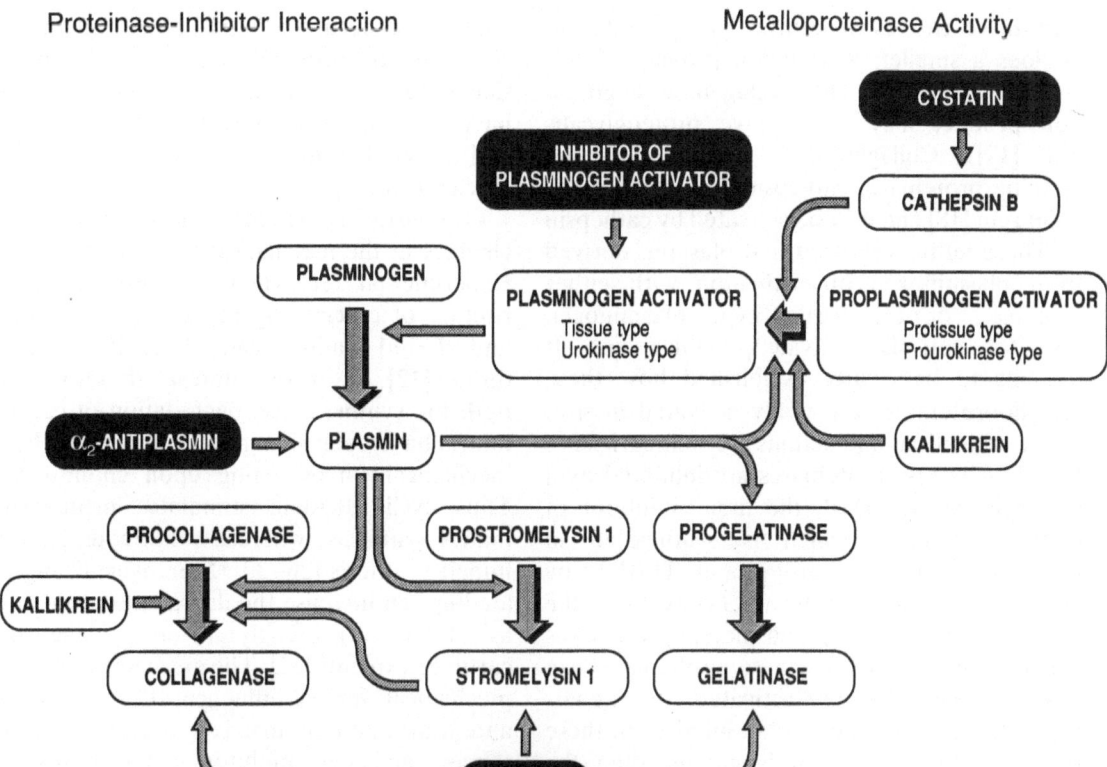

Fig. 5. The proteinases involved in the degradation of cartilage matrix and the regulation of their activities. The metalloproteinases, collagenase and stromelysin, can degrade type II collagen. Stromelysin can also degrade types IX and XI collagens and the proteoglycan aggrecan. Gelatinase cleaves denatured type II collagen α chains. TIMP is the tissue inhibitor of metalloproteinases: there are two kinds, TIMP 1 and 2. Other proteinases involved in the activation of latent prometalloproteinases are shown together with their inhibitors. (From [34], with permisson)

the fibrillar organization is not only responsible for the strength of cartilage (and other soft connective tissues such as skin, tendons, ligaments, and the sclera of the eye) but also because it acts, as indicated above (Fig. 1), as the framework about which the rest of the cartilage matrix molecules are organized.

Type II collagen can be cleaved in its triple helical domain by only one enzyme, which is called collagenase. This is one of three types of metalloproteinases (Fig. 5) which are synthesized and secreted as latent proenzymes. Collagenase can be fully activated outside the cell by another metalloproteinase called stromelysin which is probably primarily responsible for the degradation of cartilage proteoglycans, including decorin, and type II collagen attached to collagen fibrils. Stromelysin can also cleave

type II collagen in its non-helical N-telopeptide region close to where type IX collagen is covalently attached [15]. Therefore, stromelysin is a very potent enzyme. The relative involvement of collagenase versus stromelysin in the damage caused to type II collagen in osteoarthritis remains to be established. However, recent studies of adult human articular cartilages have revealed that, compared with the mRNA for collagenase, the concentration of mRNA for stromelysin is much increased in cartilage undergoing degradation [16]. Moreover, these authors also found that interleukin-1 stimulates a much larger increase in stromelysin mRNA. This may indicate that of these two proteinases, stromelysin is synthesized and secreted in greater quantities. A third metalloproteinase called gelatinase makes up this trio of enzymes.

Gelatinase cleaves denatured type II collagen, as does a smaller degradation product of collagenase (Fig. 5). This collagenase degradation product may also cleave proteoglycans (see [17]). Collagenase is activated by the cysteine proteinase, cathepsin B, as well as by kallikrein [18] and may be activated by cathepsin L. These authors showed that plasmin, derived from plasminogen on activation with either urokinase or the tissue- type plasminogen activator, can also activate procollagenase. It remains to be clearly established how these metalloproteinases are really activated in situ. These activations and actions are summarized in Fig. 5. All these proteinases are inhibited by a molecule called TIMP, the tissue inhibitor of metalloproteinases which is synthesized in two distinct forms, TIMP1 and TIMP2, by chondrocytes, as well as by other cells. Thus, the balance between TIMP and metalloproteinases will determine whether these proteinases can function, once they are activated. In osteoarthritis there is evidence for an increase in these metalloproteinases which is greater than the increase observed for TIMP, indicating the potential for net proteinase activity [19,20]. A recent review by one of the authors [17] should be consulted for a general review of proteolytic involvement in cartilage degradation in arthritis.

The transcription of these proteinases and of their inhibitors are, however, differently regulated. Transforming growth factor-β (TGF-β) can stimulate the synthesis of TIMP in fibroblasts but down regulates synthesis of metalloproteinases [17]. Interleukin-1 α and β can stimulate both TIMP and metalloproteinase synthesis [17]. It is not known whether the limited intra-articular inflammation observed in osteoarthritis may result in the production of sufficient interleukin-1 to influence the metabolism of chondrocytes. Like interleukin-1, tumor necrosis factor α also stimulates the synthesis of these proteinases and their inhibitor.

Chondrocytes can also produce significant quantities of hydrogen peroxide [21]. Since free radicals, such as the hydroxyl radical, can be produced from hydrogen peroxide, for example, by transition metal catalysis in the Fenton reaction [22], these free radicals may cause degradation of proteoglycans and link proteins. They have been shown to be capable of degrad-

ing these molecules in vitro [23,24]. Site-specific cleavages of proteoglycans and link protein that occur in ageing human articular cartilage have been ascribed in part to stromelysin [25] and may also involve free radical-mediated mechanisms.

Osteoarthritis is thought to result from changes in the mechanical loading of cartilage. Experimental removal of meniscal cartilages, rupture of cruciate ligaments, joint instability, and altered loading, can all result in osteoarthritis [12]. It is of interest, therefore, that both the synthesis and degradation of cartilage matrix have been shown to be influenced by the mechanical forces acting upon chondrocytes. Thus cyclic loading stimulates proteoglycan matrix synthesis, whereas continuous load can impair synthesis [26–30]. Moreover, changes in loading can increase the degradation (measured as release) of proteoglycans and collagen from cartilage explants [31]. The mechanisms whereby mechanical forces influence the transcription and translation of matrix molecules and proteinases and their inhibitors is not known.

Conclusions

The changes that occur within articular cartilage in human osteoarthritis reflect a response of this tissue to changing environmental factors. Altered articulation can result in degenerative changes in spite of continued synthesis. It is believed that chondrocytes are pre-programmed to respond to normal articulation. Their responses to changes in articulation result in an imbalance between synthesis and degradation.

Recent studies have revealed that in the early disease process (Mankin grades 2–6), evidence of degradation is most apparent at and close to the articular surface. Here, collagen fibrils are damaged and the proteoglycan aggrecan and the smaller proteoglycans are lost. In contrast, synthesis of new larger aggrecan molecules occurs. These contain different structures in their glycosaminoglycan chains which can be detected by monoclonal antibodies. The small proteoglycans, decorin and biglycan, are lost from superficial cartilages and appear in the deep zone. There is also evidence for increased type II collagen synthesis.

The newly synthesized proteoglycans and

collagen seem most concentrated in the deeper layer of the cartilage closer to the calcified layer. Thus, as the more superficial cartilage degenerates, the deeper layers regenerate. Later the degenerative process involves all the cartilage and, with extensive damage to collagen fibrils throughout the cartilage, aggregating proteoglycans are lost, even from the deep zone. The mechanical strength of this tissue is so weakened by the damage to collagen and the loss of proteoglycan that it starts to disintegrate as a result of the mechanical damage caused by articulation. Eventually, most of the cartilage disappears from the joint. To control this process, we need to detect these changes much earlier, before they present clinically, and to learn how to arrest progressive degradation and further stimulate the attempt at cartilage repair. With our new knowledge of the physiology and pathobiology of articular cartilage and with the wealth of new technology now at our disposal, we are better prepared now than ever before to address this challenge.

References

1. Mayne R (1989) Cartilage collagens. What is their function, and are they involved in articular disease? Arthritis Rheum 32:241–246
2. Mendler M, Eich-Bender SG, Vaughan L, Winterhalter KH, Bruckner P (1989) Cartilage contains mixed fibrils of collagen types II, IX and XI. J Cell Biol 108:191–197
3. Benninghoff A (1925) Form und Bau der Gelenkknorpel in ihren Beziehungen zur Funktion. Der Aufbau des Gelenkknorpels in seinen Beziehungen zur Funktion. Z Mikrosk Anat Forsch 2:783–862
4. Zambrano NZ, Montez GS, Shigihara KM, Sanchez EM, Junquiera LCV (1982) Collagen arrangement in cartilages. Acta Anat (Basel) 113:26–38
5. Rosenberg L, Choi HU, Neame PJ, Sasse J, Roughley PJ, Poole AR (1990) Proteoglycans of soft connective tissues. In: Leadbetter WB, Buckwalter JA, Gordon SL (eds) Sport-induced inflammation. American Academy Orthopedic Surgeons, Park Ridge, pp 171–188
6. Stockwell RA, Meachim G (1979) The chondrocytes. In: Freeman MAR (ed) Adult articular cartilage, 2nd edn. Pitman Medical, London, pp 69–144
7. Witter J, Roughley PJ, Webber C, Roberts N, Keystone E, Poole AR (1987) The immunologic detection and characterization of cartilage proteoglycan degradation products in synovial fluids of patients with arithritis. Arthritis Rheum 30:519–529
8. Dodge GR, Poole AR (1989) Immunohistochemical detection and immunochemical analysis of type II collagen degradation in human normal, rheumatoid, and osteoarthritic articular cartilages and in explants of bovine articular cartilage cultured with interleukin 1. J Clin Invest 83:647–661
9. Mow VC, Setton LA, Ratcliffe A, Howell DS, Buckwalter JA (1990) Structure function relationships of articular cartilage and the effects of joint instability and trauma on cartilage function. In: Brandt KD (ed) Cartilage Changes in Osteoarthritis. Indiana University School of Medicine and Ciba Gelgy Co, New Jersey, pp 22–42
10. Mankin HJ, Dorfman H, Lippiello L, Zarins A (1971) Biochemical and metabolic abnormalities in articular cartilage from osteoarthritic human hips. J Bone Joint Surg [Am] 53-A:523–537
11. Sweet MBE, Thonar EJ-MA, Immelman AR, Solomon L (1977) Biochemical changes in progressive osteoarthrosis. Ann Rheum Dis 36:387–398
12. Poole AR (1986) Changes in the collagen and proteoglycan of articular cartilage in arthritis. Rheumatology 10:316–371
13. Rizkalla G, Bogoch ER, Poole AR (1991) Proteoglycans in osteoarthritic cartilage: Evidence for increased degradation and increased synthesis. Trans. Orthop Res Soc 16:254
14. Poole AR, Rizkalla G, Ionescu M, Rosenberg LC, Bogoch E (1991) Increased content of the C-propeptide of type II collagen in osteoarthritic human articular cartilage. Trans. Orthop Res Soc 16:343
15. Wu J-J, Lark MW, Chun LE, Eyre DR (1991) Sites of stromelysln cleavage in collagen types II, IX, X and XI of cartilage. J Biol Chem 266:5625–5628
16. Nguyen O, Mort JS, Roughley PJ Preferential mRNA expression of prostromelysin relative to procollagenase and in situ localization in human articular cartilage. J Clin Invest In press.
17. Poole AR (1990) Enzymatic degradation: Cartilage destruction. In: Brandt KD (ed) Cartilage changes in ostoearthritis. Indiana University School of Medicine, Ciba-Geigy Corporation, New Jersey, USA pp 63–72
18. Eeckhout Y, Vaes G (1977) Further studies on the activation of procollagenase, the latent precursor of bone collagenase: Effects of lysosomal cathepsin B, plasmin, and kallikrein

and spontaneous activation. Biochem J 166: 21–31

19. Dean DD, Martel-Pelletier J, Pelletier J-P, Howell, DS, Woessner JF Jr (1989) Evidence for metalloproteinase and metalloproteinase inhibitor imbalance in human osteoarthritic cartilage. J Clin Invest 84:678–685

20. Yamada H, Nakagawa T, Stephens RW, Nagai Y (1987) Proteinases and their inhibitors in normal and osteoarthritic articular cartilage. Biomed Res 8:289–300

21. Tiku ML, Liesch JB, Robertson FM (1990) Production of hydrogen peroxide by rabbit articular chondrocytes. Enhancement by cytokines. J Immunol 145:690–696

22. Halliwell B, Gutteridge JMC (1984) Oxygen toxicity, oxygen radicals, transition metals, and disease. Biochem J 219:1–14

23. Roberts CR, Mort JS, Roughley PJ (1987) Treatment of cartilage proteoglycan aggregate with hydrogen peroxide. Relationship between observed degradation products and those that occur naturally during ageing. Biochem J 247: 349–357

24. Roberts CR, Roughley PJ, Mort JS (1989) Degradation of human proteoglycan aggregate induced by hydrogen peroxide. Protein fragmentation, amino acid modification, and hyaluronic acid cleavage. Biochem J 259:805–811

25. Nguyen Q, Murphy G, Roughley PJ, Mort JS (1989) Degradation of proteoglycan aggregate by a cartilage metalloproteinase. Evidence for the involvement of stromelysin in the generation of link protein heterogeneity in situ. Biochem J 259:61–67

26. De Witt MT, Handley CJ, Oakes BW, Lowther DA (1984) In vitro response of chondrocytes to mechanical loading. The effect of short term mechanical loading. The effect of short term mechanical tension. Connect Tiss Res 12:97–109

27. Palmoski MJ, Brandt KD (1984) Effects of static and cyclic compressive loading on articular cartilage plugs in vitro. Arthritis Rheum 27:675–681

28. Van Kampen GPJ, Veldhuijzen JP, Kuijer R, Van de Stadt RJ, Schipper CA (1985) Cartilage response to mechanical force in high-density chondrocyte cultures. Arthritis Rheum 28: 419–424

29. Veldhuijzen JP, Huisman AA, Vermeiden JPW, Prahl-Andersen B (1987) The growth of cartilage cells in vitro and the effect of intermittent compressive force. A histological evaluation. Connect Tiss Res 16:187–196

30. Sah R L-Y, Kim Y-J, Doong J-Y H, Grodzinsky AJ, Plaas AHK, Sandy JD (1989) Biosynthetic response of cartilage explants to dynamic compression. J Orthop Res 7:619–636

31. Sah, R L-Y, Doong J-Y H, Grodzinsky AL, Plaas AHK, Sandy JD (1991) Effects of compression on the loss of newly synthesized proteoglycans and proteins from cartilage explants. Arch Biochem Biophys 286:20–29.

32. Poole AR, Pidoux I, Reiner A, Rosenberg L (1982) An immunoelectron microscope study of the organization of proteoglycan monomer, link protein, and collagen in the matrix of articular cartilage. J Cell Biol 93:921–937

33. Vogel KG, Koob TJ, Fisher LW (1987) Characterization and interactions of a fragment of the core protein of the small proteoglycan (PG II) from bovine tendon. Biochem Biophys Res Commun 148:658–663

34. Poole AR (to be published) Cartilage. In: McCarty DJ, Koopman W (eds) Arthritis and allied conditions. A textbook of rheumatology, 12th edn. Lea and Febiger, Philadelphia

Pathophysiology of Osteoarthritis

Daniel J. McCarty[1]

Summary. The etiopathogenesis of osteoarthritis is complex. Genetic factors may influence the macromolecules constituting cartilage and other joint tissues. The normal tissue remodeling process may be altered by mechanical factors, by hormones, or by particulates such as wear particles and/or crystals which have biological influences on cells. These factors may accelerate the catabolic arm of tissue remodeling to the point where anabolic synthesis is overwhelmed, producing irreversible or only partially reversible damage, which is perceived clinically as joint degeneration.

Key words. Osteoarthritis — Etiology — Collagen gene mutation — Cartilage

Introduction

The pathophysiology of osteoarthritis (OA) is complex because the term represents a group of different diseases each leading to degeneration of hyaline articular cartilage with eventual proliferation of bone at joint margins [1]. Primary or "nodal" OA has strong hereditary features with a distinctive pattern of joint involvement: distal interphalangeal (DIP), proximal interphalangeal (PIP), first carpometacarpal, knee, and metatarsophalangeal (MTP) [2]. Secondary (non-nodal) OA can develop as a result of trauma, occupational overuse, surgery, obesity, joint instability, mechanical dyscongruity, or deposition of homogentisic acid, iron, or crystals in cartilage.

[1] The Arthritis Institute and Division of Rheumatology, Department of Medicine, Medical College of Wisconsin, Milwaukee WI 53226, USA

Normal Tissues [3]

Hyaline articular cartilage is a gel composed of water-imbibing proteoglycan aggregates restrained by a network of type II collagen and containing chondrocytes responsible for the turnover of its constituent molecules. Cartilage is anchored to a *plate of compact bone* which in turn is supported by a scaffolding of *trabecular bone*. Some joints contain intrasynovial fibrocartilages which are important for their stability. Hyaline cartilage functions as a self-renewing bearing which provides nearly frictionless movement of the levers (bones) which it articulates.

The muscles moving the bones provide most of the shock absorbing, but the subchondral bone deforms under pressure and absorbs some of the force generated during movement. The rarity of OA in osteopenic women has been postulated as due to the greater deformability of less dense bone. Conversely, microfractures often occur in the heavily mineralized bone of osteoarthritic patients both in the subchondral plate and in the trabeculae [1]. Articular cartilage is only a few mm thick and consequently has almost no shock absorbing capability.

Pathogenesis of OA

Heredity — Primary OA often affects multiple members of a family — such hereditary tendencies have been noted by experienced clinicians for many years. Restriction enzyme analysis of DNA from two families has disclosed an autosomal dominant trait with variable degrees of penetrance [4,5]. A point mutation resulting in substitution of cysteine for arginine in type II collagen, the major collagen of hyaline articular cartilage, has recently been described by Prockop and his collaborators as occurring in one of these families [6].

Collagen molecules are very large. The type II gene codes for about 30000 base pairs. Mistakes in the code are poorly tolerated. The frequently repeating tripeptide sequences containing the inflexible bonds of proline and hydroxyproline and the highly flexible glycine bonds are needed to permit the formation of the triple helix by a process resembling crystallization and called *nucleated growth* [7]. The posttranslational hydroxylation of proline and lysine, plus glycosylation and galactosylation of the latter amino acid occur before the 3 C terminal propeptides associate by hydrophobic and electrostatic interaction followed by disulfide bonding. After the ends of the three polypeptide strands are aligned, the triple helix is rapidly propegated to the N terminus in zipper-like fashion. These soluble molecules, like tiny ropes entwined and knotted at each end, are secreted from the cell of origin. The C and N propeptides are then enzymatically cleaved, producing a decrease in solubility of several orders of magnitude. These molecules then self aggregate into a *collagen fibril*, overlapping each other by one quarter of the length of a molecule, again by a process of *nucleated growth*. The molecules are then welded together through cross-linking covalent bonds.

Amino acid substitutions occurring as a result of mutation have profound effects on one or more of this remarkable series of events. If the procollagen polypeptide chains cannot intertwine (like a broken zipper), both the normal and abnormal peptide chains will be proteolytically degraded, a phenomenon called "procollagen suicide" and associated with lethal mutations. If the chain containing the mutant amino acid substitution does intertwine with normal chains it may produce a molecule that is "kinked". Such crooked molecules produce fibrils that appear branched or frayed. Worse, such fibrils produce tissues of less than normal resilience and strength.

Thus type I collagen mutations can be lethal or can produce various degrees of osteogenesis imperfecta or Ehlers-Danlos syndrome, type II mutations, premature osteoarthritis, and type III mutations, vascular aneurysms. It is likely that the mutant type II collagen, due to a cysteine substitution, was not adequate to sustain the integrity of articular cartilage over time, leading to premature changes of osteoarthritis, and in the reported family, mild epiphyseal dysplasia. What percentage of osteoarthritis patients have underlying defects in collagens or other cartilage molecules remains uncertain, but mutations are being sought avidly.

Trauma Including that of Use/Overuse

Motion is clearly implicated in causing or accentuating the signs and symptoms of osteoarthritis. Heberden's nodes are less well formed in paralyzed .extremities and accentuated in fingers subjected to overuse. The old idea of "wear and tear" was too simplistic but should not be abandoned completely as a contributory factor. The post meniscectomy knee, the hip after an untreated slipped femoral capital epiphysis, or shoulder joint degeneration after loss of the rotator cuff are all examples of mechanical problems producing degeneration of joint tissues. The mechanism of transduction of a mechanical force into biochemical events is completely unknown, and is a major "missing link" in any scheme of pathogenesis of degeneration of joint tissues.

Metabolic Abnormalities

The deposition of homogentisic acid in cartilage in ochronosis, cartilage hypertrophy stimulated by growth hormone in acromegaly, or deposition of microcrystals of monosodium urate monohydrate (MSUM) or calcium pyrophosphate dehydrate (CPPD) in gout and pseudogout respectively, represent examples of osteoarthritis occurring as a result of a metabolic derangement resulting in altered tissue metabolism [1].

Particulate Matter of Synovial Fluid

In addition to MSU or CPPD crystals, aggregates of ultra-microscopic calcium phosphate crystals commonly occur in joint fluid and their presence correlates with the degree of degeneration as assessed radiographically [8,9]. By fourier-transform infrared spectrophotometry these are composed of varying combinations of carbonate substituted hydroxyapatite and octacalcium phosphate and (rarely) tricalcium phosphate [10]. As these are basic, as opposed to acidic, compounds, we have named them generically "BCP" (basic calcium phosphate) crystals. These are uniformly associated with particulate collagens, which probably gain access to the joint space as wear particles from the exposed degenerating cartilages. Both BCP crystals and wear particles have biological activities which are still being explored. Most of these activities are proinflammatory and probably lead to acceleration of the degenerative process. BCP crystals are nearly always present if the X-rays show joint space narrowing with underlying bony changes. We believe that, unlike MSUM or CPPD crystals, BCP mineral develops in degenerating cartilage as an epiphenomenon.

Metabolic Decompensation of Cartilage

Like all tissues, hyaline cartilage matrix is turned over by a balanced process of molecular breakdown and synthesis. An excellent account of the reasons for the increased water content, net loss of proteoglycan, and disruption of the collagen network in osteoarthritis is provided by Robin Poole elsewhere in this volume. The disturbed metabolism is accompanied by loss of function, such as decreased cartilage compliance and loss of its lubricating function.

Biological Effects of BCP Crystals in Joints

These have been investigated most intensely in association with a condition resulting in loss of shoulder function, with lysis of the rotator cuff, in elderly women (Milwaukee Shoulder Syndrome) [11,12]. Complete needle drainage of the rather large effusions often present in these cases did not appear to change the measured levels of BCP crystals. The level of crystals (usually 5–50 mg/ml as assessed by (^{14}C)

diphosphonate binding) was nearly identical in fluids removed at monthly intervals, suggesting some degree of homeostatic control. Electron microscopic examination of the synovium in these cases showed phagocytosed aggregates of BCP crystals [13,14]. Injection of (^{85}Sr) labelled BCP or CPPD crystals into rabbit joints was followed by rapid clearance (~1 day) from the joint fluid due to uptake by phagocytic synovial living cells [15,16]. All measurable crystal dissolution took place in these cells; none occurred extracellularly.

Addition of synthetic BCP (or CPPD) crystals uniformly labelled with ^{45}Ca to synovial cells in monolayer culture resulted in endocytosis and gradual dissolution by the hydrogen ions entering the phagolysosome by action of an ATP driven proton pump in the phagolysosomal membrane [17,18]. This pump maintains the pH in the sac at about 4 in a macrophage and at about 5 in a fibroblast. Antimalarials such as chloroquine are weak bases which diffuse across cell membranes, gaining access to the phagolysosome where they are protonated and can't diffuse out again. Chloroquine, $NH4^+$ and other weak bases are called lysosomotropic agents. They raise the pH and block the dissolution of calcium-containing crystals in a dose-dependent fashion.

Synthetic or natural BCP or CPPD crystals fed to cultured human or canine synovial cells resulted in their phagocytosis with subsequent release of collagenase, neutral protease, and prostaglandins (PG)E_2 and $F_2\alpha$ into the culture medium [19]. It was hypothesized that the joint degeneration observed in these cases was due to enzymatic "strip-mining" of crystals from synovium or cartilage with subsequent synovial cell endocytosis and further enzyme induction and release, a vicious cycle [20]. Crystal aggregates were demonstrated in synovial cells by transmission electron microscopy (EM) in all cases where synovium was obtained [13,14]. Particulate collagens, types I, II, and III, were identified in the synovial pellet in each fluid examined [11]. These too could result from partial tissue digestion and serve as a stimulus for synovial cell protease release. But in follow-up studies neither we nor others have found active collagenase in most joint fluids from patients with Milwaukee Shoulder Syndrome. The impressive dissolution of collagenous structures in these patients almost certainly implicates collagenase. As in rheumatoid arthritis, this enzyme is probably activated in a microenvironment. Many factors can release the zinc atom in the active site of collagenase from the Cys^{73} which binds it, causing activation [21].

BCP and CPPD crystals both occur in cartilage. Chondrocytes in primary culture exposed to crystals released proteases and prostaglandins much as did synovial cells [22]. As crystals have been noted in human chondrocytes, albeit rarely, it is possible that autolysis of cartilage may occur directly without crystals first shedding into the synovial fluid.

The syndrome of "Milwaukee Shoulder" is becoming somewhat clearer with additional clinical experience [12]. It is largely a disease of women (22/30 cases) in mid or late life (mean age 72 years with range 54–90 years). The dominant shoulder is nearly always involved and the clinical, radiologic, and biochemical severity is always greater on the dominant side when bilateral involvement occurs, as it commonly does in two-thirds of cases. The condition is clearly not confined to the shoulder, as 16 of our 30 cases had a destructive arthropathy of one or both knees associated with microspheroidal aggregates of BCP crystals and low levels of collagenase, neutral protease, and particulate collagens. Symptoms of shoulder pain after use and at night are typical, but patients with severe pain at rest and even asymptomatic patients have been noted. On examination, the affected shoulders are either stiff or unstable. The radiologic appearance is clearly distinct from osteoarthritis (OA). In the shoulder, rotator cuff dissolution is usually massive and bony destruction of the humeral head is marked, but osteophytosis is rarely prominent. According to Neer, OA of the glenohumeral joint is *not* associated with loss of the rotator cuff and produces big osteophytes [23]. The radiologic appearance of the degenerative knee joints in MSS patients is also somewhat distinctive, resembling that associated with CPPD crystals rather than that in primary OA. The destructive process is most severe in the patellofemoral and lateral tibiofemoral compartments, rather than in the medial tibiofemoral compartment, as in primary OA [9]. This pattern is of interest in that CPPD and BCP crystals frequently co-exist [8,9].

Robert Adams, an Irish surgeon, published an atlas on arthritis in 1857 containing an excellent description of the gross anatomical features of "Milwaukee Shoulder" [24]. He recognized that, unlike a traumatic tear, the (usually) bilateral dissolution of the rotator cuff was due to a disease process. He called the condition "chronic rheumatic arthritis of the shoulder". His documentation of complete loss of the *Intrasynovial* portion of the tendon of the long head of the biceps with reattachment of the unaffected extra-articular portion is a convincing argument for the action of collagenase.

Molecular Mechanism of the Biologic Activity of Crystals Containing Calcium

Synovial cell hyperplasia was noted in each of our cases [14], perhaps related to the mitogenic properties of BCP crystals [25]. These, as well as CPPD, calcium urate, calcium carbonate, calcium diphosphonate, and other calcium-containing crystals, but not crystals or particulates that did not contain calcium such as sodium urate, diamond, silicon dioxide, or latex beads, were capable of substituting for serum growth factors such as platelet derived growth factor (PDGF). Crystal-induced mitogenesis was reduced in a dose-dependent fashion by lysosomotropic agents, but mitosis stimulated by serum or PDGF was unaffected. Endocytosis was a prerequisite both for crystal dissolution and for mitogenesis [18,26]. Crystals containing calcium act as a "competence factor" enabling anchorage-dependent cells in G_0 to enter the G_1 phase of the cell cycle. Progression factors, such as insulin-like growth factor (somatomedin C), are then needed for progression through late G_1 and S phase [27]. Somatomedin C is present in nearly all pathologic synovial fluids. These data are consistent with the formulation that intracellular crystal dissolution is associated with a rise in intracellular calcium, a known stimulus to cell division.

Addition of BCP crystals to fibroblasts resulted in rapid expression of the proto-oncogene message for c-*fos* with maximal expression in 30 min, exactly mimicking the effects of PDGF [28]. Similarly, BCP crystals and PDGF each stimulated c-*myc* transcription within 1 h with maximal effect at 3 h, although elevated levels were still easily detected at 5 h. BCP crystals induced inositol-1 phosphate formation in [³H] inositol labelled synovial cells within 1 min, a reaction peaking at 60 min. Increased [³²P] inositol, mono, bis, an trisphosphates were formed from cells labelled with [³²P] after BCP addition [29]. Clearly the crystals stimulated phospholipase C. As phosphatidylinositol is broken down into inositol trisphosphate (IP3) and diacylglycerol (DAG), which activates protein kinase C (PKC), which then translocates to the inner cell membrane, the role of the latter in mitogenesis induced by BCP crystals was explored. (Some mitogenic stimuli are dependent on PKC; others, such as epidermal cell growth factor [EGF] or PDGF, are not.) PKC was depleted from cultured cells by tumor-promoting phorbol diester (TPA) which activates PKC directly as a DAG analogue. This down regulation of PKC persists for many hours, rendering the cells relatively unresponsive to further stimulation by TPA. The expected stimulation of (³H) thymidine incorporation by BCP crystals was abrogated in PKC-depleted cells, but that stimulated by PDGF was not [30]. The increased expression of c-*fos* and c-*myc* mRNA induced by BCP crystals and PDGF was no different in control cells, but in PKC-depleted cells, PDGF stimulated c-*fos* and c-*myc* normally, whereas the response to BCP crystals, like that to TPA itself, was markedly inhibited. Full expression of BCP crystal-stimulated proto-oncogene activation and mitosis is mediated in part through protein kinase C. As already outlined, crystal endocytosis and dissolution with Ca²⁺ release are also necessary for mitogenesis.

In summary, mitosis stimulated in anchorage-dependent cells by crystals containing calcium is a two stage event: 1. a rapid stimulation of membrane phospholipase C with protein kinase C activation via DAG, and 2. a slower intracellular event dependent on intraphagolysosomal crystal dissolution with release of calcium.

Induction of Protease Synthesis and Secretion

Not only calcium-containing crystals but also sodium urate and non crystalline particulates such as latex beads undergo endocytosis by cultured cells, stimulating a five- to eightfold increased synthesis and secretion of several proteases including collagenase [31,32]. Such stimulation persists until the ingested particles are biodegraded. Northern blot analysis of mRNA in cells stimulated with BCP crystals showed a dose-dependent stimulation of collagenase mRNA, evident at 4 h and persisting relentlessly for at least 24 h. Unlike mitogenesis, protease induction and release was not dependent on intracellular dissolution of calcium-containing crystals.

Stimulation of Prostaglandin Synthesis

As mentioned already, a massive release of prostaglandin (PG) E₂ followed exposure of cultured synovial cells to various particulates including latex beads, sodium urate, or CPPD or BCP crystals [19,33]. Unlike mitogenesis, but like the induction of enzyme synthesis, this phenomenon was not dependent on intracellular dissolution when crystals containing calcium were used as the stimulus. Indomethacin, 10^{-6} M, blocked the formation of PGE₂ by BCP crystals almost completely without any effect or induction of collagenase synthesis or mitogenesis.

References

1. Hough AJ, Sokoloff L (1989) Pathology of osteoarthritis. In: McCarty DJ (ed) Arthritis and allied conditions, 11th edn. Lea and Febiger, Philadelphia, pp 1571–1594
2. Moskowitz RW (1989) Clinical and laboratory findings in osteoarthritis. In: McCarty DJ (ed) Arthritis and allied conditions, 11th edn. Lea and Febiger, Philadelphia, pp 1605–1630
3. Mankin HJ, Radin E (1989) Structure and function of joints. In: McCarty DJ (ed) Arthritis and allied conditions, 11th edn. Lea and Febiger, Philadelphia, pp 189–206
4. Palotie A, Vaisanen P, Ott J, Ryhanen L, Elima K, Vikkula M, Cheah K, Vuorio E, Peltonen L (1989) Predisposition to familial osteoarthritis linked to type II collagen gene. Lancet I:924–927
5. Knowlton RG, Katzenstein PL, Moskowitz RW, Weaver EJ, Malemud CJ, Pathria MN, Jimenez SA, Prockop DJ (1990) Genetic linkage of a polymorphism in the type II procollagen gene (COL2A1) to primary osteoarthritis associated with mild chondrodysplasia. N Engl J Med 322: 526–530

6. Ala-Kokko L, Baldwin CT, Moskowitz RW, Prockop DJ (1990) Single base mutation in the type II procollagen gene (COL2A1) as a cause of primary osteoarthritis associated with a mild chondrodysplasia. Proc Natl Acad Sci USA 87: 6565–6568

7. Prockop DJ (1990) Mutations that alter the primary structure of type I collagen. J Biol Chem 265:1–5

8. Halverson PB, McCarty DJ (1979) Identification of hydroxyapatite crystals in synovial fluid. Arthritis Rheum 22:389–395

9. Halverson PB, McCarty DJ (1986) Patterns of radiographic abnormalities associated with basic calcium phosphate and calcium pyrophosphate dihydrate crystal deposition in the knee. Ann Rheum Dis 45:603–605

10. McCarty DJ, Lehr JR, Halverson PB (1983) Crystal populations in human synovial fluid. Identification of apatite, octacalcium phosphate and beta tricalcium phosphate. Arthritis Rheum 26:1220–1224

11. Halverson PB, Cheung HS, McCarty DJ, Garancis J, Mandel N (1981) "Milwaukee shoulder"; association of microspheroids containing hydroxyapatite crystals, active collagenase and neutral protease with rotator cuff defects. II. Synovial fluid studies. Arthritis Rheum 24: 474–483

12. Halverson PB, Carrera GF, McCarty DJ (1990) Milwaukee shoulder/knee syndrome: 15 additional cases and a description of contributing factors. Arch Intern Med 150:677–682

13. Garancis JC, Cheung HS, Halverson PB, McCarty DJ (1981) "Milwaukee shoulder": association of microspheroids containing hydroxyapatite, active collagenase and neutral protease with rotator cuff defects. III. Morphologic and biochemical studies of an excised synovium showing chondromatosis. Arthritis Rheum 24:484–491

14. Halverson PB, Garancis JC, McCarty DJ (1984) Histopathologic and ultra-structural studies of Milwaukee Shoulder syndrome — a basic calcium phosphate crystal arthropathy. Ann Rheum Dis 43:734–741

15. McCarty DJ, Palmer DW, James C (1979) Clearance of calcium pyrophosphate dihydrate (CPPD) crystals in vivo. II. Studies using triclinic crystals doubly labelled with ^{45}Ca and ^{85}Sr. Arthritis Rheum 22:1122–1131

16. Palmer DW, McCarty DJ (1984) Clearance of ^{85}Sr labelled calcium phosphate crystals from rabbit joints. Arthritis Rheum 27:427–432

17. Cheung HS, McCarty DJ (1985) Mitogenesis induced by calcium-containing crystals: role of intracellular dissolution. Exp Cell Res 157:63–70

18. Borkowf A, Cheung HS, McCarty DJ (1987) Endocytosis is required for the mitogenic effect of basic calcium phosphate crystals in fibroblasts. Calcif Tissue Int 40:173–176

19. Cheung HS, Halverson PB, McCarty DJ (1981) Release of collagenase, neutral protease and prostaglandins from cultured mammalian synovial cells by hydroxyapatite and calcium pyrophosphate dihydrate crystals. Arthritis Rheum 24:1338–1344

20. McCarty DJ, Halverson PB, Carrera GF, Brewer BJ, Kozin F (1981) "Milwaukee shoulder": association of microspheroids containing hydroxyapatite crystals, active collagenase and neutral protease with rotator cuff defects. I. Clinical aspects. Arthritis Rheum 24:464–473

21. Springman EB, Angleton EL, Birkedal-Hansen H, Van Wart E (1990) Multiple modes of activation of latent human fibroblast collagenase: Evidence for the role of a Cys 73 active-site zinc complex in latency and a "cysteine switch" mechanism for activation. Proc Natl Acad Sci USA 87:364–368

22. Cheung HS, Halverson PB, McCarty DJ (1983) Phagocytosis of hydroxyapatite or calcium pyrophosphate dihydrate crystals by rabbit articular chondrocytes stimulates release of collagenase, neutral protease and prostaglandins E_2 and F_2 Proc Soc Exp Biol Med 173:181–189

23. Neer C (1983) Cuff tear arthropathy. J Bone Joint Surg [Am] 65A:1232–1244

24. McCarty DJ (1989) Robert Adams' rheumatic arthritis of the shoulder or Milwaukee Shoulder revisited. J Rheumatol 16:668–670

25. Cheung HS, Story M, McCarty DJ (1984) Mitogenic effects of hydroxyapatite and calcium pyrophosphate dihydrate crystals on canine synovial cells in culture. Arthritis Rheum 27: 668–674

26. Owens JL, Cheung HS, McCarty DJ (1986) Endocytosis precedes dissolution of basic calcium phosphate crystals by murine macrophages. Calcif Tissue Int 38:170–174

27. Cheung HS, Van Wyk JJ, Russell WE, McCarty DJ (1986) Mitogenic activity of hydroxyapatite: requirement for somatomedin C. J Cell Physiol 128:143–148

28. Cheung HS, Mitchell PG, Pledger WJ (1989) Activation of proto-oncogenes by BCP crystals: effect of beta-interferon. Cancer Res 49:134–138

29. Rothenberg RJ, Cheung HS (1988) Rabbit synoviocyte inositol phospholipid metabolism is stimulated by hydroxyapatite. Am J Physiol 254: (Cell Physiol)(23):C554–C559

30. Mitchell PG, Pledger WP, Cheung HS (1989)

Molecular mechanism of basic calcium phosphate crystal-induced mitogenesis: Role of protein kinase C. J Biol Chem 264:14071–14077

31. Werb Z, Reynolds JJ (1974) Stimulation by endocytosis of the secretion of collagenase and neutral proteinase from rabbit synovial fibroblasts. J Exp Med 140:1482–1497

32. Brinckerhoff CE, Gross RH, Nagase H, Sheldon L, Jackson RC, Harris ED (1982) Increased level of translatable collagenase messenger ribonucleic acid in rabbit synovial fibroblasts treated with phorbol myristate acetate or crystals of mono-sodium urate monohydrate. Biochem J 21: 2674–2679

33. McCarty DJ, Cheung HS (1985) Prostaglandin (PG) E_2 generation by cultural canine synovial fibroblasts exposed to microcrystals containing calcium. Ann Rheum Dis 44:316–320

Pathology of Osteoarthrosis*

B. Tillmann and M. Schünke[1]

Summary. The pathogenesis of mechanically induced arthrosis is due to a disproportion between the
physiological resistance of the supporting tissue and
the compressive stress developing in the joint. Those
mechanical factors contributing to an increase in
articular pressure are (1) a rise in the magnitude of
the resultant force during movement, (2) a reduction of the pressure-transmitting articular surface,
and (3) an eccentric position of the resultant force.
Cluster formation, subchondral bone sclerosis, and
osteophyte formation are reparation attempts made
in the course of osteoarthrosis. Osteophytes are of
chondral osteogenesis and they are subjected to stress
by compressive forces. In considering the problem of
the etiopathogenesis of osteoarthrosis, STR/1N-mice
are included in current investigations because in
this arthrosis model there are two different types of
osteoarthrosis; one due to a biomechanically-induced
instability (patellar luxation) and one due to biochemical changes (absence of keratan sulfate) in the
articular cartilage. Polychrome sequential labeling is
used to study the dynamics of subchondral bone
sclerosis during developing osteoarthrosis in the knee
joints of STR/1N-mice. The results indicate that
subchondral sclerosis is caused by cartilage lesion,
and that even slight changes of hyaline cartilage may
initiate proliferation of the subchondral bone.

Key words. Osteoarthrosis — Articular cartilage —
Subchondral bone — Arthrosis model —
Proteoglycans

Introduction

If an individual lives long enough the probability
of falling ill with arthrosis is high. A large percentage of the population over 40 years of age
shows various degrees of degenerative arthrosis;
the incidence of arthrosis is 100% in those
between the age of 70 and 80 years [1].

Senile changes are not identical with degenerative processes, and in articular cartilage
they do not inevitably lead to arthrosis. Compared with young people, older persons display
typical morphologic and biochemical changes
of the articular cartilage which lack any signs of
arthrosis or clinically ascertainable disorders of
joint function. Senile changes in the articular
cartilage take place predominantly in the lower
zones. In contrast, cartilage degeneration first
appears in the surface layer. In the initial stage
one can recognize fibrillation at the articular
surface with the naked eye.

Senile Changes in Articular Cartilage

With increasing age, collagen content decreases
in relation to the dry weight of cartilage. The
proteoglycan molecules in the cartilage of older
persons are shorter than those in young people
[2,3], and consequently the water content is
also lower. The link proteins between proteoglycans and hyaluronic acid diminish with
age; moreover, their size decreases considerably. Hyaluronic acid content may increase with
age. Compared with chondroitin sulfate, the
keratan sulfate content is reported to increase
[4].

* Dedicated to Professor Dr. K. Hirohata, with compliments
[1] Institute of Anatomy, University of Kiel, Olshausenstrasse
40, 2300 Kiel, Germany

Degenerative Changes in Arthrosis

Proteoglycan loss is consistently reported in arthrosis [5]. The cause of this is a disorder of the cross-linkage between the collagen fibrils in the joint cavity. Apart from this, damage to the collagen fibril network may lead to extension of the remaining proteoglycan aggregates [6]. In the course of this process the negatively charged side chains of glycosaminoglycans separate. The physiologically underhydrated proteoglycans thus potentially can take on a large quantity of water [7]. A further result of damage to the collagen fibril network and proteoglycan loss is that, under the influence of joint pressure, water no longer moves out of the cartilage into the joint cavity and vice versa, as it does in healthy articular cartilage, but rather escapes into regions of articular cartilage which are not affected by compressive stress. Consequently, a sufficient maintenance of the cartilagenous tissue is no longer guaranteed.

In the initial stages of arthrosis very thin collagen fibrils are formed. Compared to the proteoglycan loss, the decrease in collagen fibrils is slight. Collagen degradation only becomes manifest with advanced disease.

Pathogenesis of Mechanically Induced Arthrosis

The etiology of arthrosis is controversial and unclear in many respects. However, there is wide agreement on the pathogenesis of the disease: Arthrosis is due to a disproportion between the physiological resistance of the supporting tissues and the stress developing in the joint [8]. Both the lowering of the resistance and a rise in articular pressure are responsible for the initiation and progress of the disease. Kummer [9] considers the factors contributing to a rise in articular pressure to be:

1. Rise in the total resultant force responsible for the stress
2. Shrinking of the pressure-transmitting area
3. Disproportionate stress distribution in the pressure-transmitting area due to an eccentric position of the resultant force

The absolute *magnitude of the resultant force* at the joint changes during movement. Based upon calculations by Maquet [10], the resultant force R5 at the knee joint has been found to reach much higher values during flexion as compared to extension. Consequently, the articular pressure varies depending upon the different positions of the joint. Anatomical factors, as, for example, a different neck-shaft angle of the femur, are correlated with changes in the magnitude of the articular pressure. According to Pauwels [8], the resultant force, and hence the stress, is much higher in a coxa valga than it is in a femur with a normal neck-shaft angle.

In hallux valgus, for example, the dislocation of the metatarsophalangeal joint leads to an incongruence of the articulating elements (Fig. 1). The *reduction of the pressure-transmitting articular surface* gives rise to an increase in articular stress, the result of which is arthrosis [11].

The third factor responsible for a higher articular pressure is the *eccentric position of the resultant force*. This results in a disproportional stress distribution (Fig. 2d). Corresponding to the stress distribution one observes degenerative changes in the acetabulum, most often seen at its roof [12]. In the opposite region of the articular surface, at the edge of the acetabular fossa, reparative processes are active, in the form of osteophytes (Fig. 2a,b). In the histological section through such an acetabulum one can recognize the typical changes of advanced arthrosis (Fig. 2c). In this section, the cartilage is destroyed at the acetabular rim and the subchondral bone is exposed. A large osteophyte has developed at the inner crest of the lunate surface which juts over the acetabular fossa. The osteophyte is covered with cartilage.

Reparation Attempts

In addition to cluster formation and subchondral sclerosis, *osteophyte formation* belongs to the category of reparation attempts in the course of osteoarthrosis. Osteophytes arise in the zones of the articular surface which are relatively free of stress [13]. On the femur head they most often occur at the outer crest of the articular surface (Fig. 3). The genesis of and the stress on osteophytes are controversial topics of discussion [14]. Morphological data speak in favor of a chondral osteogenesis and pressure stress

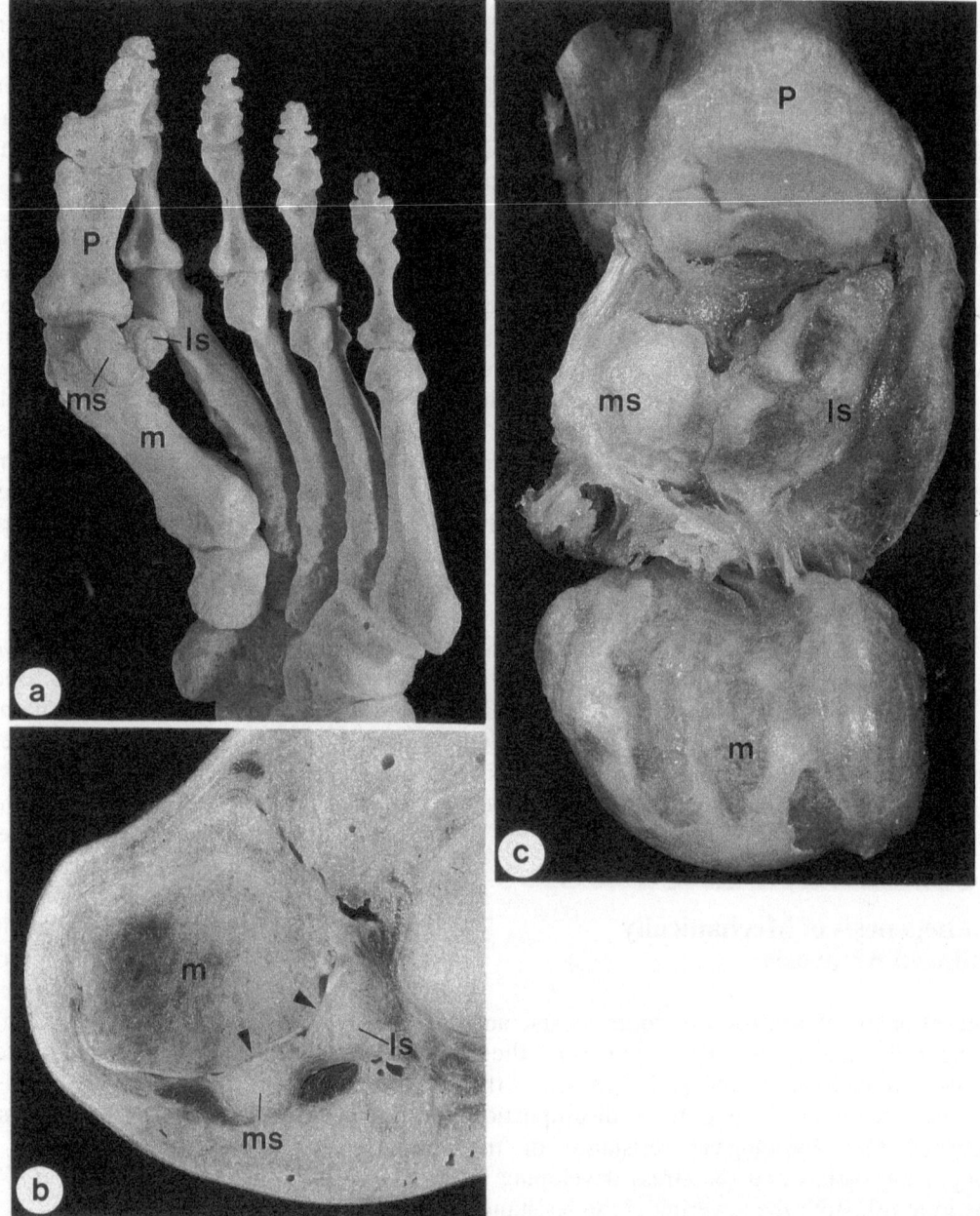

Fig. 1. a Skeleton of a left foot with hallux valgus (plantar aspect): Dislocation of the articular elements of the first metatarsophalangeal joint due to rotation of the first metatarsal bone. This leads to a reduced stress-transmitting area with concomitant degenerative changes in the articular surfaces (see c). **b** Coronal section through the first metatarsophalangeal joint of a hallux valgus showing the dislocated sesamoid bones. Degenerative changes can be seen (*arrowheads*). **c** Opened first metatarsophalangeal joint (superior aspect) from a foot with hallux valgus with arthrosis. p, first proximal phalanx; ms, medial sesamoid bone; ls, lateral sesamoid bone; m, first metatarsal bone

[15]. Not only the cartilaginous covering but also the alignment of the trabecular bone functionally explain the compressive stress (Figs. 2c, 3b). In X-rays of a bone section one can recognize the vertical radiation of the bony trabeculae within the osteophytes in the direction of the joint stress into the subchondral compact cortical bone (Fig. 3b).

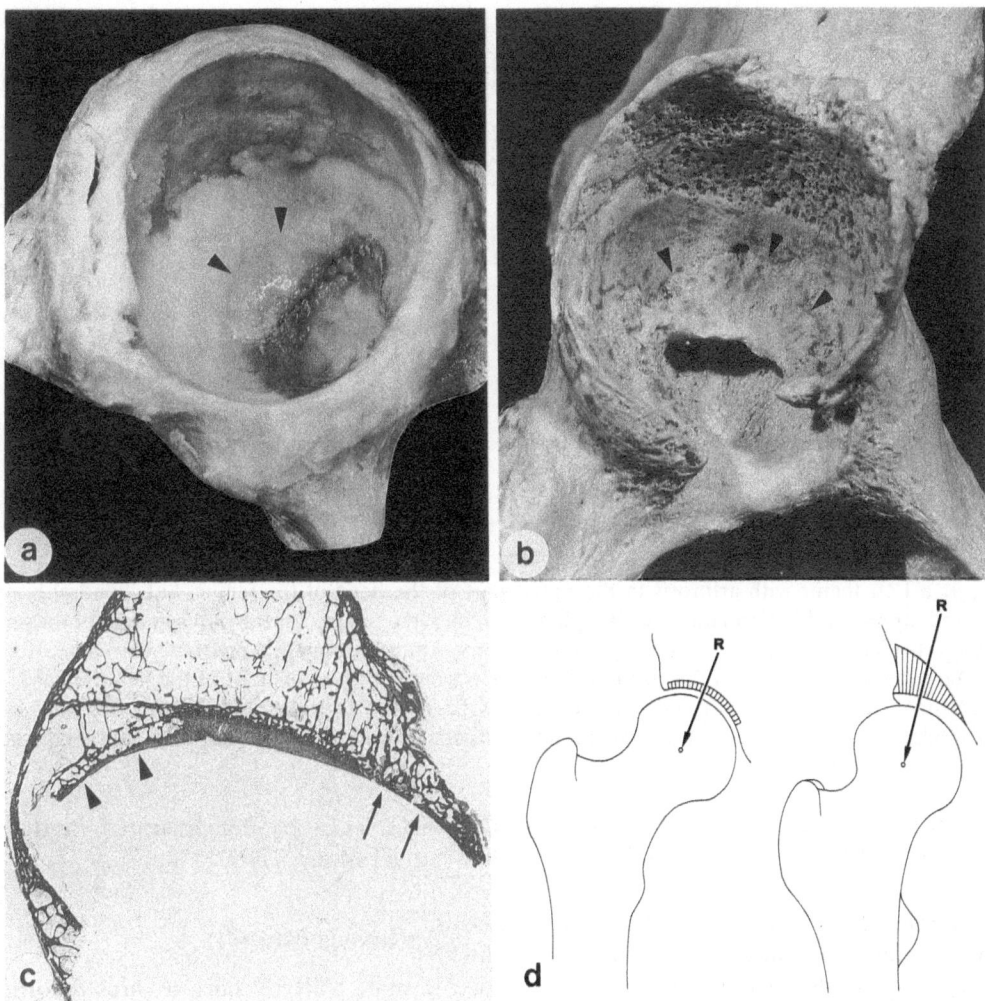

Fig. 2. a Left acetabulum with arthrosis in the socket-roof and osteophyte formation at the inner margin of the lunate surface (*arrowheads*). **b** Right macerated acetabulum. Exposure of the marrow cavities in the acetabular roof following destruction of the subchondral compact bone. Osteophyte formation at the inner margin of the lunate surface is in the form of a "double socket-bottom" (*arrowheads*). **c** Histological section (coronal plane, 10 µm, Azan) through a left acetabulum with degenerative changes (*arrows*) in the acetabular roof. Osteophyte formation at the inner edge of the lunate surface covers the acetabular fossa. Osteophytes (*arrowheads*) are covered by hyaline cartilage. Bony trabeculae radiate rectangularly into the subchondral compact bone. **d** Stress diagrams of the hip joint, showing the resultant force R, according to Pauwels [8]; equal stress distribution due to a centric position of R is shown on the *left* and unequal stress distribution due to an eccentric position of R is shown on the *right*

Etiological Aspects

In examining a very large number of joints the observation has been made that some joints, for example, hip and knee, very often exhibit degenerative changes, while other joints, for example, the ankle, are almost never affected, excluding, however, the secondary arthrosis of the younger generation following ligament in-juries that occur during athletic activities [16]. Now the question follows as to the reason for this observation. Neither the mode nor the magnitude of articular joint stress can be causes for this phenomenon, as they exhibit no deci-sive qualitative or quantitative differences in the joints mentioned. The key to understanding the morphological findings may be found in the varying composition of extracellular matrix in

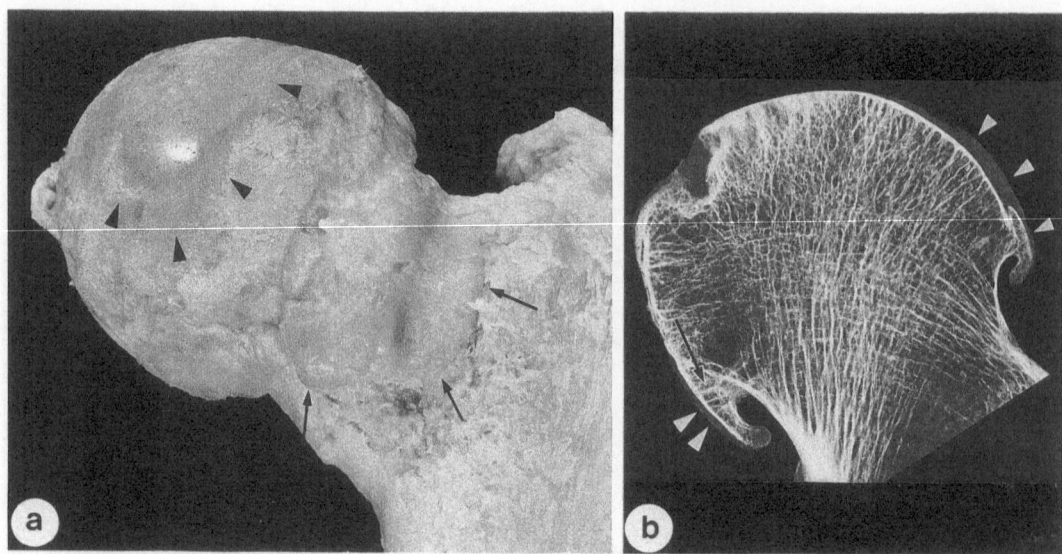

Fig. 3. a Left femur with arthrosis in the upper part of the head of the femur. Subchondral bone is partly exposed (*arrowheads*). Formation of osteophytes can be seen (*arrows*) at the outer margin of the anterior part of the articular surface. **b** X-ray of a section (thickness, 3 mm) through the proximal extremity of a left femur with coxarthrosis. Sclerosis of the subchondral bone is seen in the cranial part of the femoral head. Remnants of cartilage (*arrowheads*) are seen at the outer area of the articular surface covering the osteophytes. Trabecular spongiosa in the osteophytes radiate rectangularly (*arrow*) into the subchondral compacta

the articular cartilage of the affected joint, which is directly related to the stress tolerated by the tissue.

Therefore, not only the functional "external causes" named, but also the "internal causes" in the cartilage itself must be regarded as causes of the development of degenerative changes. Both factors can be demonstrated in the arthrosis model of the STR/1N mouse.

Arthrosis Model

In male STR/1N mice a varus deformity arises in the region of the femorotibial joint within

Fig. 4. a Frontal section of the left knee joint of a 5-month-old male STR/1N mouse. *Black arrows* indicate arthrotic lesions on the medial tibial condyle. F, femur; TP, tibial plateau; P, displaced patella (Kossa-stain, *Bar* = 470 μm). **b** Radiograph of the left knee joint in an anterior-posterior ray path. *Arrows* indicate subchondral bone sclerosis (*Bar* = 800 μm). **c** Clusters of chondrocytes at the facies patellaris femoris (Toluidine blue stained, *Bar* = 40 μm). **d** Significant loss of cartilage with partially exposed calcified layer. TP, tibial plateau (Toluidine blue stained, *Bar* = 56 μm). **e** Fibrillation of cartilage (Toluidine blue stained, *Bar* = 25 μm). **f** Numerous fissures reaching the tidemark (Toluidine blue stained, *Bar* = 25 μm). **g** Articular surface (*arrows*) consists of bone (Toluidine blue stained, *Bar* = 73 μm). **h** Polychrome sequential labeling of subchondral bone in a healthy C_3H mouse using four different coloured fluorochromes. Newly formed bone is arranged concentrically around individual marrow cavities (*MC*) (*Bar* = 40 μm). **i** In an arthrotic knee joint of a male STR/1N mouse, fluorescent bands (*1–4*) are arranged excentrically and are directed towards the cartilage lesion. Each of the different fluorochromes were injected twice at 7-day intervals. 4, xylenol orange; 3, calcein; 2, alizarine complexone; 1, tetracycline (*Bar* = 40 μm). **j** Immunohistochemical staining of keratan sulfate in the tibial articular cartilage of a male STR/1N mouse. Note the keratan sulfate-positive chondrocytes (*arrows*) (*Bar* = 27 μm). **k** eight-month old STR/1N mouse. Below the arthrotic lesion (*arrows*) fluorescent bands are arranged excentrically, in areas with normal articular cartilage (*AC*) next to the sclerotic region, however, the growth rate is unaffected (*Bar* = 80 μm)

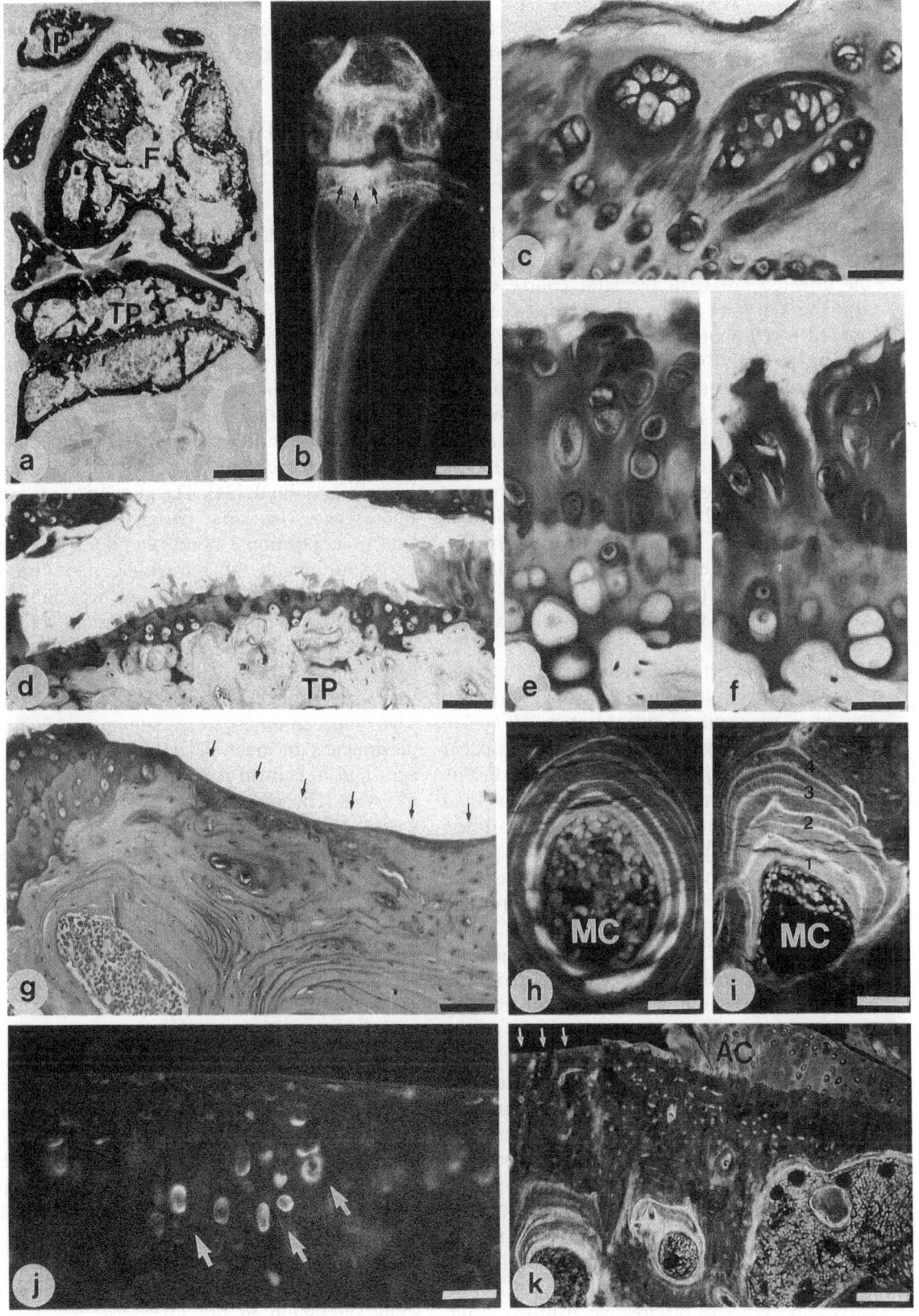

the course of spontaneously occurring osteoarthrosis of the knee; this results in a dislocation of the patella (Fig. 4a) with degenerative changes of the patellar surface of the femur [17].

The functionally caused arthrosis in the femoropatellar joint in the mouse is morphologically similar to that found in humans. The joint surface is slightly fibrillated in the initial stage and the previously mentioned clusters appear (Fig. 4c). Collagen fibrils are exposed in the affected areas. In the later course of this arthrosis the joint surface is eventually covered only by a cell-poor fibrillar tissue.

In male STR/1N mice spontaneous osteoarthrosis of the knee in the medial section of the femoral tibial joint is initiated without any identifiable mechanical cause. The course of arthrosis can be broken into four stages [18,19]. In the initial stage surface fibrillation occurs (Fig. 4e). Stage 2 is characterized by vertical fissures extending down to the tide-mark (Fig. 4f). In stage 3 the cartilage is degenerated to the mineralized zone (Fig. 4d) and in stage 4 the subchondral bone is, to a large extent, exposed and sclerosed (Fig. 4g).

The difference in appearance of degenerative changes in these two joint areas is not limited to the form of cartilage degeneration alone. In contrast to the degenerative changes that occur in the patellar surface of the femur, no clusters form during arthrosis in the femorotibial joint [20]. Thus, attempts to repair the joint cartilage are absent in this joint area.

In attempts to answer the question of the cause of spontaneous arthrosis in the femorotibial joint, the extracellular matrix has been examined, using lectins, and other agents. Immunohistochemical examinations of this matrix have also been carried out. From the lectin binding experiments it is concluded that keratan sulfate and/or hyaluronic acid occur in only small quantities, or are absent altogether, in the tibial plateau cartilage [17]. This suspicion could be confirmed by the immunohistochemical findings. The absence of this glycosaminoglycan throughout the entire thickness of cartilage could be demonstrated with an antibody against keratan sulfate (Fig. 4j). In contrast, chondroitin sulfate was normally distributed. The deficiency of keratan sulfate is regarded as the cause of the early appearance of progressive arthrosis in the femorotibial joint. These results agree with quantitative biochemical data [21,22] that show a deficiency of keratan sulfate.

Experimental Investigations Concerning Subchondral Sclerosis

Changes in the articular bones, which can be radiologically detected, also occur in STR/1N mice, as they do in arthrosis in humans. One can recognize the narrowing of the articular space and the sclerosis of the subchondral bone in X-rays [23] (Fig. 4b). X-rays and conventional histologic investigations only suggest a metaplastic process in the subchondral bone tissue in arthrosis; qualitative and quantitative evidence of the dynamics of bone growth is collected with the aid of polychromatic sequential marking in laboratory animals [24]. The method of repeated fluorescence marking permits the visualization of appositional bone accretion, using the chromatic bands of intravitally administered fluorochromes, which are incorporated as Ca^{2+}-complex producers in locations of new mineralization. The distance between two adjoining chromatic bands is a measure of the rate of bone accretion between two injections. The fluorochromes were administered intraperitoneally in male STR/1N mice of different ages and in control mice in succession at 7-day intervals. The duration of the experiment was 10 weeks.

In control joints the chromatic bands were arranged concentrically around the marrow cavity (Fig. 4h). They occurred so close together that differentiating individual markings was often achieved only with great difficulty. The rate of appositional bone accretion was between 25 and 50 µm in 10 weeks [23].

The findings in arthrotic knee joints differ in several aspects from findings in control animals: in arthrotic knee joints the chromatic bands are eccentrically arranged and aligned toward the defect on the joint surface (Fig. 4i). Individual bands can be clearly separated from each other. In early stages of arthrosis, rates of bone accretion of up to 250 µm were measured within an experimental period of 10 weeks.

Whether subchondral bone sclerosis is a result or a cause of arthrosis is the subject of some discussion in the literature. Radin and Rose [25], for example, are of the opinion that degenerative cartilage changes are the result of a preceding subchondral bone accretion. Most investigators view the hyaline joint cartilage as the location of primary damage [26,27]. The present findings confirm this idea. So subchondral bone accretion is seen to be the response to a locally increased stress which occurs as a consequence of cartilage destruction resulting from the inadequate or totally absent shock-absorbing function of the joint cartilage. The finding that normal bone growth occurs in the direct vicinity of the sclerosed area supports the biomechanical hypothesis that arthrosis represents a locally restricted and not a generalized event (Fig. 4k).

Outlook

Regarding bone regeneration in arthrosis, the question is posed as to the way in which the reactions are mediated in the tissue. Related to this, the effect of growth factors must be taken into consideration; these growth factors may stimulate not only increased bone accretion, but also, for example, the generation of osteophytes or the proliferation of joint cartilage both in the form of clusters and at the synovial membrane [28]. Meanwhile several bone tissue growth factors are already known [29]. The majority of these are polypeptides derived from the bone tissue itself or from adjoining structures. The effects of growth factors on the increase and differentiation of bone tissue are clear. As regulators they have a local but not a systemic effect. Whether the growth factors are released under elevated stress or whether they originate from the destroyed cartilage tissue itself is the subject of some discussion.

Acknowledgments. The authors wish to thank Mrs. A. Haupt, Mrs. R. Worm, Mrs. H. Waluk, and Mr. S. Kunkel for technical assistance and Mrs. B. Schierhorn for typing the manuscript.

References

1. Wagenhäuser FJ (1968) Die Rheuma-Morbidität, eine klinisch-epidemiologische Untersuchung. Huber, Bern
2. Roughley PJ, Mort JS (1986) Aging and the aggregating proteoglycans of human articular cartilage. Clin Sci 71:331–344
3. Thonar EJMA, Bjornsson S, Kuettner KE (1986) Age-related changes in cartilage proteoglycans. In: Kuettner K, Schleyerbach R, Hascall VC (eds) Articular cartilage biochemistry. Raven, New York, pp 273–291
4. Gyarmati J, Földer I, Kern M, Kiss I (1987) Morphological studies on the articular cartilage of old rats. Acta Morphol Hung 35:111–124
5. Bayliss MT (1986) Proteoglycan structure in normal and osteoarthrotic human cartilage. In: Kuettner K, Schleyerbach R, Hascall VC (eds) Articular cartilage biochemistry. Raven, New York, pp 295–310
6. Poole AR (1986) Proteoglycans in health and disease: structure and functions. Biochem J 236: 1–14
7. Muir H (1977) Molecular approach to the understanding of osteoarthrosis. Ann Rheum Dis 36: 199–208
8. Pauwels F (1976) Biomechanics of the normal and diseased hip. Springer, Berlin Heidelberg New York
9. Kummer B (1969) Die Beanspruchung der Gelenke, dargestellt am Beispiel des menschlichen Hüftgelenkes. Verh Dtsch Ges Orthop, Enke, pp 301–311
10. Maquet PGJ (1976) Biomechanics of the Knee. Springer, Berlin
11. Tillmann B, Tichy P, Schleicher A (1986) Biomechanik des Vorfußes unter besonderer Berücksichtigung des Hallux valgus. In: Blauth (Hrsg) Der Hallux valgus. Springer, Berlin Heidelberg New York Tokyo, pp 27–36
12. Tillmann B (1978) A contribution to the functional morphology of articular surfaces. In: Bargmann W, Doerr W (eds) Normale und Pathologische Anatomie, vol 34. Thieme, Stuttgart
13. Grasset EJ (1960) La Coxarthrose. Masson, Paris
14. Bombelli R (1976) Osteoarthritis of the hip, Springer, Berlin Heidelberg New York
15. Carstens C, Tillmann B (1983) Zur Beanspruchung der Osteophyten bei der Coxarthrose. Verh Anat Ges 77:319–320
16. Tillmann B, Schünke M (1991) Struktur and Funktion extrazellulärer Matrix. Verh Anat Ges 84:23–36
17. Schünke M, Tillmann B, Brück M, Müller-Ruchholtz W (1988) Lectin-binding in normal and osteoarthrotic articular cartilage from STR/1N-mouse knee joints. Virchows Arch [Cell Pathol] 54:327–333
18. Walton M (1977) Degenerative joint disease in the mouse knee: histological observations. J Pathol 123:109–122
19. Wilhelmi G (1981) Morphological observations on proliferation and regeneration processes in

spontaneous osteoarthrosis in the C57 black mouse. In: Peyron JG (ed) New research developments in osteoarthrosis. Huber, Bern

20. Schünke M, Tillmann B, Brück M, Müller-Ruchholtz W (1988) Morphologic characteristics of developing osteoarthrotic lesions in the knee cartilage of STR/1N mice. Arthritis Rheum 31: 898–905

21. Venn G, Mason RM (1985) Absence of keratan sulfate from skeletal tissues of mouse and rat. Biochem J 228:443–450

22. Rostand KS, Baker JR, Caterson B, Christner JE (1986) Articular cartilage proteoglycans from normal and osteoarthritic mice. Arthritis Rheum 29:95–105

23. Benske B, Schünke M, Tillmann B (1988) Subchondral bone formation in arthrosis. Polychrome labeling studies in mice. Acta Orthop Scand 59: 536–541

24. Rahn BA (1976) Die polychrome Sequenzmarkierung des Knochens. Nova Acta Leopoldina 44:249–255

25. Radin EL, Rose RM (1986) Role of subchondral bone in the initiation and progression of cartilage damage. Clin Orthop 213:34–40

26. Maroudas A (1976) Balance between swelling pressure and collagen tension in normal and degenerated cartilage. Nature 260:808–809

27. Tillmann B (1980) Pathomechanics of articular surfaces. In: Gastpar H (ed) Biology of the articular cartilage in health and disease. Schattauer, pp 155–171

28. Hulth A (1988) Growth factors in arthrosis. Acta Orthop Scand 59(5):594

29. Canalis E, McCarthy T, Contrella M (1988) Growth factors and the regulation of bone remodeling. J Clin Invest 81:277–281

Mechanical Factors in the Pathogenesis of Osteoarthritis

T. Derek V. Cooke, R. Allan Scudamore, and Tim Bryant[1]

Summary. A comparison of hip and knee osteoarthritis (OA) cases in Japan and North America supports the involvement of abnormal joint mechanics in most. Yet differences in patterns of subluxation (hip) and alignment (knee), as defined by standardized radiographs in the populations, plus occurrence of OA in seemingly normally formed joints, makes it very likely that biological factors are involved. Models of joint wear (loss of cartilage) are described in OA (as contrasted to age related changes), in which unsound factors, mechanical and biological, may add to each other and thereby contribute to progression.

Key words. Osteoarthritis — Hip — Knee mechanical and biological factors

Introduction

Mechanical attrition in osteoarthritis (OA) is supported by the focal nature of the joint pathology, slowly progressive changes, and time dependency [1]. When joint disease is associated with imperfect anatomy or malalignment, these geometric aberrations generate locally high stresses and promote subluxation. Such conditions support the cartilage damage as being due to excessive compressive and shear forces [2]. In Japan, OA of the hip is uncommon, but when seen it is associated with dysplasia or subluxation and is evident mainly in females (Table 1). However, another mechanism for cartilage destruction is that of an inherent weakness in the tissue such that it does not stand up to loads normally. That many apparently normal joints develop OA supports the potential that the tissue may be weaker [1]. In contrast to hip disease patterns in Japan, hip OA in North America is more prevalent and the patterns of change are quite different and less well explained; those due to subluxation are much less frequent than in Japan (Table 1) [3].

When one examines patterns of other more commonly involved joints than the hip, such as the knee, gonarthrosis in Japan is found predominantly in women, with a nearly exclusive pattern of varus alignment (Table 1). In North America the varus orientation is also a more often encountered pattern, but the ratio is close to even (more OA in cases with apparent normal alignment); also it is much less female dominated [4] (Tables 2, 3). Features suggesting a local malformation of the joint may be found, but many cases remain unexplained (idiopathic or primary disease). (Tables 1, 2).

These racial and sex-related variations argue for the involvement of non-mechanical factors in pathogenesis. Environmental influences may be involved but genetic factors could also provide a predisposition for tissue weakness [1].

The action of mechanical factors as a causative lesion for cartilage damage is well exemplified by the geometric aberration of the hip in Japan. But a causative role for deformity at the knee is less clear; focal loss of joint space readily changes alignment.

---

[1] Surgery Arthritis Laboratory and Clinical Mechanics Group, Department of Surgery and Mechanical Engineering, Queen's University, Kingston, Ontario, Canada

Table 1. Patterns of hip and knee osteoarthritis in Japan and North America

	Hip			*Knee*		
Patterns %	Japan	N. America	Patterns[a]	Japan	N. America	
Perthes	3	5	Male/female	1:9	2:3	
Head tilt	NA	13				
Protrusio	NA	6	Polyarticular	NYD	80%	
Axillary	2	1				
Superomedial	NA	42	Mean age	70	65	
Superolateral	17	17				
Dysplasia	60	6	Varus/valgus	8:1	3:2	
Dislocation	18	NA				
Other	NA	10				

[a] Attending orthopedic clinics
NA, not available; NYD, not yet diagnosed

Investigations

In our studies of this question — whether deformity or cartilage damage comes first — we have employed standardized computer-based radiographs (x-rays) of the knees to assess large numbers of OA cases presenting with knee symptoms and to characterize their alignment and geometry [5,6]. The angles examined are shown in Fig. 1a,b. For comparison, we examined young healthy adults (a group of 25 males and 24 females) who had no knee complaints [4]. Alignment in these young healthy adults (YHA) revealed a pattern of load bearing from the centre of the femoral head to the ankle passing very close to the center of the knee [4] (Table 2). The angle of the joint bearing surfaces varied considerably, as measured by femoral condylar

Table 2. Comparison of coronal alignment between young · healthy adults (YHA) and symptomatic osteoarthritics (OA) in N. America

Angular parameter	YHA (n = 44)	OA (n = 170)
Hip-knee-ankle	−1.5 (2.8)	−4.0 (7.8)[a]
Condylar-hip	3.8 (2.3)	1.9 (3.3)[b]
Plateau-ankle	−3.5 (2.2)	−2.4 (4.1)

Values in parentheses are SD
[a] $P < 0.05$, [b] $P < 0.001$

rotation to the hip (condylar hip angle) and tibial plateau rotation of the ankle (Fig. 1). To maintain the joint surfaces more parallel (condylar plateau angle) in the coronal plane, it appeared that condylar rotation (of the femur) in one direction was balanced by the plateau rotation (of the tibia) in the other (Table 2). Yet

Table 3. Comparison of angular geometry of males and females with arthritic or healthy knees Symptomatic osteoarthritis

	Hip-Knee-Ankle	Condylar-Hip	Plateau-Ankle
Males n = 76	−6.0	0.6[a]	−2.5
Females n = 91	−2.4	2.9	−2.4

Male/female difference   [a] $P < 0.001$

Young healthy adults

	Hip-Knee-Ankle	Condylar-Hip	Plateau-Ankle
Males n = 23	−0.4	3.0	−3.2
Females n = 21	−0.3	4.7	−3.9

Male/female difference—not significant (*NS*)

Fig. 1a,b. Features of long limb alignment in the knee. Figure 1 illustrates the angles subtended in a varus limb with loading, and illustrates the joint space narrowing medially, depicted by the condylar plateau angle, and the varus limb position, depicted by the hip-knee-ankle angle (*CMTS*). The coronal rotation of the femur to the hip is defined as the condylar hip angle and that of the plateau to the ankle is the plateau-ankle angle. *CMXC*, capitomidcondylar-transcondylar angle; *TPTS*, tibial plateau-tibial shaft angle

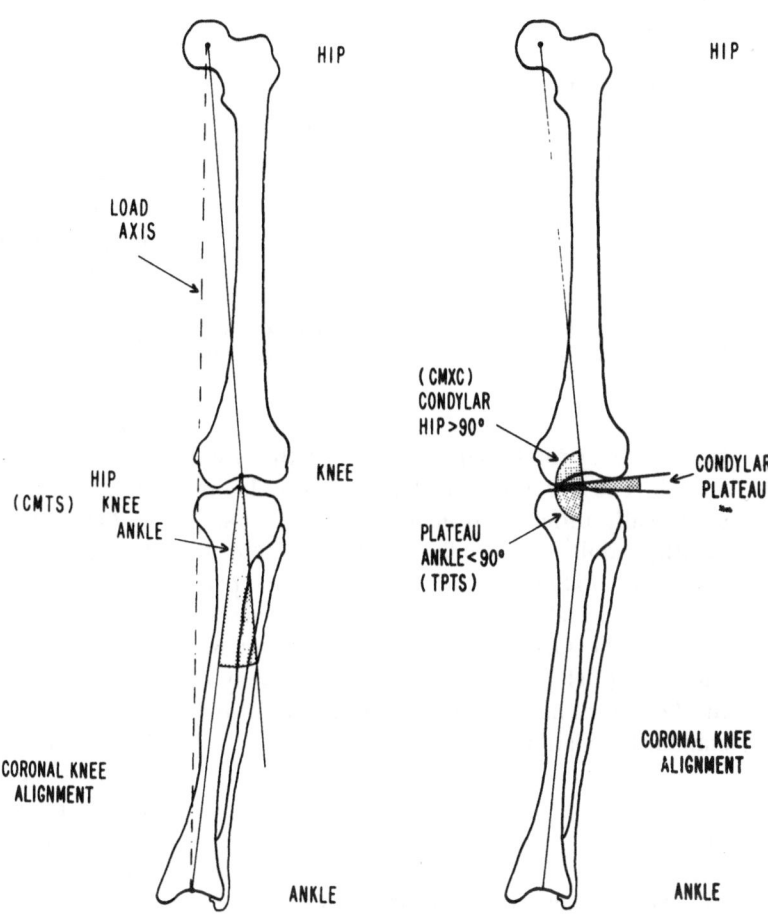

significant variations in coronal knee joint angle geometry were a feature of the young healthy adult population, as seen by the high standard deviations (Table 2). Geometric variations of similar kind and extent in adult non-arthritic skeletons were seen in separately done anatomical studies [7–9]. These geometric variations in non-arthritic joints triggered our interest to look closely at the nature of angular changes associated with OA. The postulate was that specific angular features may predispose for abnormal joint loading of excessive compression and shear force.

Standardized radiographs have been most useful; they allowed us to define specific alignment disorders in which progressive functional disability and arthritis was common. The patterns identified included a varus form of knee dysplasia [10], valgus deformities due mainly to condylar femoral valgus [1] and rotary ab-

normalities of the proximal tibia, lending an insquinting appearance to the knee [11].

Results

Analysis of the OA radiographic findings have been interesting as compared to YHA (Tables 2, 3, 4). Of interest were patterns that originated

Table 4. Joint angle and spaces for patients with osteoarthritis (OA) and young healthy adults (YHA) in North America

Parameter	YHA	OA
Condylar plateau	−1.8 (1.4)	−3.5 (4.3)[a]
Lateral joint space	5.4 (1.3)	6.3 (3.7)
Medial joint space	4.9 (0.8)	3 (1.9)[a]

Values in parentheses are SD
[a] $P < 0.001$

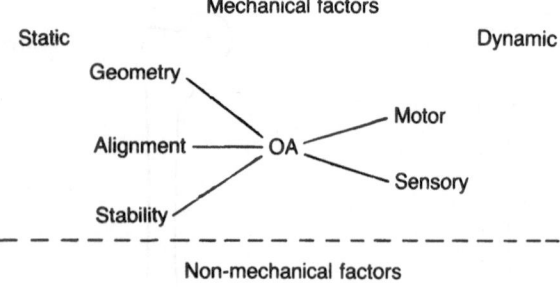

Fig. 2. The interface between static, dynamic, and biological factors in the genesis of osteoarthritis of the knee

from coronal rotational variations of the distal femur. These rotational changes were highly statistically different from those in the young healthy adults, especially as they related to condylar rotation to the hip and joint space angles. They also differed significantly among sexes in the OA population — a feature not shown in (YHA) (Table 3). However, many of the OA cases had alignment within that of one standard deviation of YHA.

Discussion

To explain these relationships of OA in normally aligned joints, one needs to consider factors beyond static mechanics (Fig. 2). Dynamic factors may produce excessive motor overload to the joint; such could be due to sensory disturbances, especially deficits in proprioception [1]. These may be an important potential mechanism, since many OA joints do not have much pain [12,13].

However, another important mechanism may be inherently weak tissues (due to biological factors). Many of these influences are not obvious to general inspection [14,15] and include genetic predisposition or defective genes for collagen formation [16].

In a sequential series of OA patients coming to hip and knee arthoplasty in Canada some 80% showed evidence of polyarticular involvement [17]. Doherty et al. [18] demonstrated that in patients who had had a meniscectomy many years before, the most severe damage for OA in the traumatized joint was in patients exhibiting polyarticular hand changes. These patients also had significantly more OA evident in the

opposite non-traumatized knee. Polyarthritis may thus be evidence of a systemic marker for tissue weakness. Past studies in our laboratory demonstrated immune deposits in cartilage of most poly OA cases, with a variety of inflammatory infiltrates in osteoarthritic synovia [19]. Taken together, these features may indicate that the polyarticular patterns of OA have multiple causative elements in their etio-pathogenisis whose net result in a given joint is weaker tissue [1].

Conclusions

One way to model the pathogenetic mechanisms in OA may be to suggest that an excessive destructive wear process occurs in the joint when more than one noxious element interacts locally. Thus *unsound* biological factors in combination with *unsound* mechanical factors will invariably lead to OA (Fig. 3); whereas one unsound factor alone may not increase the rate of damage sufficiently to provoke symptoms. Wear may ordinarily occur as an age-related phenomenon, with changes correlating with increasing years. These changes include chondromalacia, joint space narrowing, and shape change, and have been well reviewed by Sokoloff [20] (Fig. 4). But accelerated wear that exemplifies OA comes via the interaction between factors creating a more rapidly progressive situation [1]. Thus, the more factors that are involved the more rapid will be the destructive changes. Inflammatory arthritis in a malaligned limb represents the extreme of biological factors, with a mechanical aberration acting to destroy cartilage weakened by inflammation in the face of normal mechanical stresses. In Fig. 4, the rate change of these scenarios is depicted, with the width of each panel being the dynamic range of over- or underload shown by various cases [20].

Future Directions

These concepts may provide the opportunity to define those mechanical factors in pathogenisis whose treatment will tend to stabilize and reduce the rate of damage in the joint. OA occurring without an obvious mechanical dis-

	Biological	
	Sound B+	Unsound B−
Mechanical — Sound M+	Group 1	Group 2
Mechanical — Unsound M−	Group 3	Group 4

Fig. 3. Interaction between sound and unsound biological and mechanical factors. *Group 1* here represents age-related changes in joints that do not progress to osteoarthritis. *Groups 2 and 3* represent aberrations in joints which may lead to pathologic change, but on their own may not give rise to symptoms unless the penetrating factor of their activity is very strong. *Group 4* represents the interaction of both unsound mechanical and biological factors which at some time or other will always give rise to abnormal changes

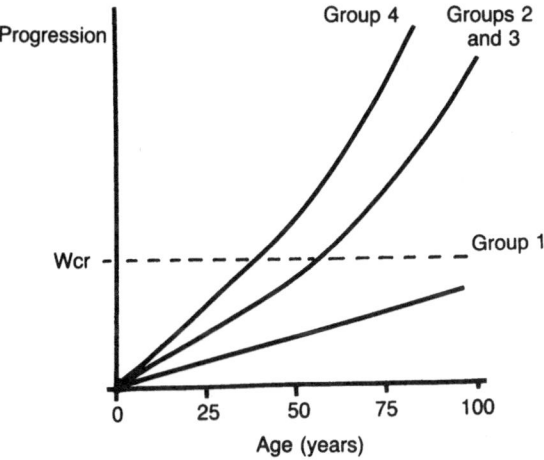

Fig. 4. Age-related changes in joints with progressive wear. The *bottom panel* represents the age-related attrition of joint cartilage and thinning that may accompany most joints with time but do not progress. *Groups 2 and 3* represent successive additions of abnormal factors, with *Group 4* representing the most advanced features of at least two and/or more abnormal factors promoting progressive damage in the joint. *Wcr* represents the critical level of wear beyond which mechanical stresses and the wear process is accelerated

order is likely, by definition, to have major or multiple unsound biological influences. The means to separate mechanical from biological influences in etiopathogenesis may be the key to understanding progression and rationalizing treatment.

Acknowledgements. The author thanks Mrs. Julie Carty and Mrs. Kim Clark for their careful work in preparing this manuscript and the MRC for their past support of this research.

References

1. Cooke TDV (1985) Pathogenetic mechanisms in polyarticular osteoarthritis. Clin Rheum Dis: Osteoarthritis 11(2): 203–238
2. Radin EL (1976) Mechanical aspects of osteoarthritis. Bull Rheum Dis 26:862–65
3. Hoagland FT, Shiba R, Newberg AH, Leung YK (1985) Diseases of the hip. J Bone Joint Surg [Am] 67:1376–1383
4. Cooke TDV, Bryant JT, Scudamore RA, Britten M (1991) Comparative analysis of static biomechanics in young healthy adults and symptomatic osteoarthritis patients. Transactions of the 37th Annual Meeting of the Orthopaedic Research Society 16(2):582
5. Siu D, Cooke TDV, Broekhoven LD, Lam M, Fisher B, Saunders G, Challis TW (1991) A standardized technique for lower limb radiography: Practice applications and error analysis. J Invest Radiol 26(1):71–77
6. Cooke TDV, Scudamore RA, Bryant JT, Sorbie C, Siu D, Fisher B (1991) Quantitative approach to radiography of the lower limb. J Bone Joint Surg [Br] Vol 73-B, No. 5, 715–720
7. Yoshioka Y, Siu D, Cooke TDV (1987) The anatomy and functional axes of the femur. J Bone Joint Surg [Am] 69(6):873–880
8. Yoshioka Y, Siu D, Scudamore RA, Cooke TDV (1989) Tibial anatomy and functional axes. J Orthop Res 7:132–137
9. Yoshioka Y, Cooke TDV (1987) Femoral anteversion: Assessment based on function axes. J Orthop Res 5:86–91
10. Cooke TDV, Pichora D, Siu D, Scudamore RA, Bryant JT (1989) Surgical implications of varus deformity of the knee with obliquity of joint surfaces. J Bone Joint Surg [Br] 71(4):560–565
11. Cooke TDV, Price N, Fisher B, Hedden D (1990) The insquinting knee: An unrecognized problem of external rotational malalignment. Clin Orthop 260:56–60
12. Jorring K (1980) Osteoarthritis of the hip. Acta Orthop Scand 51:523–530
13. Lawrence JS, Bremner JM, Bier F (1966) Osteoarthrosis. Prevalence in the population and rela-

tionship between symptoms and x-ray changes. Ann Rheum Dis 25:1–24

14. Dieppe PA, Doyle DV, Huskisson EC, Willoughby DA, Crocker PR (1978) Mixed crystal deposition disease and osteoarthritis. Br Med J [Clin Res] 1:150

15. Ehrlich GE (1972) Inflammatory osteoarthritis: I. The clinical syndrome. J Chronic Dis 25:317–328

16. Knowlton RG, Katzenstein, PL, Moskowitz RW, Weaver EJ, Malemud CJ, Pathria MN, Jimenez SA, Prockop DJ (1990) Genetic linkage of a polymorphism in the type II procollagen gene (COL2A1) to primary osteoarthritis associated with mild chondrodysplasia. N Engl J Med 322: 526–530

17. Cooke TDV (1983) The polyarticular features of osteoarthritis requiring hip and knee surgery. J Rheumatol 10(2):288–290

18. Doherty M, Watt I, Dieppe P (1983) Influence of primary generalized osteoarthritis on development of secondary osteoarthritis. Lancet II:8–11

19. Cooke TDV, Bennett EL, Ohno O (1980) The deposition of immunoglobulins and complement components in osteoarthritic cartilage. Int Orthop 4:211–217

20. Sokoloff L (1983) Aging and degenerative disease affecting cartilage. In: Hall BK (ed) Cartilage, vol 3, Biomedical Aspects. Academic, New York pp 109–141

Immunopathology of Rheumatoid Synovium

MORRIS ZIFF[1]

Summary. The character of the immunologically stimulated chronic inflammatory infiltrate is to a considerable extent determined by nonspecific factors governing mononuclear cell traffic. The volume, composition, and distribution of this traffic is strongly dependent on an initial adhesive interaction between circulating mononuclear cells and the EC of the postcapillary venules (PCV) of the involved tissues. The emigration of lymphocytes from the PCV is preceded by binding of the lymphocytes to the endothelial lining cell. This binding is enhanced by lymphokines (IFN-γ, TNF-β, IL-4) and monokines (IL-1, TNF-α), secreted by perivascular inflammatory cells and acting on the EC. This enhancement may permit an initial, immunologically generated small focus of mononuclear cells to amplify itself to a larger infiltrate. Two general mechanisms appear to be operative in chronic inflammation: (1) a specific mechanism in which an antigen stimulates an immune response with an initial secretion of cytokines, and (2) a nonspecific mechanism in which the cytokines released mediate a largely nonspecific infiltration of chronic inflammatory cells. The specific mechanism may determine the site of the inflammatory response and the nature of the antibodies which may be locally synthesized. The nonspecific mechanism creates the conventional pattern of chronic inflammation observed in variable sites in a number of diseases.

Introduction

The rheumatoid synovial membrane is infiltrated with chronic inflammatory cells. Although the pattern of infiltration in rheumatoid arthritis,

as in other chronic synovitides, is largely nonspecific, certain characteristic configurations of the mononuclear cell infiltrates may be discerned. There are, in some synovial membranes, lymphocyte-rich areas in which small lymphocytes are densely aggregated. We have referred to these as lymphocyte-rich areas [1]. Such areas often make a transition at their borders, to areas made up of macrophages, lymphocytes and plasma cells. In such areas, immunoglobulins and rheumatoid factors are synthesized. We have referred to these as transitional areas [1].

There is an interesting relationship between the appearance of the endothelium of the postcapillary venules, from which the mononuclear cells emigrate, and the composition of the perivascular mononuclear cell population. Electron microscopic measurements of the endothelial cells (EC) of these vessels disclosed a highly significant positive correlation between the tallness of the EC and the percentage of lymphocytes in the surrounding infiltrate [2]. In contrast, the correlation was highly negative when EC tallness was compared to the percentage of macrophages, plasma cells, and fibroblasts in the immediate perivascular region. As such cells increased in percentage, the endothelium tended to be flatter. The intimate relationship observed between tall endothelium and the presence of large numbers of small lymphocytes in the perivascular tissue has been previously noted in the paracortical areas of lymphoid tissue [3] and in the salivary glands of patients with Sjogren's syndrome [4]. The mechanism underlying the relationship between the tallness of the endothelium, with its associated cuboidal

[1] The University of Texas Southwestern Medical Center, Dallas, TX 75235, USA

or columnar morphology, and the cellular compositions of the surrounding infiltrate has been a subject of considerable interest. It has been observed that depletion of afferent lymphatics to lymph nodes leads to flattening of the EC and this has been attributed to a depletion of macrophages from the lymphoid tissue [5–7]. Recent evidence has pointed to a role of a monokine in the development of tall endothelium [8]. Evidence obtained in our laboratory suggests that this monokine is tumor necrosis factor (TNF)-α, and that lymphotoxin, TNF-β, is also active in this respect [9].

Effect of Cytokines on T Cell to Endothelial Cell Binding

The emigration of lymphocytes from the blood into the perivascular tissue space is critically dependent on the endothelial cell (EC). There are three essential steps in the emigration of the lymphocyte (1) binding of the lymphocytes to the EC, (2) migration of the lymphocyte through the endothelium and basement membrane into the perivascular space, and (3) migration or ecotaxis of the lymhocyte to its appropriate microenvironment along a chemotactic gradient. In our laboratory, we have studied these three steps with particular regard to rheumatoid inflammation.

On the assumption that the binding of T cells to EC might be influenced by cytokines liberated by cells of the adjacent chronic inflammatory infiltrate, we studied the effect of cytokine-containing supernatants, such as PHA-stimulated peripheral blood mononuclear cell culture supernatants or mixed lymphocyte reaction culture supernatants, on the binding of T lymphocytes to human umbilical vein EC, using ^{51}Cr-labelled T cells to measure binding [10]. Following incubation of such supernatants with EC, a significant increase in the capacity of the EC to bind T cells was observed. This was demonstrated to be due to an effect on the EC and not on the T cell, since preincubation of the supernatants with T cells produced no increase in binding. In view of the stimulatory activity of the supernatants, four cytokines thought to be present in such supernatants were investigated for their capacity to activate binding. It was observed that increased binding of T cells to EC was stimulated in dose-dependent fashion when the EC were incubated with interferon-γ (IFN-γ) [11], interleukin 1β (IL-1β) [12], and TNF [13]. Maximal effect was noted with as little as 10 U/ml of IFN-β, 0.1 U/ml of IL-1β, and 1 U/ml of TNF.

Effect of Lipopolysaccharide on Binding

Large increases in T-EC adhesion were also observed after preincubation of EC with nanogram quantities of bacterial lipopolysaccharide (LPS) isolated from a variety of gram-negative organisms [14]. This effect was also exerted on the EC and not on the T cell. This action of LPS is probably responsible for the rapid onset of lymphopenia which occurs in gram-negative infection.

Chemotaxis in Lymphocyte Emigration

It appears likely that chemotaxis plays a role in the movement of lymphocytes through the endothelium and underlying basement membrane of the postcapillary venules (PCV) and in their movement in the perivascular space. For this reason, we have investigated the role of cytokines in the chemotaxis of lymphocytes. Using a modified Boyden chamber technique, we initially observed that IL-1 was an effective chemotactic agent for T cells and B cells, though these experiments were carried out with the ultrapurified and not with a recombinant preparation [15]. It was further observed that rheumatoid synovial fluid had a chemotactic action on lymphocytes and that this effect was expressed in a concentration-dependent manner [16]. IL-8 has also been demonstrated to be chemotactic for T lymphocytes [17]. The macrophage inflammatory protein-1 (MIP-1) and TGFB are also chemotactic for lymphocytes.

The Integrin Family of Adhesion Molecules

Emigration of leukocytes from the blood requires initial binding of these cells to the EC of PCV. Following emigration, the mononuclear cells adhere to each other and to matrix components. Adhesion of mononuclear cells to matrix proteins facilitates their movment toward inflammatory foci and their retention in such foci. Recognition of these phenomena has stimulated intensive study of the role of adhesion molecules in the immune response and in chronic inflammation. From these studies, evidence has emerged for the existence of a supergene family of adhesion molecules, the integrins, which to a considerable extent carry out the adhesive functions of the leukocytes of the body.

The integrin family, as it occurs on nucleated cells, consists of three subfamilies of glyco-protein heterodimers made up of α and β chains. In each of these, the α chains vary in com-position and the β chains are constant [18,19]. These subfamilies are as follows (1) the CD11/CD18 Family, a group of three glycoprotein heterodimers expressed on hematopoietic cells which contain a common β2 variety of β chain. This family is responsible for the binding of leukocytes to EC prior to emigration from the blood and for the adhesive interactions of the extravascular cells which participate in the tissue cellular immune response, (2) the VLA-Fibronectin Receptor Family, a group of heterodimers containing a common β1 chain, which is present on a variety of cells, and whose main function is to mediate the adhesion of these cells to extracellular matrix proteins, and (3) the Vitronectin Receptor Family, a group of heterodimers containing a cmmon β3 chain, present on a variety of cells, which also has the function of attachment of these cells to their surroundings by reaction with proteins in the extracellular matrix.

The baseline binding of T cells to HUVEC monolayers is largely achieved by the LFA-1 receptor, as indicated by blocking experiments in which monoclonal antibodies to the α and β chains of this heterodimer inhibited up to 90% of the binding [10]. Binding was increased fol-lowing stimulation of the T cell with phorbol ester, and the majority of the increase was due to heightened expression of LFA-1. The ligand on the EC for LFA-1 is the intercellular adhesion molecule-1 (ICAM-1), a single chain glycoprotein expressed on cells from various sources [20–22].

As mentioned above, four cytokines, gamma interferon (IFN-γ), IL-1, TNF-α, and TNF-β increased the binding activity of HUVEC and dermal microvascular EC [23]. Recently, IL-4 has been shown to have similar activity. In experiments carried out to identify the ligand on

the EC which was responsible for the increase in T cell binding, antibodies to LFA-1, which markedly inhibited lymphocyte binding by un-stimulated EC, had little effect on the increased binding induced by IL-1 [10], suggesting that the EC ligand induced was not ICAM-1. Dustin and Springer have also observed increased lymphocyte binding on EC stimulated by cytokines [24], and in their experiments, this was accompanied by upregulation of ICAM-1 on the EC. However, only a portion of the increase in binding could be attributed to increased expression of this ligand. These results have suggested the presence of other ligands for lymphocyte binding on cytokine-stimulated EC. Recent evidence has demonstrated the EC ligands VCAM-1 and ELAM-1, which also bind lymphocytes to the EC.

T Cell Diversity in the Rheumatoid Synovial Infiltrate

Accepting the strong likelihood that the cellular response in rheumatoid synovitis is immu-nologically induced, it may be assumed to begin with a specific interaction between a reactive T cell clone and an antigen. Though, initially, selective recruitment of immune T lymphocytes may occur in this type of reaction [25,26], the population of lymphocytes finally assembled is, in the main, immunologically nonspecific, only a small fraction bearing immunity to the injected antigen [26,27]. As would be predicted from this, most analyses of the T cell receptors of the lymphocytes of rheumatoid synovial fluid and tissue have failed to demonstrate clonality among the infiltrating T cells (28–30). It appears likely that a major factor in the development of the T cell receptor diversity of the synovial T cell is the upregulation of EC binding of these cells by cytokines leading to binding of activated T cells in an immunologically nonspecific manner.

Greater Responsiveness to Antigen of Synovial Fluid Mononuclear Cells Compared to Peripheral Blood Mononuclear Cells

Recent observations have shown that the T4 cells of the chronic inflammatory synovial membrane and synovial effusion, and of a number of lesions in other chronic inflammatory diseases, are mainly helper-inducer (HI) memory cells, i.e., CD4+CDw29+ HI T cells, which are identified by the 4B4 antibody [31] and the similar UCHL1 antibody [31,32]. Only small numbers of the naive T4 cell subset (CD4+CD45RA+ suppressor-inducer (SI) T cell, reacting with 2H4 antibody [33] are found. Pitzalis et al. [34] observed that 93.8% of rheumatoid synovial fluid T cells were 4B4+. Thus, most of the T4 cells in the rheumatoid effusion were memory cells; the memory to naive cell ratio was 16.8. Emery et al. [35] found this ratio to be 9.5. These ratios markedly exceeded those measured in the peripheral blood. The above findings have recently been confirmed by others [36]. In rheumatoid synovial tissue, Duke et al., using immunohistological techniques, found a similar excess of the HI subset of T cells [37], and Pitzalis et al. [34], staining isolated rheumatoid synovial membrane cells, found that while 90% of the T cells were UCLH1+, only 7.1% carried the 2H4 marker.

Recently, the rheumatoid synovial fluid studies of Pitzalis et al. were extended to other inflammatory arthritides, and a similar elevated ratio of memory (CD4+4B4+UCLH1+) to naive (CD4+2H4+) T cells was observed [38]. In parallel experiments, Morimoto et al. [39] compared the percentages of CD4+4B4+ and CD4+2H4+ lymphocytes in the peripheral blood and synovial fluid of patients with rheumatoid arthritis (RA), psoriatic arthritis, ankylosing spondylitis, and Reiter's syndrome. The findings in the four conditions were similar. While the ratio of the HI to SI cell subset was 1.5 in the blood, in the synovial fluid it was 8.5. In a group of miscellaneous chronic pleural and peritoneal effusions, Pitzalis et al. [31] also found a marked excess of UCHL+ (CDw29+) over UCHL1− (CD45RA+) cells. Similar findings have also been obtained in the thyroid tissues in Graves' disease [40] and in atopic dermatitis [41]. Finally, an elevated 4B4+ to 2H4+ ratio has been found in the plaques and adjacent white matter of the central nervous system tissue of patients with multiple sclerosis. Thus, the predominance of the CDw29+, HI memory T cell seems to be characteristic of a miscellany of chronic inflammatory conditions.

An important characteristic of the T cells accumulated in synovial effusions may be explainable by the excess of CD4+CDw29+ T cells present, i.e., their active responses to antigens to which the hosts might be expected to be immunized, either in association with their disease (*chlamydia*, mycoplasma, enteric bacteria, *Borrelia*, Yersinia, influenza, and *herpes simplex*) or, in the case of other antigens, as a result of previous contact with the antigen [41–48]. Active responsiveness to soluble antigens is highly characteristic of the HI (memory) T cell.

References

1. Ishikawa H, Ziff M (1976) Electron microscopic observations of immunoreactive cells in the rheumatoid synovial membrane. Arthritis Rheum 19:1–14
2. Iguchi T, Ziff M (1986) Electron microscopic study of rheumatoid synovial vasculature: Intimate relationship between tall endothelium and lymphoid aggregates. J Clin Invest 77:355–361
3. Gowans JL, Knight EJ (1964) The route of recirculation of lymphocytes in the rat. Proc R Soc Lond (Biol) 159:257–282
4. Freemont AJ, Jones CJP (1983) Endothelial specialization of salivary gland vessels for accelerated lymphocyte transfer in Sjogren's syndrome. J Rheumatol 10:801–804
5. Hendriks HR, Eestermans IL, Hoefsmit ECM (1980) Depletion of macrophages and disappearance of postcapillary high endothelial venules in lymph nodes deprived of afferent blood vessels. Cell Tissue Res 211:375–389
6. Hendriks HR, Eestermans IL (1983) Disappearance and reappearance of high endothelial venules and immigrating lymphocytes in lymph nodes deprived of afferent vessels: A possible regulatory role of macrophages in lymphocyte migration. Eur J Immunol 13:663–669
7. Drayson MT, Ford WL (1984) Afferent lymph and lymph-born cells; their influence on lymph node formation. Immunobiology 168:362–379
8. FitzGerald OM, Hess EV, Chance A, Highsmith RF (1987) Quantitative studies of huma monokine-induced endothelial cell elongation. J Leukocyte Biol 41:421–428
9. Cavender D, Edelbaum D, Ziff M (1989) Endothelial cell activation induced by tumor necrosis factor and lymphotoxin. Am J Pathol 134:551–560

10. Haskard D , Cavender D, Beatty P, Springer T, Ziff M (1986) T lymphocyte adhesion to endothelial cells: Mechanisms demonstrated by anti-LFA-1 monoclonal antibodies. J Immunol 137:2901–2906

11. Yu C-L, Haskard DO, Cavender D, Johnson AR, Ziff M (1985) Human gamma interferon increases the binding of T lymphocytes to endothelial cells. Clin Exp Immunol 62:554–560

12. Cavender D, Haskard DO, Joseph B, Ziff M (1986) Interleukin-1 increases the binding of human B and T lymphocytes to endothelial cell monolayers. J Immunol 136:203–207

13. Cavender D, Saegusa Y, Ziff M (1987) Stimulation of endothelial cell binding of lymphocytes by tumor necrosis factor. J Immunol 139:1855–1860

14. Yu C-L, Haskard DO, Cavender DE, Ziff M (1986) Effects of bacterial lipopolysaccharide on the binding of lymphocytes to EC monolayer. J Immunol 136:569–573

15. Miossec P, Yu C-L, Ziff M (1984) Lymphocyte chemotactic activity of human interleukin 1. J Immunol 133:2007–2011

16. Miossec P, Dinarello CA, Ziff M (1986) Interleukin 1 lymphocyte chemotactic activity in rheumatoid synovial fluid. Arthritis Rheum 29:352–357

17. Larsen CG, Anderson AO, Apella E, Oppenheim JJ, Matsushima K (1989) The neutrophil-activating protein (NAP1) is also chemotactic for T lymphocytes. Science 243:1464–1466

18. Hynes RO (1987) A family of cell surface receptors. Cell 49:549–554

19. Hogg N (1989) The leukocyte integrins. Immunol Today 10:111–114

20. Rothlein R, Dustin ML, Marlin SD, Springer TA (1986) A human intercellular adhesion molecule [ICAM-1] distinct from LFA-1. J Immunol 137:1270–1274

21. Marlin SD, Springer TA (1987) Purified intercellular adhesion molecule-1 [ICAM-1] is a ligand for lymphocyte function-associated antigen 1 (LFA-1). Cell 51:813–819

22. Makgoba MW, Sanders ME, Luce GEG, Dustin ML, Springer TA, Clark EA, Mannoni P, Shaw S (1988) ICAM 1, a ligand for LFA-1 dependent adhesion of B, T, and myeloid cells. Nature 331:86–88

23. Haskard DO, Cavender D, Fleck RM, Sontheimer R, Ziff M (1987) Human dermal microvascular endothelial cells behave like umbilical vein endothelial cells in T cell adhesion studies. J Invest Dermatol 88:340–344

24. Dustin ML, Springer TA (1988) Lymphocyte function-associated antigen-1 [LFA-1] interaction with intercellular adhesion molecule-1 (ICAM-1) is one of at least three mechanisms for lymphocyte adhesion to cultured endothelial cells. J Cell Biol 107:321–331

25. Lipscomb MF, Lyons CR, O'Hara RM, Stein-Streilein J (1982) The antigen-induced selective recruitment of specific T lymphocytes to the lung. J Immunol 128:111–116

26. McCluskey RT, Benacerraf B, McCluskey JW (1963) Studies on the specificity of the cellular infiltrate in delayed hypersensitivity reactions. J Immunol 90:466–477

27. Scheper RJ, van Dinther-Janssen ACHM, Polak L (1985) Specific accumulation of haptene reaction T cells in contact sensitivity reaction sites. J Immunol 134:1333–1336

28. Keystone EC, Minden M, Klock R, Poplonski L, Zalcberg J, Takadera T, Mak TW (1988) Structure of T cell antigen receptor chain in synovial fluid cells from patients with rheumatoid arthritis. Arthritis Rheum 31:1555–1557

29. Douby AD, Sinclair AK, Osborne-Lawrenc SL, Zeldes W, Kan L, Fox DA (1989) Clonal heterogeneity of synovial fluid T lymphocytes from patients with rheumatoid arthritis (abstract). Arthritis Rheum 32:B44

30. Dier DL, Roessner KD, Cooper SM (1989) Diversity of rheumatoid tissue T cells by T cell receptor analysis (abstract). Arthritis Rheum 32:B43

31. Morimoto C, Letvin NL, Boyd AW, Hagan M, Brown HM, Kornracki MM, Schlossman SF (1985) The isolation and characterization of the helper-inducer T cell subset. J Immunol 134:3762–3769

32. Smith SH, Brown MH, Rowe D, Callard RE, Beverley PCL (1986) Functional subsets of human helper-inducer cells defined by a new monoclonal antibody, UCHL-1. Immunology 58:53–70

33. Morimoto C, Levin NL, Distaso JA, Aldrich WR, Schlossman SF (1985) The isolation and characterizatio of the human suppressor inducer T cell subset. J Immunol 134:1508–1515

34. Pitzalis C, Kingsley G, Murphy J, Panayi G (1987) Abnormal distribution of the helper-inducer and suppressor-inducer T lymphocyte subsets in the rheumatoid joint. Clin Immunol Immunopathol 45:252–258

35. Emery P, Gentry KC, Mackay IR, Muirden KD, Rowley M (1987) Deficiency of the suppressor inducer subset of T lymphocytes in rheumatoid arthritis. Arthritis Rheum 30:849–856

36. Gerli R, Bertotto A, Rambotti P, Barbieri P, Ciompi ML, Bombardieri S (1988) T cell immunoregulation in rheumatoid arthritis. Arthritis Rheum 31:1075–1076

37. Duke O, Panayi GS, Bofill M, Poulter L, Janossy G (1986) Evidence for a deficiency of the suppressor-inducer T cell subset in the synovial membrane in rheumatoid arthritis (abstract). Br J Rheumatol 25 (Suppl 65):38

38. Kingsley GH, Pitzalis C, Kyriazis N, Panayi GS (1988) Abnormal helper-inducer/suppressor-inducer T cell subset distribution and T cell activation status are common to all types of chronic synovitis. Scand J Immunol 28:225–232

39. Morimoto C, Romain PL, Fox DA, Anderson P, Dimaggio M, Levine H, Schlossman SF (1988) Abnormalities in CD4+ lymphocyte subsets in inflammatory rheumatic diseases. Am J Med 84:817–825

40. Ishikawa N, Eguchi K, Otsubo T, Ueki Y, Fukuda T, Tezuka H, Matsunaga M, Kawabe Y, Shimomura C, Izumi M, Ban Y, Ito K, Nagataki S (1987) Reduction in the suppressor-inducer T cell subset and increase in the helper T cell subset in thyroid tissue from patients with Graves' disease. J Clin Endocrinol Metab 65:17–23

41. Lever R, Turbitt M, Sanderson A, MacKie R (1987) Immunopathology of the cutaneous infiltrate and of the mononuclear cells in the peripheral blood in patients with atopic dermatitis. J Invest Dermatol 89:4–7

42. Ford DK, Da Roza D (1987) Further observations on the response of synovial lymphocytes to viral antigens in rheumatoid arthritis. J Rheumatol 13:113–117

43. Ford DK, Da Roza D, Shah P (1980) Cell-mediated immune responses of synovial mononuclear cells to sexually transmitted enteric and mumps antigens with Reiter's syndrome, rheumatoid arthritis and ankylosing spondylitis. J Rheumatol 8:220–232

44. Ford DK, DaRoza DM, Reid GD, Chantler JK, Tingle AJ (1981) Synovial mononuclear cell responses to rubella antigen in rheumatoid arthritis and unexplained persistent knee synovitis. J Rheumatol 9:420–423

45. Ford DK, DaRoza D, Schulzer M, Reid GD, Denegri JF (1987) Persistent synovial lymphocyte responses to cytomegalovirus antigen in some patients with rheumatoid arthritis. Arthritis Rheum 30:700–704

46. Gaston JSH, Life PF, Granfors K, Merilahti-Palo R, Bailey L, Consalvey S, Toivanen A, Bacon PA (to be published) Synovial T lymphocyte recognition of organisms which trigger reactive arthritis

47. Padula SJ, Pfister RD (1988) Lyme disease synovial fluid cells show significantly greater response to *Borrelia Burgdorferi* antigens than peripheral cells (abstract). Clin Res 36:535 A

48. Sigal LH, Steere AC, Freeman DH, Dwyer JM (1986) Reactivity to *Borrelia burgdorferi* antigens is greater in joint fluid than in blood. Arthritis Rheum 29:761–769

Interaction of Pannus and Rheumatoid Cartilage

K. FEHR[1]

Summary. The destruction of rheumatoid joint cartilage by pannus is reviewed. The final result of the destruction is the collaborative result of interacting cells and enzymes. These are mainly located in cell nests at the pannus-cartilage junction which are related to early vascularization of the cartilage surface. The most important cells at sites of erosion are macrophages, fibroblasts, mast cells, granulocytes, and chondrocytes. Thus, external and internal destruction of rheumatoid arthritis (RA)-cartilage can be distinguished. Besides the highly destructive granulocyte elastase and cathepsin G, most enzymes involved are neutral metalloproteinases. Recent work has focused on metalloproteinase-3 (stromelysin) which has multiple functions and a most deleterious effect on cartilage. An additional potentially very destructive enzyme is cathepsin B, from chondrocytes, which highly resists inactivation by neutral pH and thus can function outside the cell.

Knowledge of cartilage destruction is still limited and research into this field is of significant importance.

Key words. Rheumatoid arthritis — Pannus — Cartilage destruction — Cells and enzymes involved in cartilage destruction.

Introduction

It is generally accepted that the growth of pannus in rheumatoid arthritis (RA) begins from the synovial recessus at the cartilage border (Fig. 1). It then may overgrow the cartilage surface and damage it to varying extents.

An additional attack on cartilage may begin from the subchondral bone and again damage the cartilage to varying extents. At a later stage destructive pannus may become nondestructive, poor in inflammatory cells, and rich in fibroblasts, which synthesize collagen and thus try to repair the damage.

Structure of Destructive Pannus

Destructive pannus overgrowing rheumatoid cartilage has a somewhat similar structure to synovial tissue, with synoviocytes at the surface and subsynovial fibrous tissue; the cartilage-pannus junction with cell-nests contains various types and amounts of leukocytes (Fig. 2). A prominent feature of such pannus is its highly developed vascularization (Fig. 3). The resulting blood flow brings leukocytes to the pannus-cartilage junction, nourishes outgrowing or invading fibroblasts and allows for the attack of appropriate cell types against the cartilage (Fig. 4). The most aggressive spots in these outgrowing small blood vessels are the above-mentioned cell nests consisting of at least one small blood vessel and cells which destroy the cartilage (Fig. 4) To date it is not clear why small blood vessels overgrow rheumatoid cartilage.

Such macroscopically still intact cartilage is often depleted of proteoglycans and contains many damaged chondrocytes. Preliminary data show that hydrogen superoxide (H_2O_2) might be the main actor in depleting hyaluronate from intact cartilage and damaging the chondrocytes (T. Matsubara (1990), personal communica-

[1] Department of Rheumatology, University Hospital, Gloriastrasse 25, CH-8091 Zurich, Switzerland

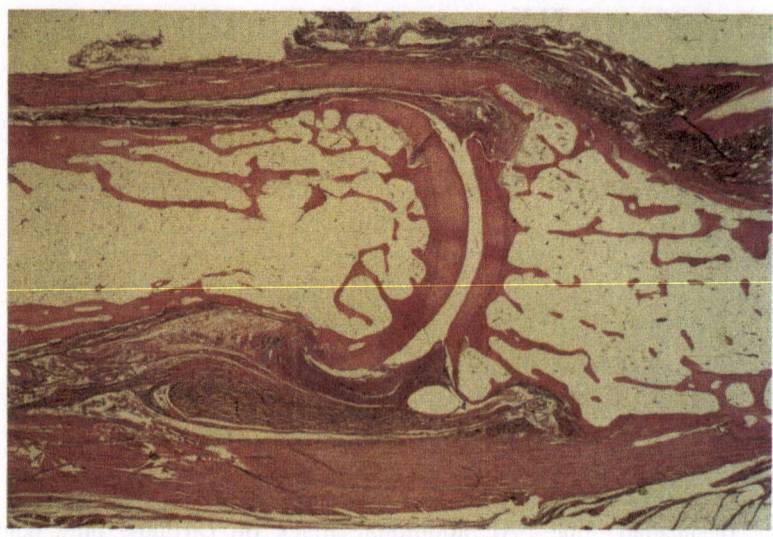

Fig. 1. Aggressive pannus in a finger joint of a patient with RA. The pannus attacks the border of the joint cartilage including the adjacent bone

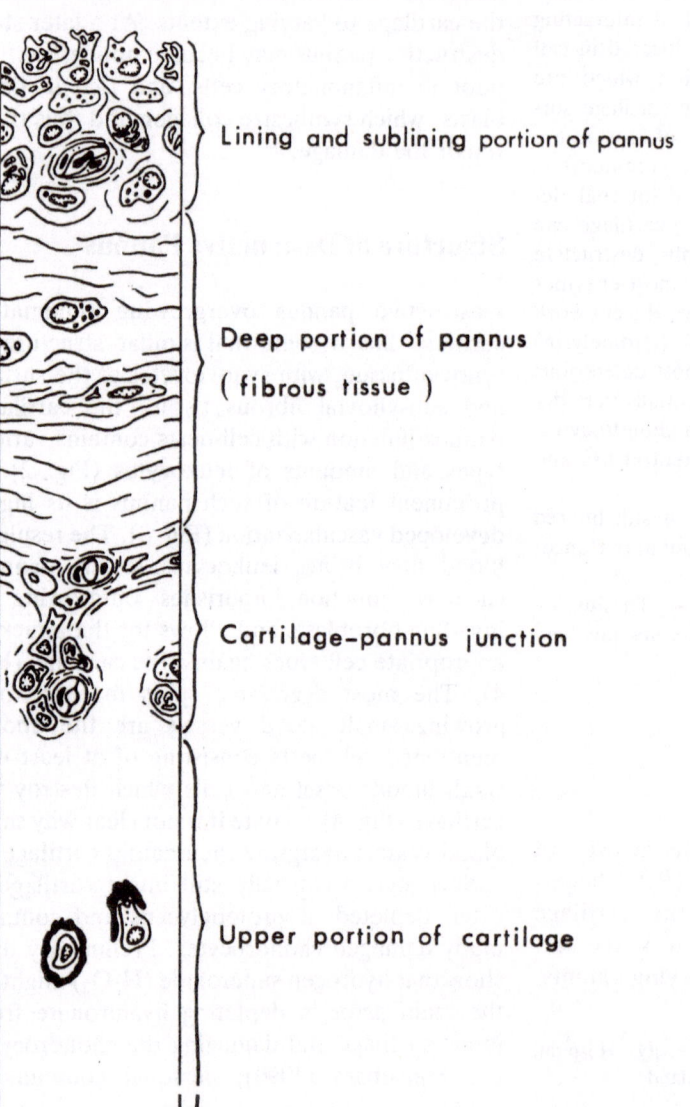

Lining and sublining portion of pannus

Deep portion of pannus
(fibrous tissue)

Cartilage-pannus junction

Upper portion of cartilage

Fig. 2. Structure of pannus according to the electron-microscopic findings of Kobayashi and Ziff [4]

Fig. 3. Pannus in RA according to the electronmicroscopic findings of Kobayashi and Ziff [4] 1975. The importance of early vascularization

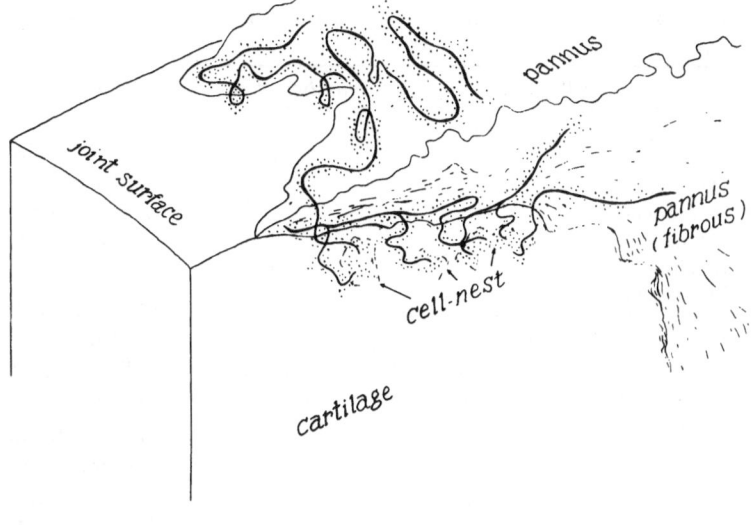

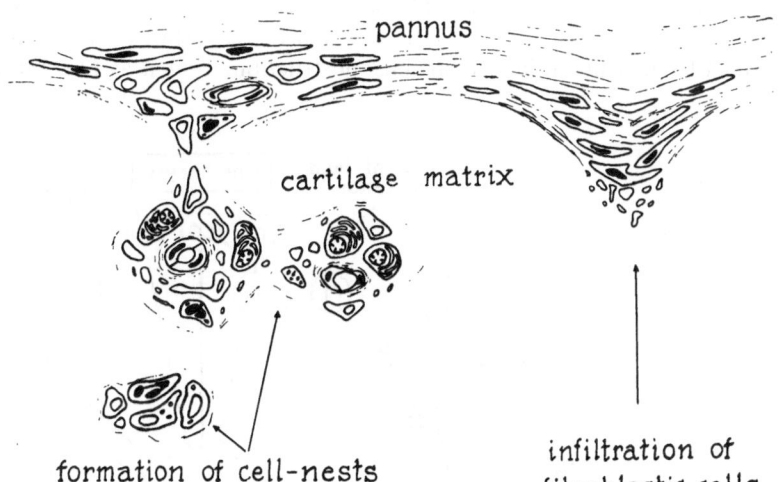

Fig. 4. Pannus in RA according to the electronmicroscopic findings of Kobayashi and Ziff [4] The formation of cell nests

tion). Hyaluronate in turn seems to act as an important promoter of angiogenesis.

An indirect indication of increased angiogenesis in rheumatoid pannus is provided by the studies of Matsubara et al., which were carried out in synovial tissue. In one approach, blood vessels were analyzed with specific antibodies against fibronectin [1] while in the other, antibodies against type four collagen were used [2]. In both cases the resulting immunoelectronmicroscopic pictures showed a clearly pronounced multilamellarity of the capillaries which was explained by increased death of endothelial cells. Newly grown endothelial cells synthesized new lamellas, thus showing hyperactivity in

the endothelial cells of small blood vessels. In addition, Mohr [3], and Kobayashi and Ziff [4], have well documented the hypervascularization in aggressive pannus.

Cells Involved in the Destruction of Articular Cartilage

In this situation the important question is which cells destroy rheumatoid cartilage. Table 1 shows the frequency of various cell types at the pannus-cartilage junction. It is clear that macrophages and fibroblasts play by far the most important role. In addition, mast cells and

Table 1. Predominant cell types at sites of cartilage erosion in rheumatoid arthritis[a]

Predominant cell type[b]	Number of cases[c]
Macrophages	10
Fibroblasts	9
Mast cells	3
Neutrophils	2
Plasma cells	1
Dendritic cells	1
Not classified	2

[a] according to Bromley and Woolley [9]
[b] Characterization by histochemistry (choloroacetate esterase, naphthyl acetate esterase, aminocaproate-esterase) and electronmicroscopy
[c] $n = 25$

granulocytes are not infrequently found to play a role in the damage. These cell types, in addition to the chondrocytes, will be discussed with respect to their potential for cartilage destruction.

Cartilage-Destroying Enzymes

Any discussion of cartilage destroying enzymes has to focus on proteoglycanases and collagenases able to work at neutral pH. In general it has to be stressed that there is a large range of interactions between cells and enzymes which attack cartilage. These interactions are schematically outlined in Fig. 5, in which only the most important interrelations are taken into account.

From Fig. 5 it becomes clear that most relevant enzymes are latent metalloproteinases which have to be activated in order to become active enzymes able to attack cartilage. Exceptions are the serinproteinases, elastase and cathepsin G, from granulocytes. The most broadly active activator of the latent enzymes is plasmin, which in turn is activated by plasminogen activator. As shown, this activator is secreted by mutiple cells such as fibroblasts, macrophages, granulocytes,

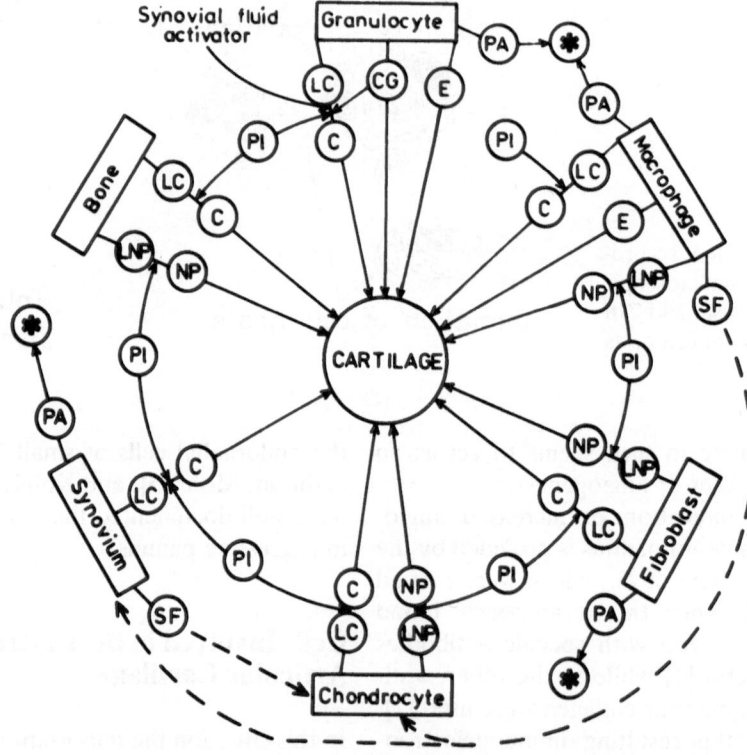

Fig. 5. Some important interrelations between cells and enzymes involved in cartilage breakdown, according to A. Baici [21], and A. Baici [10] E, elastase; CG, cathepsin G; SF, soluble factor; LC, latent collagenase; C, active collagenase; LNP, latent neutral metal-dependent proteoglycanase; NP, active neutral metal-dependent proteoglycanase; PA, plasminogen activator; PI, plasmin; *, PA → Plasminogen → PI; →, Protein-protein interaction

Table 2. Granulocytes: Possible role of neutral proteinases in cartilage damage[a]

Proteinase	Effect on cartilage
Collagenase	Latent form; activated mostly by cathepsin G and plasma-kallikrein, poorly by plasmin, also by oxygen radicals[b]
	Cleaves collagen(s) at the typical domain
Elastase	Cleaves collagen(s) (Type II, IX, probably XI)[c]
	Cleaves proteoglycans
	Activates stromelysin[d]
Cathepsin G	Cleaves collagen(s) at the telopeptide region
	Cleaves proteoglycans
	Activates latent collagenase
	Activates stromelysin[d]
Plasminogen activator	Activates plasminogen to plasmin

[a] from A. Baici [10]
[b] from Weiss et al. [11]
[c] from R. Mayne [12] and Okada et al. [13]
[d] from Okada and Nakanishi [14]

and also chondrocytes. However, a latent enzyme is not activated by only one mechanism, but most probably by several biological mechanisms. Thus, for example, latent collagenase from granulocytes is most efficiently activated by cathepsin G and plasma kallikrein, and also by oxygen radicals (Table 2).

In Fig. 5 the soluble factors able to activate the chondrocytes or fibroblasts are not specified. It is well known that — for instance — the soluble factors from macrophages are interleukin-1 (IL-1) and tumor necrosis factor (TNF) [5].

At present, the destruction of joint cartilage is defined as either external or internal destruction.

External destruction is brought about by enzymes from cells which attack the cartilage from the outside. Internal destruction is brought about by the chondrocytes themselves. In this respect a proteolytic destruction may take place or the chondrocytes may be lacking in the appropriate matrix synthesis. In the following section, we focus mostly on the proteolytic destruction although — as mentioned above — chondrocyte damage, including cell death, seems to be a very prominent feature in the decay of rheumatoid cartilage.

Table 3. Fibroblasts: Possible role of neutral proteinases in cartilage damage

Proteinase	Effect on cartilage
Metalloproteinase-1 = collagenase	Latent form, activated by plasmin
	Fully activated by stromelysin via plasmin[a]
	Stimulated by rIL-1β[b]
	Cleaves collagen(s) at the typical domain
Metalloproteinase-3 = stromelysin (proteo = glycanase)	Latent form
	Activated by plasmin, neutrophil elastase and cathepsin G[c]
	Stimulated by IL-1β[b]
	Cleaves proteoglycans, hyaluronic acid-binding region and linkprotein[d]
	Cleaves type IX collagen[e]
	Helps to activate collagenase via plasmin[a]
Plasminogen activator	Activates plasminogen to plasmin

[a] from Chengshi et al. [15]
[b] from Frisch and Ruley [16] and Saus et al. [17]
[c] from Okada and Nakanishi [14]
[d] from Nguyen et al. [18]
[e] from Okada et al. [13]

Table 4. Mast cells: Possible role in cartilage damage[a]

Mediators	Effect
Tryptase	Not inhibited by plasma antiproteinase
	Cleaves proteoglycans
Chymotryptase	Cleaves proteoglycans
Heparin	Involved in angiogenesis
Cell extracts	Strongly stimulate production of[b] collagenase in human cultures of adherent synovial fibroblasts
Cell extracts	Stimulate production of collagenase[b] and neutral proteinase in chondrocytes
Cell products	Stimulate macrophages to produce[b] more IL-1
Histamine	Stimulates PGE synthesis in fibroblasts and chondrocytes by interaction with H1-histamine receptors

[a] from K. Fehr [5]
[b] from Yoffe et al. [19]

In the Tables 2–6 actual knowledge of the cell enzymes directly or indirectly involved in cartilage destruction is roughly summarized, and some relevant literature is given below the

Table 5. Macrophages: Possible role of neutral proteinases in cartilage damage[a]

Proteinase	Effect on cartilage
Collagenase	Latent form, activated by plasmin
	Cleaves collagen(s) at the typical domain
Proteoglycanase	Latent form, activated by plasmin
	Cleaves proteoglycans
Elastase	Cleaves proteoglycans in addition to elastin
Plasminogen activator	Activates plasminogen to plasmin
IL-1 and TNF[b]	Stimulate synthesis of collagenase and stromelysin in fibroblasts and chondrocytes

[a] from A. Baici [10]
[b] from Frisch and Ruley [16] and Saus et al. [17]

Table 6. Chondrocytes: Possible role of neutral proteinases in cartilage damage[a]

Proteinase	Effect on cartilage
Metalloproteinase-1 = collagenase	See fibroblasts; probably very similar or same enzyme
Metalloproteinase-3 = stromelysin	See fibroblasts; same or very similar enzyme. Immunologically identical[b]
Plasminogen activator	Activates plasminogen to plasmin
Cathepsin B[c]	Specialized form, very resistant to alkaline pH
	Cleaves proteoglycans extensively
	Cleaves collagen(s) at the telopeptide region

[a] from A. Baici [10]
[b] from Gunja-Smith et al. [20]
[c] from A. Baici et al. [6]

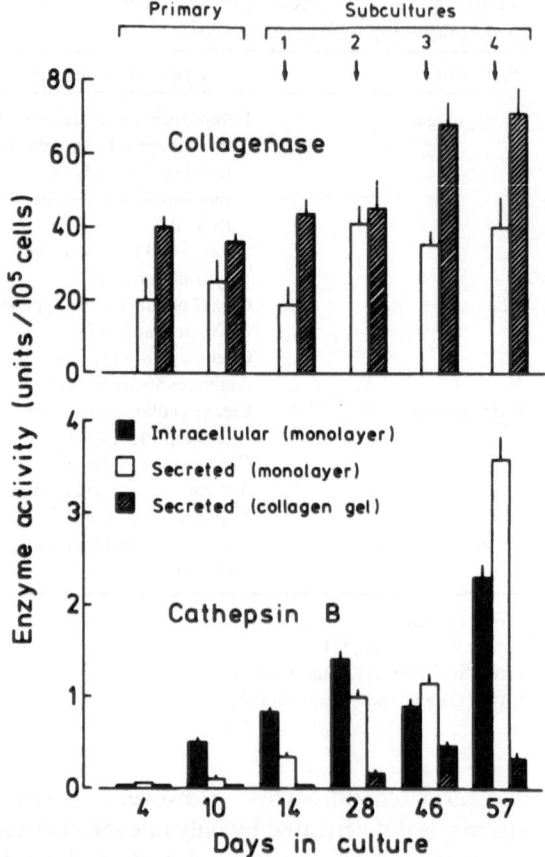

Fig. 6. Collagenase and cathepisn B produced by cultured rabbit articular chondrocytes. The *hatched columns* represent enzyme activities secreted by cells cultured in monolayers for the periods shown, transferred to collagen cultures, left to adhere to the collagen matrix overnight, and further cultured by this technique for 48 h. The *columns* represent mean values of five to seven different culture preparations and *bars* indicate one SD. (From Baici et al. [6] with permission)

Tables. Although the research into these enzymes has only recently become more intensive, some important new insights have been gained. The metalloproteinases of connective tissue cells are now characterized as metalloproteinase-1 (= collagenase), metalloproteinase-2 (= gelatinase) and metalloproteinase-3 (= stromelysin). The newly characterized stromelysin is a highly potent enzyme able to destroy not only proteoglycans, but also link proteins and hyaluronic acid binding protein, as well as collagen type IX. It, furthermore, is indirectly involved in the full activation of collagenase after the action of plasmin (Table 3). As is now known, the cleavage of collagen type IX is shared only by granulocyte elastase, which probably also degrades cartilage collagen type XI (Table 2). Collagen type IX — in holding together the collagen type II fibrils — seems to be very important for the intact structure of joint cartilage.

Stromelysin synthesis is highly stimulated by recombinant IL-1β on fibroblasts. This stimula-

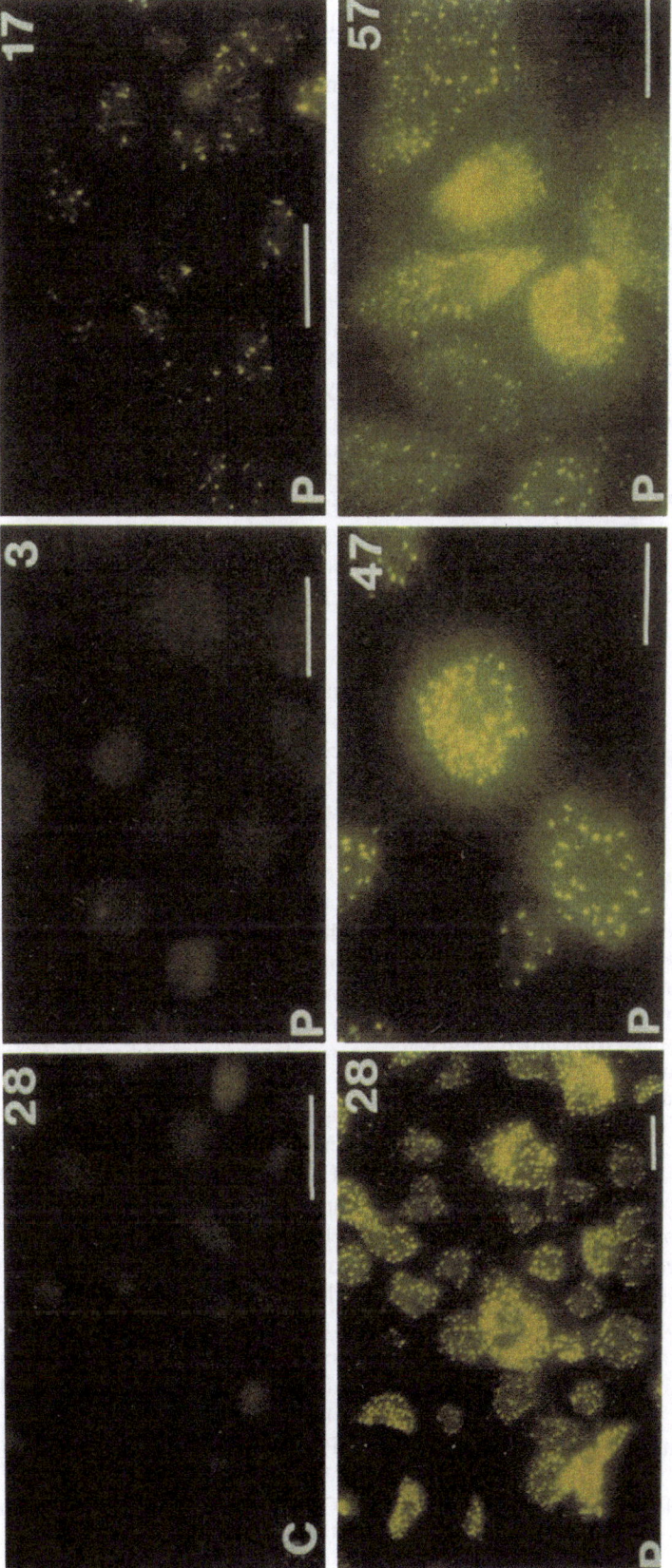

Fig. 7. Fluorescence microscopic demonstration of cathepsin B in cultured rabbit articular chondrocytes. The fluorescent granules represent enzyme activity visualized by coupling 4-methoxy-β-naphthylamide, liberated by hydrolysis of the cathepsin B specific substrate Z-Ala-Arg-Arg-4MβNA, to 5-nitrosalicylaldehyde. C, controls obtained by including in the incubation solution 2.5 µM leupeptin, a cathepsin B inhibitor; P, positive staining. *Bars* = 50 µm. The *numbers in the upper right hand corner of the individual figures* represent the days in culture (From Baici et al. [6] with permission)

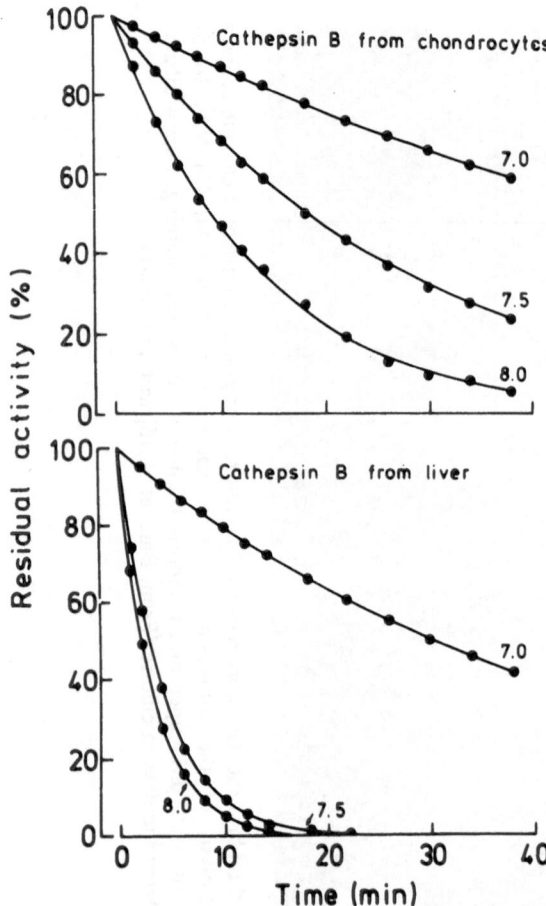

Fig. 8. pH-induced inactivation of cathepsin B from rabbit liver and cultured rabbit articular chondrocytes. The buffer system used was 0.1 M Na$^+$/K$^+$ phosphate containing 2 mM edetic acid and 2 mM dithiothreitol at the three pH values indicated (numbers labelling the curves). The data are shown as a first derivative plot obtained from progress curves. Points are experimental and the curves represent best fit values to a first order equation. (From Baici et al. [6] with permission)

tion by gene expression parallels the effect of IL-1 on collagenase synthesis, so that the synthesis of both enzymes seems to be interrelated. Stromelysin from synovial fibroblasts is immunologically identical with stromelysin from chondrocytes (Tables 3 and 6). Furthermore, it can be assumed that TNF — a well known stimulator of the synthesis of collagenase in fibroblasts — is also able to stimulate collagenase synthesis in chondrocytes.

With respect to stromelysin, the multiplicity of biological activation is again visible. It is not only activated by plasmin, but also by granulocyte elastase and cathepsin G (Tables 2 and 3).

Rabbit chondrocytes have recently been shown by Baici et al. [6] to synthesize a special form of cathepsin B in monolayer cultures. Primary and secondary cultures begin to synthesize this highly active proteoglycanase and collagenase in a manner that is strictly dependant on the time of culture (Figs. 6 and 7). In contrast to cathepsin B from rabbit liver, the enzyme is very resistant to alkaline pH (Fig. 8) and is thus an important candidate for causing cartilage destruction outside the chondrocytes. It still has to be shown if this enzyme is synthesized by human chondrocytes and if its increased synthesis also depends on cytokines. Synthesis of cathepsin B is stimulated by IL-1: [A. Baici, personal communication (1991)] If the cells in the monolayers are reintegrated into a network of collagen (or another three dimensional system) they adopt their original chondrocyte morphology and stop the synthesis of the specialized enzyme.

The information in Table 4 suggests that the mast cell is not only an inactive bystander in cartilage destruction. The number of mast cells increases manyfold in synovitis, with increased vascularization. It has been suggested that one of the main activities of the mast cell may be its stimulation of angiogenesis by heparin, but the information in Table 4 suggests that it might also be directly involved in the degradation of proteoglycans, and indirectly, in matrix destruction through the stimulation of other cells capable of destroying cartilage through the external or internal pathway. The stimulation of PGE synthesis in chondrocytes by histamine reduces their capacity to participate in matrix synthesis.

In conclusion, it can be pointed out that, of the many enzymes possibly involved in the destruction of rheumatoid cartilage, only three have been caught directly at work at the pannus-cartilage junction by immunohistochemical methods:

1. Rheumatoid synovial collagenase (by Woolley et al. [7]).
2. Granulocyte elastase and cathepsin G (by Velvart and Fehr [8]) (Fig. 9).

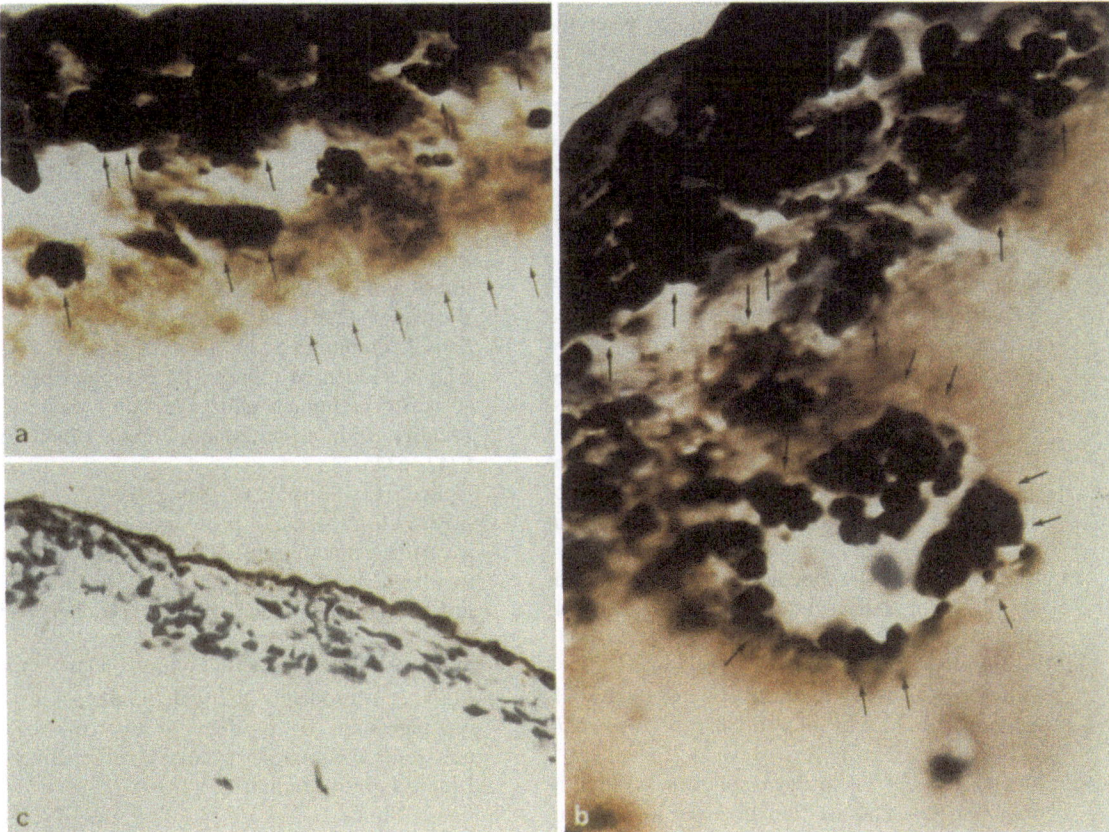

Fig. 9a–c. Light micrographs of pannus-covered ■ AC from a patient with seropositive RA. AC was immunostained with specific antibodies using the indirect peroxidase-anti-peroxidase method (*brown color*). Counterstaining with H **a** Staining with specific antibodies to cathepsin G. The surface of the cartilage is covered by pannus, which is richly infiltrated with PMN. Cathepsin G deposits in and around the PMN can be seen (*arrows*). Large amounts of cathepsin G are located in the cartilage matrix adjacent to the pannus (*arrows*) (×425). **b** Adjacent section stained with specific anti-elastase antibodies. The surface of the cartilage is covered by pannus which is deeply protruding into the matrix. Elastase is detectable in and around the PMN (*arrows*) which are localized in pannus tissue and at the sites of cartilage matrix erosion. Large elastase deposits are seen in the cartilage matrix adjacent to the PMN (*arrows*) (×425). **c** Adjacent section stained with specific anti-IgG antibodies. At the cartilage-pannus junction, no IgG deposits are seen (×170). In addition, in the whole area of **a** and **b** no deposits of C3. α_1-PI or α_2-MG were found

References

1. Matsubara T, Spycher MA, Rüttner JR, Fehr K (1983) The localization of fibronectin in rheumatoid arthritis synovium by light and electron microscopic immunohistochemistry. Rheumatol Int 3:153–159
2. Matsubara T, Trüeb B, Fehr K, Rüttner JR, Odermatt BF (1984) The localization and secretion of type IV collagen in synovial capillaries by immunohistochemistry using a monoclonal antibody against human Type IV collagen. Exp Cell Biol 52:159–169
3. Mohr W (1984) Gelenkkrankheiten. Diagnostik und Pathogenese makroskopischer und histologischer Strukturveränderungen. Thieme, Stuttgart, pp 74–165
4. Kobayashi I, Ziff M (1975) Electron microscopic studies of the cartilage-pannus junction in rheumatoid arthritis. Arthritis Rheum 18:475–483
5. Fehr K (1989) Aetiologie und Pathogenese der chronischen Polyarthritis. In: Fehr K, Miehle W,

Schattenkirchner M, Tillmann K (eds) Rheumatologie in Praxis und Klinik. Georg Thieme Verlag, Stuttgart pp 7.10–7.69

6. Baici A, Lang A, Hörler D, Knöpfel M (1988) Cathepsin B as a marker of the dedifferentiated chondrocyte phenotype. Ann Rheum Dis 47: 684–691

7. Woolley DE, Crossley MJ, Evanson JM (1977) Collagenase at sites of cartilage erosion in the rheumatoid joint. Arthritis Rheum 20:1231–1239

8. Velvart M, Fehr K (1987) Degradation in vivo of articular cartilage in rheumatoid arthritis and juvenile chronic arthritis by cathepsin G and elastase from polymorphonuclear leukocytes. Rheumatol Int 7:195–202

9. Bromley M, Wolley DE (1984) Histopathology of the rheumatoid lesion. Identification of cell types at sites of cartilage erosion. Arthritis Rheum 27:857–863

10. Baici A (1984) Die Bedeutung der Proteinasen für die Knorpeldestruktion. Therapiewoche 34: 1038–1055

11. Weiss SJ, Peppin G, Ortiz X, Ragsdale C, Test ST (1985) Oxidative autoactivation of latent collagenase by human neutrophils. Science 227: 747–749

12. Mayne R (1989) Cartilage collagens. What is their function, and are they involved in articular disease? Arthritis Rheum 32:241–246

13. Okada Y, Konomi H, Yada T, Kimata K, Nagase H (1989) Degradation of type IX collagen by matrix metalloproteinase 3 (stromelysin) from human synovial cells. FEBS Lett 244:473–476

14. Okada Y, Nakanishi I (1989) Activation of matrix metalloproteinase 3 (stromelysin) and matrix metalloproteinase 2 (gelatinase) by human neutrophil elastase and cathepsin G. FEBS Lett 249:353–356

15. Chengshi H, Scott MW, Pentland AP, Marmer BL, Grant GA, Eisen AZ, Goldberg GI (1989) Tissue cooperation in a proteolytic cascade activating human interstitial collagenase. Proc Natl Acad Sci USA 86:2632–2636

16. Frisch St M, Ruley HE (1987) Transcription from the stromelysin promoter is induced by interleukin-1 and repressed by dexamethasone. J Biol Chem 262:16300–16304

17. Saus J, Quinones S, Otani Y, Nagase H, Harris ED, Kurkinen M (1988) The complete primary structure of human matrix metalloproteinase-3. Identity with stromelysin. J Biol Chem 263: 6742–6745

18. Nguyen Q, Murphy G, Roughley PJ, Mort JS (1989) Degradation of proteoglycan aggregate by a cartilage metalloproteinase. Evidence for the involvement of stromelysin in the generation of link protein heterogeneity in situ. Biochem J 259: 61–67

19. Yoffe JR, Taylor DJ, Woolley DE (1984) Mast cell products stimulate collagenase and prostaglandin E production by cultures of adherent rheumatoid synovial cells. Biochem Biophys Res Commun 122:270–275

20. Gunja-Smith Z, Nagase H, Woessner JF (1989) Purification of the neutral proteoglycan-degrading metalloproteinase from human articular tissue and its identification as stromelysin matrix metalloproteinase-3. Biochem J 258: 115–119

21. Baici A (1982) Neutral proteinases, cartilage breakdown and osteoarthrosis. Facts and fiction. In: Verbruggen G, Veis Em (eds) Degenerative joints. Excerpta Medica, Amsterdam, pp 35–46

Mechanism of Collagen Breakdown by Local Infiltration of Steroids

P. Balasubramaniam[1]

Summary. Breakdown of collagen in tendons after local infiltration with corticosteroids was studied under the electron microscope in the rabbit as well as in specimens of teased collagen. Corticosteroid infiltration produces a breakdown of collagen to a structureless amorphous mass. The breakdown appears to occur first by the collagen fibril unwinding into smaller ones with no periodic banding; the collagen finally becoming a structureless mass. These changes are likely to be due to a direct chemical action of corticosteroids on the intermolecular and intramolecular bonds of collagen.

Key words. Steroids — Collagen — Bonds — Breakdown — Gelatin

Introduction

Spontaneous rupture of tendons has been reported in patients receiving local steroid therapy [1–4]. Most of these ruptures occurred after muscular activity [3,4] and Sweetnam [5] has suggested that hydrocortisone plays at least some part in the tendon rupture. A previous light microscope study by us [6] showed that local infiltration of hydrocortisone into calcaneal tendons caused necrosis at the site of infiltration. This effect was seen as early as 30 min after the local injection of hydrocortisone, when the collagen showed a woolly eosinophilic appearance after losing its parallel arrangement. It was therefore postulated that the necrosis of collagen may be due to a direct action by the hydrocortisone. The present electron microscope study was undertaken to determine the nature of collagen breakdown by the local action of various types of corticosteroids.

Materials and Methods

Sixteen adult New Zealand white rabbits weighing between 2.5 and 3 kg were used. The rabbits were anesthetized with ether and their calcaneal tendons were exposed by incising the skin over them. Five mg of hydrocortisone acetate in 0.2 ml of suspension was injected into the center of the exposed right calcaneal tendon with a 25 gauge needle. Clear supernatant fluid (0.2 ml) of the hydrocortisone acetate suspension was injected into the left calcaneal tendon and this was used as a control. Both calcaneal tendons of eight rabbits were excised ½ h after the injection. The tendons from the other eight rabbits were excised 1 h after the injection. The excised tendon was bisected. One-half was fixed in 4% formaldehyde and embedded in paraffin for light microscope study. The other half was used for electron microscope study. The tendon was cut into 1-mm-long cubes, fixed in 4% glutaraldehyde and c-acodylate buffer at pH 7.4 and post-fixed in 1% osmium tetroxide in collidine buffer at pH 7.4. The cubes of tendon were dehydrated through increasing grades of ethyl alcohol and were embedded in epon resin. Ultra-thin sections of about 900 angstroms were cut and stained with uranyl acetate and lead

[1] Department of Orthopaedic Surgery, National University of Singapore, Singapore 0511

hydroxide for examination under the electron microscope.

Electron Microscope Study of Lesion by the Replica Method

Sections from half of the tendon used for light microscope study were used. Sections (5-μm-thick) of the tendon embedded in paraffin were stained with hematoxylin and eosin and the lesion produced by the hydrocortisone was identified under the light microscope. The paraffin block was then trimmed down to the area of the lesion. Sections of the lesion (2-μm-thick) were cut and placed on a glass slide. The paraffin from the sections was removed by xylene and the sections were then allowed to dry at room temperature (30°C) on the glass slide. Shadow-cast of these sections with chromiun was done at an angle of 45°. The shadow-cast was floated from the glass slide with dilute hydrofluoric acid and the tissue was dissolved in 5% sodium hypochlorite. The replica was washed in water, transferred onto copper grids and examined under the electron microscope.

Electron Microscope Study with Teased Collagen

Adult rabbits were anesthetized with ether and their calcaneal tendons were excised and preserved in sterile distilled water for about 6 h at room temperature. In addition, a few tendons were fixed overnight in 4% formaldehyde. Strips of calcaneal tendon were teased on a clean, sterile glass slide under the dissecting micro-scope. The teased collagen was washed twice in sterile distilled water and then soaked in 0.01 ml of corticosteroid on a glass slide. The cor-ticosteroids used were hydrocortisone acetate suspension, aqueous solution of hydrocortisone, methyl prednisolone suspension, and aqueous solution of betamethasone. Table 1 shows the different types of corticosteroids used and their concentrations. Different batches of teased col-laged were soaked in corticosteroid for 1, 15, and 30 min. Clear supernatant fluid from the corticosteroid suspension, or distilled water, was used for soaking the collagen used as controls. Table 2 shows the number of collagen specimens used. The collagen soaked in the corticosteroid was washed twice in distilled water and spread

Table 1. Strength of corticosteroid solutions used

Type of corticosteroid used	Amount of corticosteroid (in μg) in 0.01 ml of solution or suspension
Hydrocortisone acetate suspension	250
Aqueous solution of hydrocortisone	200
Methyl prednisolone acetate suspension	400
Betamethasone solution	4

Table 2. Number of teased collagen specimens used

Substance used for soaking collagen	Number of teased collagen specimens used		
	1 min	15 min	30 min
Hydrocortisone acetate suspension	4	12	12
Aqueous solution of hydrocortisone	4	12	12
Methyl prednisolone suspension	4	12	12
Betamethasone solution	4	12	12
Clear supernatant fluid from hydrocortisone acetate suspension	4	12	12
Clear supernatant fluid from methyl prednisolone suspension	4	12	12
Sterile distilled water	4	12	12

again on a glass slide with a fine needle under the dissecting microscope. It was then allowed to dry at room temperature. Shadow-cast of the collagen was done with chromium at angle of 45°. The replica was separated, as in the previous experiment, and transferred to copper grids for viewing under the electron microscope.

Results

The findings of light microscope studies after infiltration of the tendon with hydrocortisone were similar to the results obtained in our previous study [6] (Fig. 1). The breakdown of collagen was seen in all experimental specimens after a ½ h. Electron microscope study showed that the breakdown of collagen was accom-panied by loss of its periodic banding. Where the

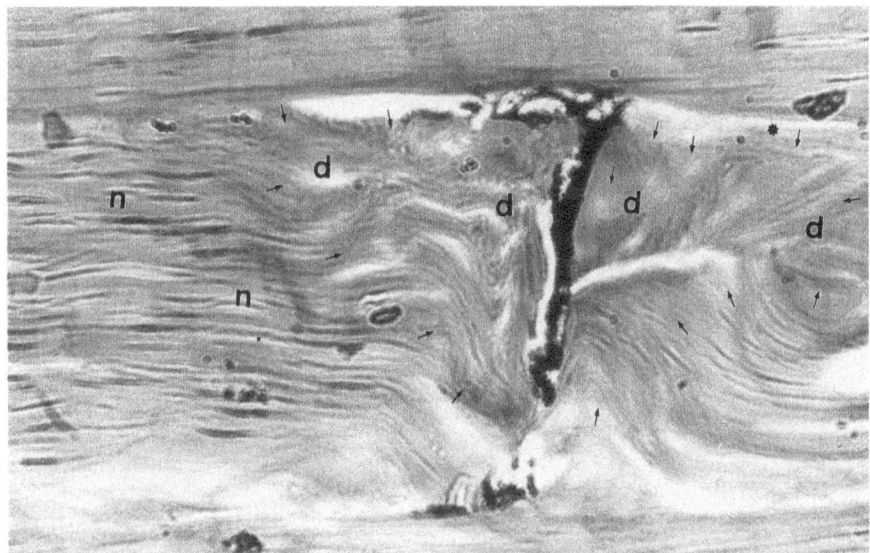

Fig. 1. Thirty min after injection of hydrocortisone into tendon. Normal collagen (*n*) fibers are seen to be continous with disorganized collagen (*d*) (*arrows*), which appears as an amorphous mass. (H and E ×240)

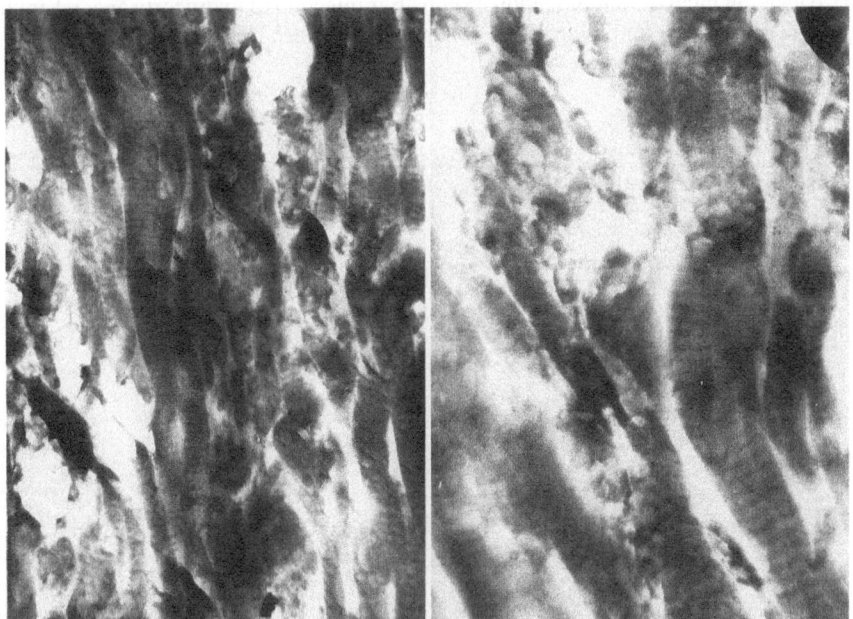

Fig. 2. Two electron micrographs of tendon 45 min after injection of hydrocortisone. The collagen fibrils which have broken down have lost their periodic bending and appear as an amorphous mass. (Uranyl acetate ×20000)

breakdown of collagen was severe it appeared as a structureless mass with empty spaces in some areas (Fig. 2). When the breakdown of collagen was not extensive the collagen fibril was seen to unravel into smaller fibrils, finally becoming a structureless mass (Fig. 3). Replicas made by chromium shadow-cast of the lesion showed the changes better. The method of identifying

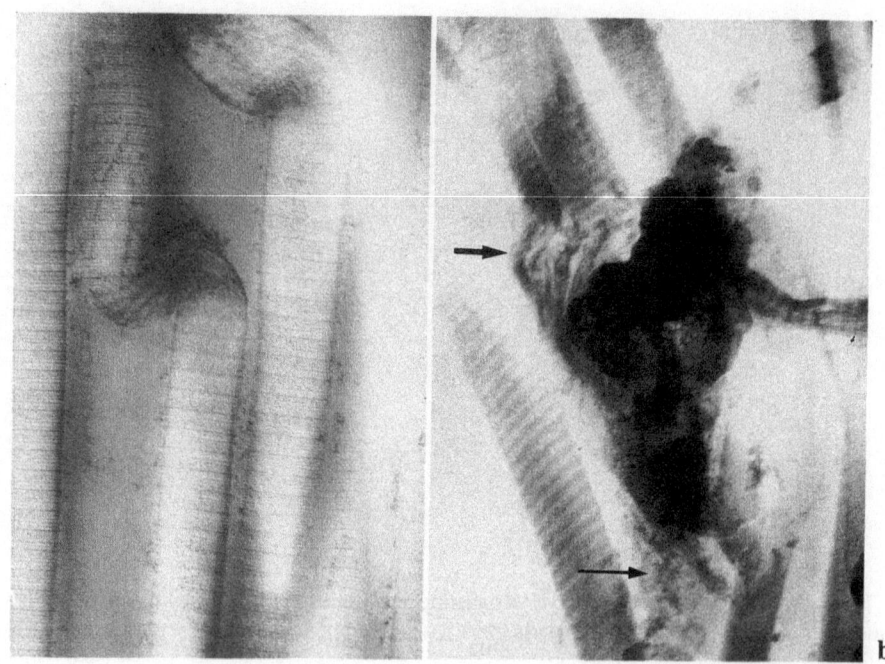

Fig. 3. Two electron micrographs of tendon 45 min after injection of hydrocortisone. **a** Kinking of two collagen fibers can be seen; **b** shows unfolding of the collagen fibers (*thick arrow*) and the formation of a structureless mass (*small arrow*). (Uranyl acetate ×30 000)

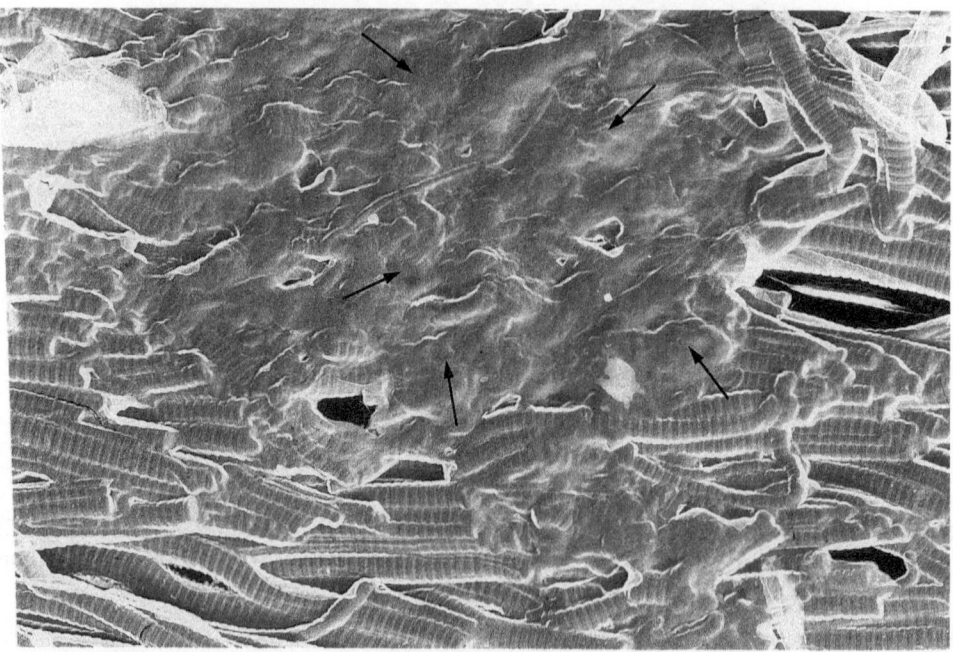

Fig. 4. Electron micrograph of shadow-cast of lesion in tendon 45 min after injection of hydrocortisone. The collagen fibrils are seen to have broken down into a structureless mass (*arrows*). (×11 000)

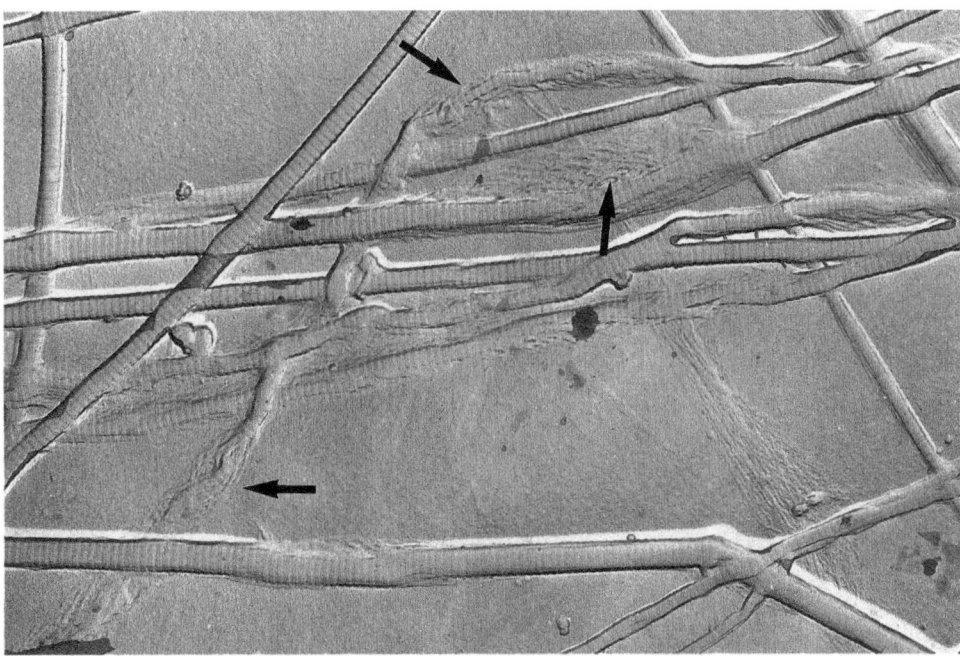

Fig. 5. Electron micrograph of shadow-cast with chromium of teased collagen soaked in methyl prednisolone for 15 min, showing the unwinding of collagen fibrils into smaller ones (*arrows*). (×11 000)

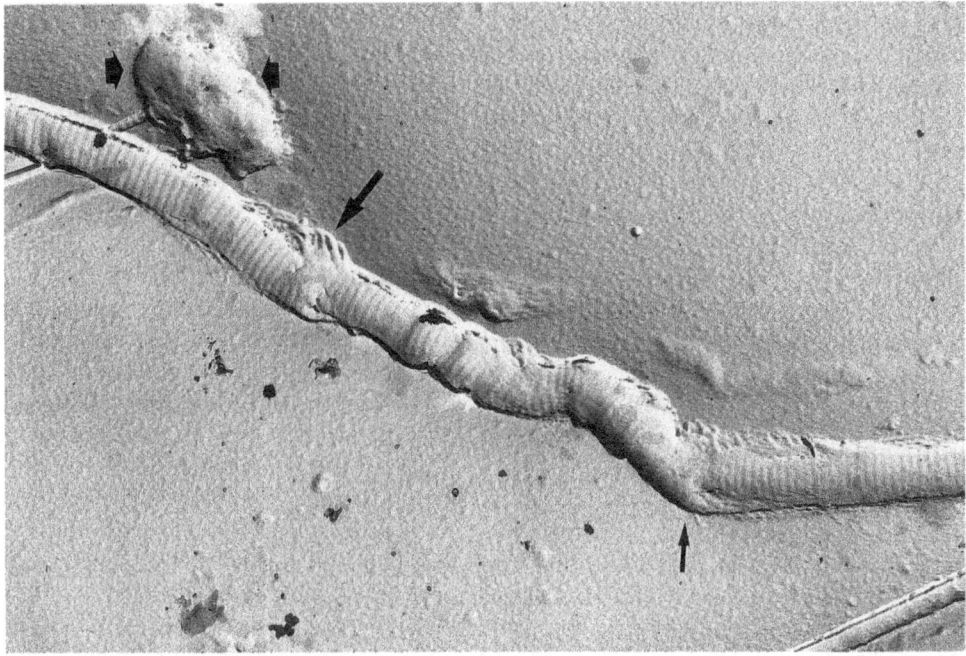

Fig. 6. Electron micrograph of shadow-cast with chromium of teased collagen soaked in betamethasone for 30 min, showing unwinding of fibril (*thick arrow*), change in direction of fiber axis (*thin arrow*), and amorphous change. (×11 000)

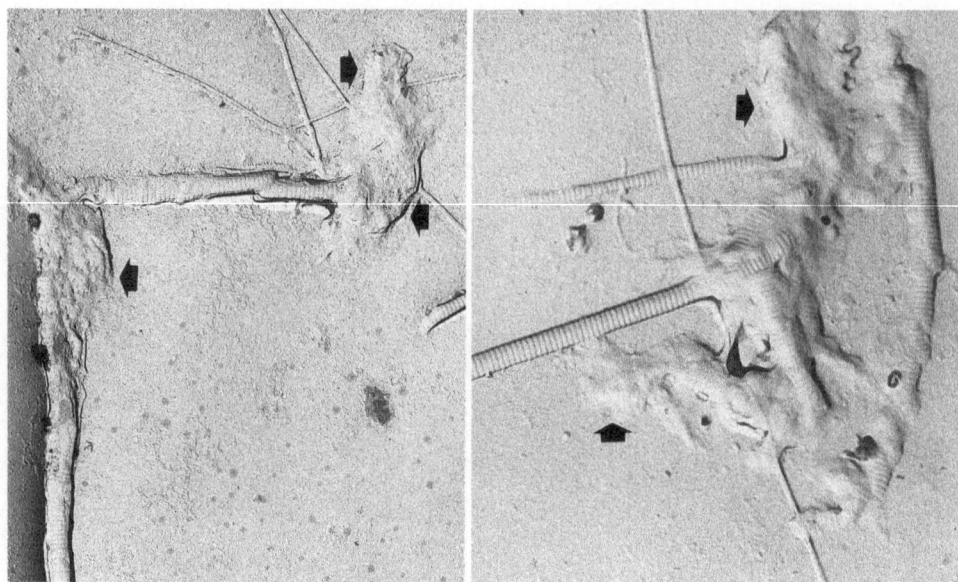

Fig. 7. Two electron micrographs of shadow-casts with chromium of teased collagen soaked in beta-methasone for 30 min, showing collagen fibrils turning into an amorphous mass (*arrows*). (×11 000)

the lesion first in paraffin sections under the light microscope and then selecting the area for electron microscope study was very useful in checking the results seen in ultra-thin sections of the tendon under the electron microscope. The chromium shadow-cast gave a three-dimensional view of the lesion where the collagen fibrils were first seen to unwind, and then break down into a structureless mass; in its midst fragments of collagen were seen with their periodic banding (Fig. 4). The lesion was continous at the periphery with normal collagen fibrils. None of the above changes were seen in any of the control tendons injected with clear supernatant fluid from the hydrocortisone suspension.

Results of Collagen Fibers Soaked in Corticosteroid

By 15 min the collagen fibril was seen to unfold into smaller fibrils like the unfolding of a coir rope (Fig. 5). This local weakening of the fibril structure resulted sometimes in a kinking and change in direction of fibril axis (Fig. 6). At the end of a ½ h the collagen fibrils which had unravelled had lost their periodic banding and had become a structureless mass (Fig. 7). Similar changes were seen in all specimens of teased collagen soaked in the different types of

corticosteroids. No similar change was seen in any of the control collagen specimens under the electron microscope. The unravelling of the collagen fibril produced by corticosteroids in the present study is very similar to the electron-micrographs obtained by Steven and Jackson [7] after chemical degradation of collagen.

Discussion

Collagen is an extracellular fibrous protein and is a structural component of many organs; it is specialized in certain areas such as bone, cartilage, and tendons. It is formed by fibroblasts from three polypeptide chains which are twisted into a triple helical trophocollagen molecule. Hydrogen bonds between the chains in the trophocollagen molecule provide stability to the triple helical structure. Many molecules of collagen line up in a staggered fashion, overlapping by one quarter of their length, to form a collagen fibril. This alignment within a fibril produces a characteristic banded appearance under the electron microscope [8].

Collagen fibrils in turn collect into fibers that can be seen under the light microscope. Intermolecular cross-links hold the polymer chains of collagen together, give it tensile strength, and act to weld the molecules into a strong rope-like unit.

Trophocollagen that has not polymerized into fibrils is soluble in cold water [9]. As time passes the solubility decreases until only acid substances will dissolve the fiber. Finally, a state of insolubility is reached in which only materials which break covalent bonds or totally destroy the fiber will bring the collagen into solution. Polymerized collagen has varying degrees of intermolecular cross-linking, with resultant stability toward heat, chemical, and enzymatic degradation [10]. The degree of polymerization affects such properties as solubility, swelling, fiber tensile strength, and metabolic turnover [10].

Collagen can be denatured by physical, chemical, and biological means by enzymes such as collagenase. Heat above 60°C, 4 molecular urea, 2 molecular potassium thiocyanate, or 5 molecular guanidine hydrochloride will denature collagen. Denaturation of collagen fibers involves breakdown into smaller fibrils, the collapse of the helical configuration of the trophocollagen, and separation into individual chains; gelatin is the end product.

The study of collagen resorption or breakdown is not a recent development. However, only in very recent years have extensive biochemical studies been made into the mechanisms of collagen breakdown [11]. Baker and Whitaker [12] and Castor and Baker [13] found that following prolonged daily local application of various corticosteroids a thinning of the skin occurred. They reported that there was a diminution of the connective tissue components of the skin. Keloids will disappear with corticosteroid treatment if it is done at certain times following the formation of the keloid [14,15]. Intralesional injection of the steroid triamcinolone acetonide produces involution of very old keloids [15]. These findings suggest that corticosteroids can bring about a dissolution of already formed collagen. The actual mechanism by which corticosteroids reduce the keloid or bring about the loss of collagen in the keloid by their local infiltration is not known.

It is well known that systemic injection of corticosteroids brings about a reduction in the amount of collagen. This effect has been ascribed to the anti-inflammatory action of corticosteroids on fibroblasts, resulting in the formation of less collagen. It has also been shown that systemic injection of steroids brings about a reduction of preformed collagen, and this has been attributed to an enzyme-mediated action by the steroids [16].

The above two explanations have also been given for the reduction in the amount collagen or scar tissue that occurs after local infiltration of corticosteroids. Though these biological mechanisms are possible, the second experiment on teased collagen in the present study shows an in vitro breakdown of fibers soaked in various types of corticosteroids. Therefore this effect of the local injection of corticosteroids into tendons or other collagenous tissue is most likely a direct chemical action and not an enzyme-mediated one.

The earliest recognizable change of kinking and unwinding of the collagen fibrils seen under the electron microscope may be due to a break in the intermolecular cross-links that is caused by a direct chemical action of corticosteroids. This results in the production of fibrils of smaller diameter and finally in the collapse of the helical configuration of the trophocollagen molecule. The word collagen means "to form glue". The ultimate disappearance of the smaller fibrils of collagen into a structureless mass, as seen under the electron microscope, may be due to a breakdown of the intramolecular cross-links of the trophocollagen molecule, resulting in separation into individual chains to form gelatin.

Conclusions

1. Local infiltration of corticosteroid into a tendon has a collagenolytic effect on it, resulting in the formation of a structureless amorphous mass.
2. The breakdown of collagen after local infiltration of corticosteroid into a tendon, as seen under the electron microscope, occurs first by the collagen fibril unwinding into smaller fibrils with no cross banding; the collagen finally becoming a structureless mass.
3. These changes may be due to a direct chemical action of corticosteroids on the intermolecular and intramolecular bonds of collagen.

References

1. Bedi SS, Ellis W (1970) Spontaneous rupture of calcaneal tendon in rheumatoid arthritis after local steroid injection. Ann Rheum Dis 29: 494–495

2. Cowan MA, Alexander S (1961) Simultaneous bilateral rupture of Achilles tendons due to triamcinolone. Br Med J [Clin Res] I:1658

3. Ismail AM, Balakrishnan R, Rajakumar MK (1969) Rupture of patellar ligament after steroid infiltration. J Bone Joint Surg [Br] 51:503–505

4. Lee HB (1957) Avulsion and rupture of the tendo calcaneus after injection of hydrocortisone. Br Med J [Clin Res] II:395

5. Sweetnam R (1969) Corticosteroid arthropathy and tendon rupture. J Bone Joint Surg [Br] 51:397–398

6. Balasubramaniam P, Prathap K (1972) The effect of hdydrocortisone injections into tendons. A morphological study in rabbits. J Bone Joint Surg [Br] 54:729–734

7. Steven FS, Jackson DS (1967) Purification and amino-acid composition of monomeric and polymeric Collagens. Biochem J 104:534–536

8. Hodge AJ (1967) Structure at the electron microscope level. In: Ramachandra GN (ed) Treatise on collagen, vol 1. Chemistry of collagen. Academic, London, p 185

9. Gross J (1964) Organisation and disorganisation of collagen. Bio phys J 4:63–68

10. Veis A (1967) Intact collagen. In: Ramachandran GN (ed) Treatise on collagen, vol. I. Chemistry of collagen. Academic, London, p 368

11. Woessner Jr JF (1969) Biological mechanisms of collagen resorption. In: Gould BS (ed) Treatise on collagen, vol 2. Biology of collagen Part B. Academic, London, p 254

12. Baker BL, Whitaker WL (1950) Interference with wound healing by the local action of adrenocortical steroids. Endocrinology 46:544–551

13. Castor CW, Baker BL (1950) The local action of adrenocortical steroids on epidermis and connective tissue of the skin. Endocrinology 47:234–241

14. Griffith BH (1966) The treatment of keloids with triamcinolone acetonide. Plast Reconstr Surg 38:202–208

15. Ketchum LD, Smith J, Robinson DW, Masters FW (1966) The treatment of hypertrophic scar, keloid and scar contracture by triamcinolone acetonide. Plast Reconstr Surg 38:209–218

16. Dougherty TF, Berlinear DL (1968) The effects of hormones on connective tissue cells. In: Gould BS (ed) Treatise on collagen, vol 2. Biology of collagen Part A. Academic, London, p 370

Pathogenesis of Steroid-Induced Avascular Necrosis and Its Response to Lipid Clearing Agent

Gwo-Jaw Wang[1]

Summary. Steroid-induced avascular necrosis of bone is a fascinating and complex disease entity. While the mechanism of the disease is controversial, previous studies in the rabbit have shown that high doses of steroids caused significant alterations in lipid metabolism. The study described here was designed to show the effects of steroid therapy on serum lipids, liver morphology, marrow volume changes, and eventually on femoral head pressure and its blood flow changes. With prolonged steroid treatment it was noted that the fat droplets that were observed in small vessels of the treated rabbits led to eventual focal occlusion of the subchondral arterioles. There was also a persistent elevation of serum cholesterol and a gradual increase of fat cell size, from 60 µm in the normal untreated rabbit to 70 µm after 7 weeks of treatment. There was a concomitant increase of femoral head pressure, from 24.6 ± 5.5 cm of water in controls, to 60 cm of water in treated rabbits at 10 weeks of treatment. Simultaneously it was observed that the blood flow of the femoral head decreased from 0.23 ml/min per g in the control to 0.16 ml/min per g after 10 weeks of steroid treatment. An anti-lipid agent was used in an attempt to reverse the on-going process. The result of simultaneous use of a steroid and a lipid clearing agent indicated that there was a slight improvement in cholesterol level, but that the intrafemoral head pressure was maintained. Measurement of blood flow also indicated that the femoral head blood flow was preserved. Concomitant study of fat vacuoles within the osteocytes revealed modification of fatty accumulation within these cells. We fell that lipid clearing agents are beneficial in preventing steroid-induced avascular necrosis.

Key words. Steroid — Avascular necrosis — Fat cell volume — Femoral head pressure — Blood flow — Osteocytes

Introduction

Avascular necrosis of the femoral head usually results from obliteration of blood supply to it, which leads to tissue death and subsequently to fracture of the subchondral trabecula. The common causes of the problem are trauma, such as fracture of the femoral neck or hip dislocation, Cason's disease, systemic diseases such as thrombocytopenia, Gaucher's disease, sickle cell disease, or prolonged increased intake of alcohol or steroids. Increased use of steroids in some instances, such as in the treatment of rheumatoid arthritis or especially in patients with kidney transplant, has resulted in increased numbers of cases of avascular necrosis of the femoral head [1–28].

Previous studies in rabbits showed that high doses of steroid caused significant alteration in lipid metabolism and that animals so treated had high levels of phospholipid and cholesterol in the serum, intravascular deposits of lipid in the lung, brain, and kidney, and fatty metamorphosis of the epithelial cells of the liver, adrenal glands, and ovaries [15,24,25].

The study described here was designed to show the effects of steroid therapy on serum lipids and liver morphology, as well as on bone marrow volume and on femoral head pressure and its blood flow.

[1] University of Virginia Medical Center, Department of Orthopaedics, Charlottesville, VA 22908, USA

Materials and Methods

Fat Cell Measurement

Initially, 45 New Zealand white rabbits were studied to determine the effect of long-term high doses of cortical steroid therapy. The rabbits received prophylactic bicillin and streptomycin twice weekly and were divided into two groups. The first group consisted of 20 immature rabbits weighing 1.6–2.3 kg, of which 16 were given daily injections of 15 mg of cortisone acetate subcutaneously and 4 were controls. The second group consisted of 25 adult rabbits weighing an average of 4.5 kg, of which 18 received weekly doses of 12.25 mg (2.7 mg per kg body weight per week) of Depomedrol (methylprednisone) and 7 served as controls. The Depomedrol dosage in the adults responded to the steroid dosage in the young rabbits corrected for body weight.

In the Group I rabbits, base-line cholesterol level was established by withdrawing 3 ml of blood before the experiment. For the first 2 weeks, blood was drawn daily from 4 of the treated young rabbits; subsequently blood was drawn at weekly intervals from all 20 rabbits for up to 22 weeks. The serum cholesterol and triglyceride levels were determined and lipoprotein electrophoresis was performed on each of these weekly samples. Of the 16 young rabbits, 1 was killed each week (from weeks 1–12) and 4 were kept for 19 weeks and then killed 2 weeks after the cortisone was discontinued. In the control group, one rabbit was killed at 0, one at 6, one at 8, and one was killed at 20 weeks. Specimens of liver, kidney, lung, and both femoral heads were obtained immediately after the rabbits had been killed. All the specimens were preserved in 10% neutral buffered formalin. A modification of the Jones and Sakovich technique for staining bone fat with oil-red-O was used [20]. In addition, a section of liver, kidney, and lung was stained for fat and with routine hematoxolin and eosin stains.

From the 25 adult Group II rabbits, blood was withdrawn once prior to treatment and once each week thereafter to determine serum cholesterol and triglyceride level and to perform lipoprotein electrophoresis. Of the 18 treated rabbits, 6 died within the first 5 weeks of treat-ment. Of the remaining rabbits in this group, 2 were killed weekly from the 3rd week to the 8th week. Similarly, of the 7 adult control rabbits, 1 was killed weekly from the 3rd to the 8th week.

The femoral head, liver, kidney, and lung obtained from these rabbits after death were prepared with the same staining methods employed in Group I, except that osmic acid was used instead of Oil-Red-O to stain for fat in the bone sections.

The analytical procedure used to determine the volumes of fat and marrow was performed in both groups according to the following methods.

Polar Planimetry

Microphotographs ($\times 25$) of whole sections of the femoral head and a small portion of the metaphyseal region were prepared, and the exact magnification factor for each photograph was calculated from overall measurements and photographs as compared with measurements of the section. Total area of the head or epiphysis and of the marrow within the head or epiphysis was measured using a planimeter which gave consistently reproducible results in measurements done by two different operators. The inter-observer differences were less than 6 parts per 1000.

Quantitative Microscopy

The size and number of marrow fat cells were determined with an eye-piece micrometer. Fat cell size was calculated as an average of the greatest diameter of 25 fat cells in four pre-selected epiphyseal locations on each histological slide. The number of fat cells was the average of the fat cells counted in at least three randomly selected fields in each epiphysis. The overall size and number of cells was the average value for each group of rabbits studied.

Volume Fraction Analysis

In an isotrophic material, the volume fraction of any component of the material (V_v^x) is equal to the fraction of that component (A_A^x) in the plane of observation. Therefore, the microscopically observed area of the fraction can be equated with the volume fraction and the expression of $V_v^x = A_A^x$, where the superscripts refer to the component (marrow or fat cells) of the material and subscripts indicate the fraction (volume or area), can be analyzed. This equality is not generally true for an anisotrophic material, such as the femoral head epiphysis, but the equation is experimentally useful for volume estimation from planar histological specimens. The marrow area fraction was calculated as the ratio of the total marrow area in the epiphysis to the total epiphyseal area obtained from polar planimetry measurements.

The fat cell area fraction in an observed microscopic field was calculated from the ratio of the area of the fat cells to the area of the observed microscopic fields which was constant at $50 \times 10^{-8} \, m^2$. The fat cell area was calculated from the average diameter and average number of fat cells in at least three observed fields in each epiphysis.

The total fat cell area in the epiphysis was then obtained as the product of the fat cell area fraction and the total epiphyseal area.

Femoral Head Pressure Measurement

Twenty-eight New Zealand white adult rabbits, weighing an average of 4.5 kg were used in this experiment. Sixteen of the animals received a weekly dose of 12.25 mg of Depo-medrol and 0.5 cc of combiotic intramuscularly twice a week to control infection. Twelve served as controls.

Baseline cholesterol level was established by withdrawing 3 ml of blood weekly. Intrafemoral head pressure was measured weekly in the control rabbits, from week 0 to week 14, and at 2-week intervals, from week 2 to week 14, in the steroid-treated rabbits. The rabbits were killed after each experiment and specimens were obtained for histological study.

Rabbits received general anesthesia with Nembutal and Azpromazine i.v., and a standard lateral approach was utilized to expose the lateral aspect of the greater trochanter. A 1-inch long conical tip 18 gauge needle was then inserted at the flare of the greater trochanter and into the femoral head. The location of the tip of the needle was confirmed by biplane x-ray. The needle was attached to an isotonic saline-filled manometer tube. The cannula in the femoral head was back-filled from a sterile reservoir and allowed to come to pressure equilibrium with the manometer. Arterial pulsations were always observed in the saline column prior to measure-ment. It was also noted that occlusion of the femoral vessels at mid thigh would increase the pressure. Intrafemoral head pressure was recorded after the saline column reached maximum height and stabilized at 30 min. The rabbits were killed after measurement. The femoral heads and livers were obtained for histological study.

Femoral Head Blood Flow

Twenty-two New Zealand white adult rabbits, weighing an average of 4.0 kg, were used. Fourteen of the animals received a weekly dose of 12.25 mg of Depo-medrol and 8 served as controls. Femoral head blood flow was established using the radioactive microsphere technique. Control and steroid-treated rabbits had measurements of femoral head flow at 6 weeks, (3 control, 4 treated) at 8 weeks (3 control, 3 treated), and at 10 weeks (2 control, 3 treated). Four treated rabbits died of systemic infection during the course of the experiment.

The rabbits were strapped in the supine position with both hind legs free of constraint. They were anesthetized with 2 mg of Azpromazine i.v. followed by pentobarbital sodium (50 mg/ml) given in increments of 0.2 ml until effective. After the left carotid artery was exposed, a DE 60 catheter filled with heparinized saline and attached to a pressure monitoring system (P2310 Gould pressure transducer) was inserted and threaded down to the left ventricle. The brachial artery, serving as a reference sample, was exposed and cannulated. The catheter was attached to a sage withdrawal pump, withdrawing at the rate of 2.0 ml per min when in use.

Once the pressure returned to normal, 0.8 ml microspheres, size $15 \pm 3 \, \mu m$ and labeled with ^{85}Sr, were injected into the left ventricle $(1.0 \times 10^6$ microspheres, activity $= 0.032 \, mci)$ in 30 s. The catheter was then flushed for 15 s with 0.5 ml of heparinized saline. To prevent possible stretching of the hip capsule, both hind legs were exercised during the injection. Withdrawal of blood from the brachial artery was started 30 s before the injection of microspheres and continued for 2.5 min. The rabbits were then killed, and the femoral heads were cut at the level of the articular cartilage. The soft tissue was stripped completely and the femoral head was weighed fresh. The radial activity of the specimen was counted for 5.0 min in a Beckmann Biogamma Counter and blood flow was computed by the following formula [29–31]:

1. Flow rate of the reference organ

$$= \frac{\text{Weight of the blood sample}}{2.5 \, \text{min}}$$

2. $\dfrac{\text{Microspheres in blood sample}}{\text{Blood flow rate of reference organ (ml/min)}}$

   $= \dfrac{\text{Microspheres in femoral head}}{\text{FHBF rate (ml/min)}}$

3. $\dfrac{\text{FHBF rate (ml/min)}}{\text{Weight of femoral head}}$

   $= \text{FHBF (ml/min per g)}$

   FHBF, femoral head blood flow

Assessment of Osteocytes

Ten New Zealand white rabbits, weighing an average of 4.5 kg, were used. The rabbits were divided into two groups. Group I was the control group and consisted of three normal, non-treated rabbits. Group II consisted of seven steroid-treated rabbits that received weekly intramuscullar injections of 12.25 mg of Depomedrol.

All the rabbits received prophylactic antibiotics to prevent systemic infection. Three steroid-treated rabbits died prematurely. Two rabbits were killed at 8 weeks (1 normal and 1 steroid treated), three at 10 weeks (1 normal and 2 steroid-treated), and 2 were killed at 12 weeks (1 normal and 1 steroid treated). After the animals were killed, femoral heads were obtained. The subchondral cancellous bone within the femoral head was removed and fixed in 10% phosphate buffered formalin and 1% glutaraldehyde for 72 h, then decalcified with ethylenediaminetetraacetate (EDTA) for 1 week. Specimens were embedded in Epon in preparation for electron microscopy. Hematoxylin and eosin staining for conventional sections were also carried out.

Results

Fat Cell Volume

All the steroid–treated rabbits in Group I lost weight. The weight of many dropped to as little as 30% of the body weight of the controls. Serum cholesterol level was elevated after steroid administration, but no significant changes were noted in the serum lipoprotein patterns. Occasional fatty droplets were visible in the kidney and lung capillaries, as was nephrocalcinosis in several kidneys. Fatty metamorphoses of the liver was presented in all steroid–treated rabbits as determined by comparison with the livers in the control group.

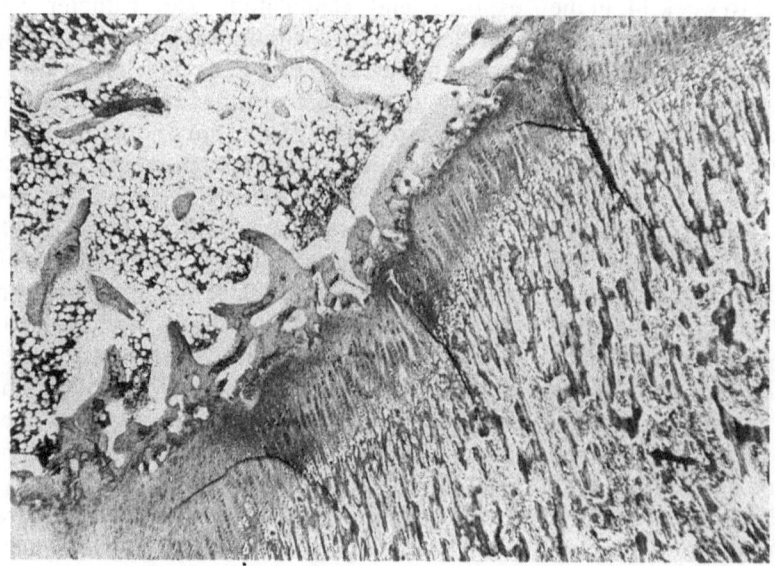

Fig. 1. Epiphyseal growth plate from the femoral head of immature rabbit at 20 weeks. Note the ratio of marrow fat to hematopoietic elements in the epiphyseal area (*upper left*), activity of the growth plate, and large number of primary bone trabecula in the metaphysis (*lower right*). (Hematoxylin and eosin, ×35)

Fig. 2. Epiphyseal growth plate from the femoral head of immature cortisone-treated rabbit at 21 weeks. Note predominance of the fat in both epiphysis (*upper left* and metaphysis, *lower right*). The growth plate appeared less active here than in the control rabbit and only rare primary trabecula are seen. (Hematoxylin and eosin, ×35)

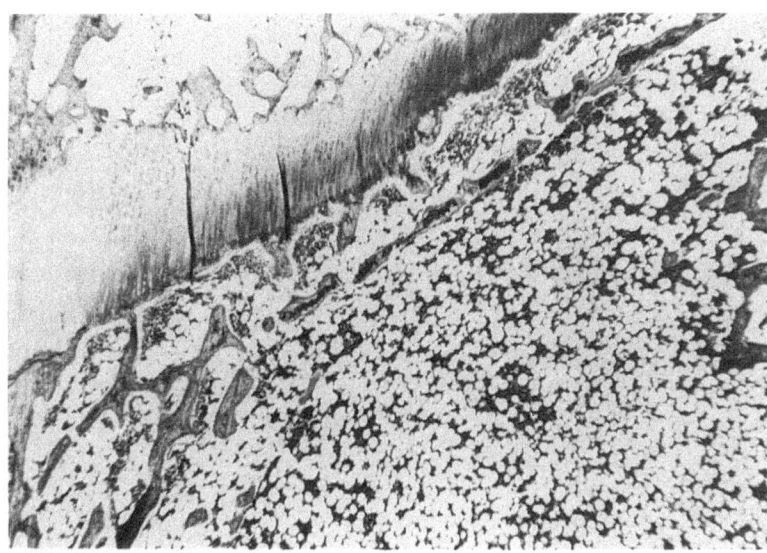

Gross examination of the femoral and humeral heads of the rabbits treated with steroid revealed significantly smaller heads than those of the controls. This failure was accompanied by a significantly smaller and less active epiphyseal growth plate, fewer primary and secondary bone trabecular cells in the metaphysis and a smaller epiphysis. The trabecular area fraction was 39% in the control rabbits and 23% in the treated rabbits; the decrease appearing to result both from decreased bone production and increased cortical resorption. The distribution of marrow fat was significantly different in the steroid-treated and control rabbits. The steroid–treated rabbits showed a considerable increase in percentage of marrow fat since their fat cell area section was 77% and that of the control was 61% (Figs. 1, 2).

The average fat cell diameter in both epiphysis and metaphysis of the steroid-treated rabbits was larger ($P < 0.001$) than that in the control rabbit. Interestingly, the difference between the epiphyseal and metaphyseal fat cell size when comparing the steroid-treated and control group rabbits was always significant ($P < 0.001$).

Fat droplets were occasionally demonstrated in the arterioles in the ligamentum Teres of the treated rabbits. In addition, by the 20th week, there appeared to be a gradual accumulation of fat droplets in the subchondral arterioles, suggesting focal occlusion of occasional vessels. After withdrawal of steroids there was no re-

solution of these intravascular fat droplets in the subchondral vessels during the period of observation.

In the Group II rabbits, weight loss and changes in serum cholesterol were similar to those in the immature rabbits. The growth plate was closed and the bone and marrow architecture was normal in the femoral and humeral heads in the control adult rabbits. The fat cell size was the same in both the epiphyseal and metaphyseal marrow areas in the controls and averaged 60 µm in diameter. The average fat cell in the steroid-treated rabbits after 1–2 weeks of treatment was 62 µm at its greatest diameter while after 3–6 weeks of treatment the average greatest diameter was close to 70 µm, and at 7 weeks it was 72 µm (Figs. 3, 4). The difference between the marrow fat cell size of the control and steroid-treated rabbits after 5 weeks of therapy was statistically significant ($P < 0.001$) (Table 1). Occasional fat droplets were identified in the subchondral vessels of all femoral and humeral heads of the treated rabbits. The femoral and humeral heads of the same rabbits also showed mild osteoporosis, with the marrow area fraction increased from 52% in the controls to 66% in the treated rabbits.

Femoral Head Pressure

There was a persistent increase in serum holesterol and intrafemoral head pressure over

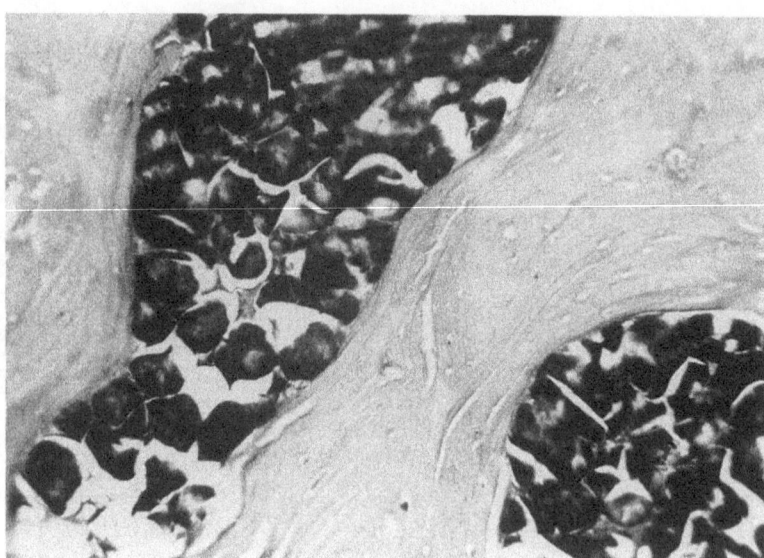

Fig. 3. Epiphyseal bone and the marrow fat from the femoral head of mature control rabbit at 7 weeks. Note the size of marrow fat cell. (Osmic acid and hematoxylin and eosin, ×240)

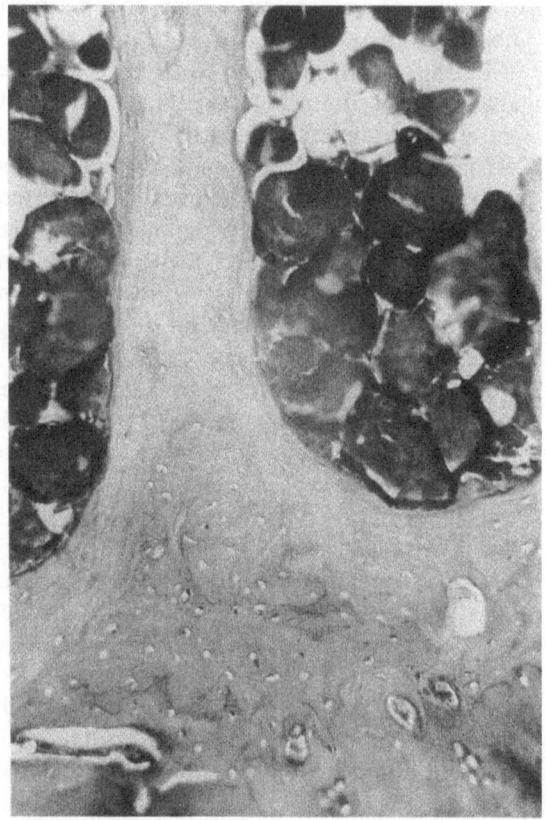

Fig. 4. Bone and marrow fat from the femoral head of mature cortisone-treated rabbit at 7 weeks. Note enlargment of many fo the marrow fat cells compared with the marrow fat cells of the control rabbits. (Osmic acid and hematoxylin and eosin, ×240)

both hips from 6 to 8 weeks after the steroid treatment. The treated group showed intra-femoral head pressure of a maximum of nearly 60 cm of water at 10 weeks in comparison to the untreated control value which remained constant throughout the experiment at 24.6 ± 5.5 cm of water (Fig. 5).

Femoral Head Blood Flow

The blood flow in the control femoral head averaged 0.204 ± 0.026 ml/min per g at 6 weeks, 0.238 ± 0.134 ml/min per g at 8 weeks and 0.292 ± 0.009 ml/min per g at 10 weeks. The average blood flow from 6 through 10 weeks was 0.239 ± 0.076 ml/min per g, with no significant difference between the left and right and $P < 0.05$ level. In the treated rabbits, the average blood flow at 6 weeks of treatment was 0.210 ± 0.078 ml/min per g on the right and 0.251 ± 0.108 ml/min per g on the left, with an average of 0.230 ± 0.090 ml/min per g. With further steroid treatment the blood flow appeared further decreased to 0.147 ± 0.097 on the right and 0.218 ± 0.193 on the left, with an average of 0.182 ± 0.142 ml/min per g between the left and right at 8 weeks after initial steroid administration. At 10 weeks of treatment the blood flow was 0.162 ± 0.039 ml/min per g on the right and 0.164 ± 0.037 on the left, with average of 0.163 ± 0.031 ml/min per g. Using two-way analysis of variance, this is statistically significant at $P <$

Table 1.[a]

	Marrow area $(A_S \times 10^{-4}m^2)^b$	Total area $(A_T \times 10^{-4}m^2)^b$	Marrow area fraction $(A_S/A_T)^b$	Av. no. of fat cells per 50 × $10^{-8}m^2$	Av. fat-cell diameter × $10^{-8}m$	Av. fat-cell area per field $(A_F \times 10^{-8}m^6)^b$	Fat-cell area fraction $(A_F/A_O)^b$	Total area × $10^{-4}m^2$	Total increase in fat-cell volume (%)
Adult control	3.8	7.5	0.52	54	60	15.2	0.30	117	
Adult treated	4.1	6.1	0.66	46	72	18.9	0.38	146	24.8
Immature control	3.1	5.2	0.61	65	53	14.3	0.29	90	
Immature treated	3.6	4.6	0.77	51	61	14.9	0.30	115	27.8

[a] Femoral epiphyseal measurements (means) from polar planimetry and fat-cell area fractions (means) from quantitative microscopy. For each value the standard deviation is less than 15%, as calculated from at least three experimental determinations.

[b] A_S is the total marrow area in the femoral capital epiphysis; A_T, the total epiphyseal area; A_F, the area of fat cells in a microscopic field; and A_O, the area of a microscopic field which was $50 \times 10^{-8}m^2$

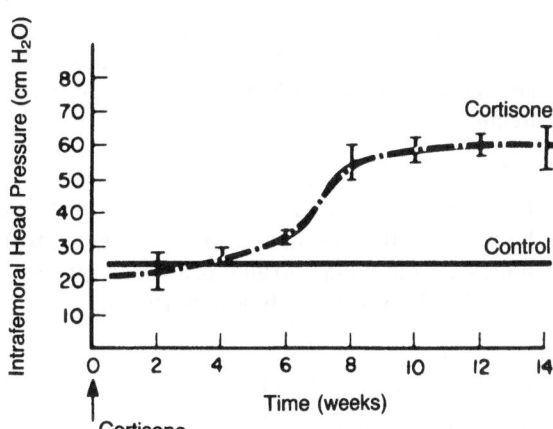

Fig. 5. Intrafemoral head pressure of control and steroid-treated rabbits. There is a gradual increase of intrafemoral head pressure after 6 weeks of steroid treatment

0.01 level of competence at 8 weeks of treatment (Fig. 6).

Osteocyte Study

Osteocytes obtained from the specimens during different stages of treatment were examined under the electron microscope. Normal osteocytes exhibited distinct cytoplastic membranes with occasional small fat globules, a few mitochondria and cytoplastic extensions. Examination of 123 osteocytes from untreated specimens revealed 80% normal appearing cells with 4% small fat vacuole cells and 16% large fat vacuole cells. In the experimental group killed before 8 weeks had elapsed, 124 cells were examined which contained 68.5% normal appearing osteocytes and 20.1% large fat vacuelo cells. From the experimental group, killed after 8 weeks, 88 steroid group cells were examined. Normal appearing osteocytes were observed in 39.7% of samples. At the same time osteocytes containing large fat vacuoles were observed in 50.3%.

With these observations, it was felt that preservation of the intrafemoral head pressure and maintenance of femoral head blood flow would be of vital interest in preventing avascular necrosis. clofibrate, an antilipidemic agent with a depressant effect on both cholesterol and triglycerides, especially on the very low density lipoprotein that is rich in triglycerides, is a medication that has been widely used previously in treating patients with hypercholesterolemia.

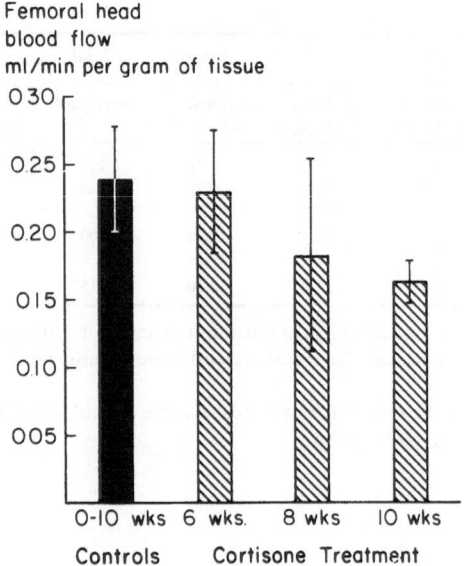

Fig. 6. Femoral head blood flow of control and steroid-treated rabbits. There is a statistically significant decreased blood flow after 8 weeks of steroid treatment

Experiments designed to test the probable beneficial effects of an antilipidemic agent, with hopes of modifing intrafemoral head pressure and blood flow, were then undertaken.

Femoral Head Pressure Study

Twenty-four adult New Zealand white rabbits, average weight 4.5 kg, were used. All received weekly 12.25 mg intramuscular injections of Depo-medrol for 14 weeks. The rabbits were divided into three groups of eight. Group I rabbits received steroid only. Group II rabbits received weekly Depo-medrol plus prophylactic clofibrate, 500 mg orally, daily. Group III rabbits were given weekly steroid but the clofibrate was not administered until 4 weeks after the beginning of steroid treatment. In the previous experiments, we noted the gradual increase of serum cholesterol, fat cell size, and increase of intrafemoral head pressure after up to 4–6 weeks of steroid treatment. Thus, Group III was given clofibrate at a time when the early change of marrow fat cell hypertrophy had already begun. The femoral head pressure was measured at 8 through 14 weeks of treatment according to previously described established methods.

Blood Flow Study

Thirty-five New Zealand white adult rabbits, weighing an average of 4.5 kg, were used. Five rabbits received no medication and were used as controls. All the others received weekly intramuscular doses of 12.25 mg of Depo-Medrol for 12 weeks. The rabbits were divided into three groups of 10 each. Group I received steroid only. Group II received weekly Depo-medrol plus prophylactic clofibrate, 500 mg daily, by mouth. Group III rabbits were given weekly steroid but clofibrate was not started until 4 weeks after the institution of steroid treatment.

Group I steroid-treated rabbits received measurements of intrafemoral head blood flow from week 6 through week 12. Group II and Group III rabbits received measurements from week 8 through week 10. The measurement of blood flow was again carried out using the established method, as described previously.

Osteocyte Study

Ten New Zealand white rabbits, weighing an average of 4.5 kg, were used. They all received 12.25 mg of Depo-medrol weekly plus clofibrate, in daily doses of 500 g, orally. One rabbit was killed at 8 weeks, three at 10 weeks and two were killed at 12 weeks. The others died prematurely.

Results

Pressure Study

In both Group I and Group II, seven of eight rabbits survived to undergo pressure measurements while one in each group died from the effect of the long-term steroid. Two of eight rabbits in Group III also died in the experiment. Data obtained from the non-treated rabbits in the previous study was used as the control. The steroid-treated rabbits showed an elevated serum cholesterol. The steroid- and clofibrate-treated rabbits showed an initial decrease of cholesterol level, but this depression did not persist.

Untreated control rabbits' intrafemoral head pressure was consistent at 24.6 ± 5 cm of saline. By 12 weeks, the steroid-treated rabbits' intra-

Fig. 7. Steroid plus time 0 clofibrate treated-rabbits showed no rise in intrafemoral head pressure

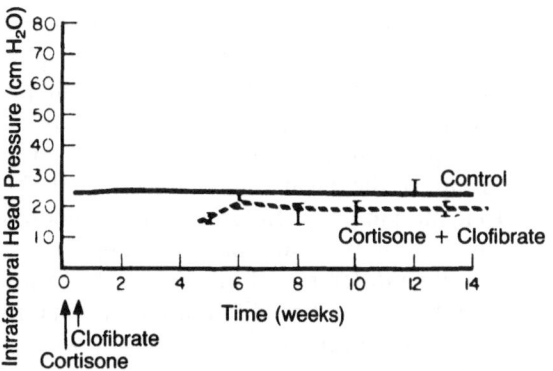

Fig. 8. Steroid plus delayed clofibrate treated rabbits showed initial increase of intrafemoral head pressure and gradual decrease to the normal after clofibrate treatment

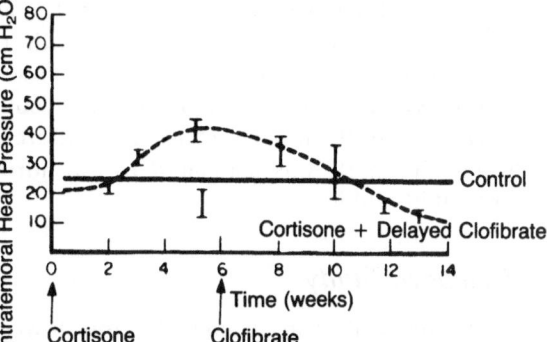

femoral head pressure had increased to 55.2 ± 5 cm of saline. Proximal tibia metaphyseal pressure was measured in fewer of the steroid-treated rabbits and no steroid induced change was observed.

In the rabbits receiving steroid plus clofibrate from day 1, there was no rise in intrafemoral

head pressure. Even after 12 weeks of steroid treatment the manometer readings were not significantly different from those of the untreated group (Fig. 7).

In rabbits receiving steroid followed by clofibrate treatment, beginning after a delay of 4 weeks, there was an initial increase in pressure, to 45 cm of saline at 4–6 weeks, and then it gradually decreased to the normal 18 ± 4 cm of saline after 8–10 weeks of clofibrate treatment (Fig. 8).

Statistical analysis, using 2-way analysis of variance, revealed that the difference between the group treated with steroid only and those treated with steroid and clofibrate was statistically significant ($P < 0.005$).

Blood Flow Study

Ten control femoral heads, 20 Group I femoral heads, 10 femoral heads from Group II, and 12 from Group III were available for study. Five rabbits in Group II and four rabbits in Group III died prematurely due to systemic infection. The average blood flow in the normal untreated rabbits was 0.239 ± 0.076 ml/min per g, with no

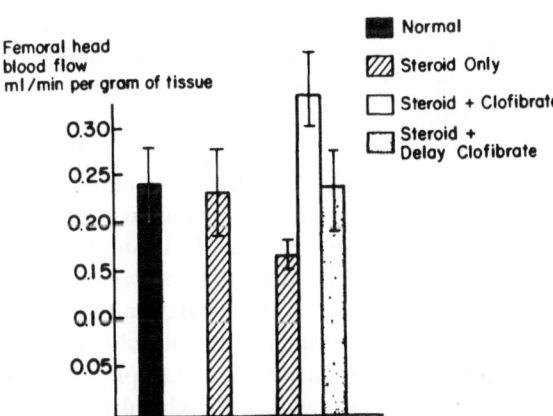

Fig. 9. Femoral head blood flow. Normal rabbits, 0–10 weeks; rabbits treated with steroids only, 6–10 weeks; rabbits administered steroid plus clofibrate and steroid plus delayed clofibrate, 10 weeks

significant difference between the left and right. In the steroid-treated rabbits, the average blood flow at 10 weeks was 0.162 ± 0.039 ml/min per g. Group I and Group II rabbits' measurements were performed between 8 and 10 weeks. In Group II the mean blood flow was 0.327 ± 0.115 ml/min per g. In Group III the blood flow was 0.212 ± 0.115 ml/min per g (Fig. 9).

Using a difference of means T-test, we found a significant statistical difference between Group II and the normal untreated group, with consistent increase of blood flow in the Group II rabbits' femoral heads. There was also a statistical difference between Group III and the Group I steroid-treated group, with the maintenance of femoral head blood flow in Group III and decreased blood flow in Group I. Furthermore, the findings showed no difference when Group III was compared to the normal untreated rabbits.

Osteocyte Study

Thirty-one cells were examined before 8 weeks had elapsed. These cells consisted of 74.1% apparently normal cells and 22.5% large fat vacuole cells. This was statistically nonsignificant when compared with the normal untreated group. From rabbits killed after 8 weeks, 215 cells were examined; 61.3% were apparently normal cells with 27.9% of large vacuole cells. This is statistically a difference of $P < 0.01$ with the steroid-treated group but no difference with the normal untreated group.

Discussion

This preliminary study of growing and adult rabbits treated with steroid was undertaken primarily to demonstrate the various morphological effects of steroid therapy on bone and bone marrow and the physiological implications of its effects.

The pathogenesis of steroid-induced osteonecrosis remains controversial. The subchondral bone is known to contain end arteries and the marrow pressure in the long bone is greater in the diaphysis, decreasing toward the epiphysis [32,33]. Considering this fact, as well as the very small diameter of the subchondral arteries and the tendency of fat droplets to adhere to the

vessel walls, it seems likely that fat emboli could collect in the terminal arterioles. It has also been suggested that fat globules can be deformed, compressed, and impacted in the terminal arterioles by the force of intramedullary blood pressure [19–21]. Other authors have suggested that this increase of fat embolization associated with steroid therapy resulted in the obstruction of these vessels and is the mechanism for the development of avascular necrosis [7,8,21]. Our observations of steroid-treated rabbits showed an initial 30% weight loss, with concomitant fatty metamorphosis of the liver, hypercholesterolemia, and increased incidence of fatty embolization resulting in some obstruction of subchondral arterioles. These changes confirmed findings by other investigators [24,25]. Although the gross appearance of the steroid-treated rabbits was similar to that noted in chronic starvation experiments, the observed increase in fat cell size was parodoxical and sharply in contrast to the general decrease in the size of fat cells during starvation.

Our steroid-treated adult rabbits showed a significant increase in the size of fat cells in the bone marrow. The average diameter was 72 μm compared with a normal diameter of 60 μm. The quantitative assessment of the histological changes involved two techniques. First, we measured epiphyseal marrow area to assess the change in the marrow volume; to find that the area marrow cavity following treatment with steroid increased 14%–16% depending on whether the rabbit was growing or mature.

Next, we determined the epiphyseal fat cell volume fraction, which showed an increase of 25%–28% following steroid treatment, again, depending on the maturity of the rabbit. We believe that the discrepancy between the large increase in marrow fat cell volume and the slight increase in marrow cavity volume (this cavity containing the fat cells) may be of significance in the development of avascular necrosis in steroid-treated individuals. In a closed chamber, such as a femoral head, an increase of volume of one cellular constituent must take place at the expense of others within the chamber, because the ultra structure cannot expand. The space required to accomodate the 25%–28% increase in marrow fat cell volume following steroid therapy is greater than that represented by the 14%–16% increase in marrow volume. This leaves more than a 10% increase in fat cell volume which must be accomodated by reduction of either the hemopoetic or the vascular sinusoidal component of the marrow space. In addition, subsequent experiments revealed an increase of intrafemoral head pressure over both hips, from 33.5 ± 2.1 cm of water at 6 weeks of treatment to 53.5 ± 4.4 cm of water at 8 weeks, with the control value remaining constant throughout the experiment, at 24.6 ± 5.5 cm of water. This seems to further confirm the study of Ficat in humans [34]. This increase of pressure of more than 20 cm of water is statistically significant, with $P < 0.001$. We feel that this significant increase in pressure may further collapse the sinusoidal system within the femoral head and impair the circulation. With additional study we further demonstrated that substantial decrease of blood flow in the femoral head indeed occurred after 8 weeks of steroid therapy, with a significant difference, at $P < 0.01$.

We believe the cause of the osteonecrosis is multifactoral [1,11,14,16,19,20,26,28,34–41]. Previous studies have shown that prolonged steroid administration will lead to systemic fatty embolization and subsequent accumulation of fatty emboli in the intraosseous arterioles, especially in the subchondral region of the femoral head [19,20]. Furthermore, concomitant fat cell hypertrophy occurs [26,28]. This leads to eventual increase in intrafemoral head pressure [42]. Studies by Wilkes and Vischer demonstrated normal bone function as a closed compartment, with normal cortex representing the nondistensible wells of a rigid cannister [43]. The increase of marrow fat cell volume and pressure should eventually lead to collapse of the sinusoidal system of the femoral head. We believe and have demonstrated experimentally that this phenomenon led to the decrease of blood flow to the femoral head in steroid-treated rabbits [44] and we believe that this phenomenon has become one of the major contributing factors in osteonecrosis of the subchondral bone.

Fatty accumulation has been demonstrated within the osteocyte, which is believed to contribute to eventual osteocyte death. Since fatty metamorphosis of the liver cells also occurs, but does not necessarily lead to cell death, we wonder whether this is merely a physiological response to increase fat within the system or whether it is actually a cause of cell death. We agree with Kawai that lipid most likely reaches the osteocyte through canaliculi and becomes a fat vacuole within the cell after further metabolic processing. Yet our ultra structural observation does not preclude this finding to be a reflection of normal cell metabolism in the hyperlipidemic state rather than the cause of cell death. Clinical and experimental observation has indicated that osteonecrosis is initially a marrow event with serial change in marrow fat cells, vascular space, and capillary endothelial cells, which precedes observable bony change. Thus, we feel that factors paramount to sustaining marrow serial constituents, such as blood flow, eventually determine the outcome of marrow and bone viability and should be the prime concern.

Joint replacement surgery has not proven to be the answer to this problem, due to the young age of many of the patients with the disease, which leads to premature wear and failure of the replaced joint [45]. Other conservative measures also have had a dismal record [12,46–49].

There is no well-accepted conservative or surgical treatment for on-going osteonecrosis. Progression of this disease will eventually lead to collapse of the femoral head within 2 years following onset of the first clinical symptoms. With this background it was felt that the maintenance of femoral head blood flow during systemic steroid administration is of vital interest in preventing avascular necrosis.

Our study here indicated that clofibrate, when given to rabbits receiving steroids, can lower the serum cholesterol and lessen fat cell size, with ultimate lowering of femoral head pressure and improvement of the femoral head blood flow. This result led us to believe that lipid clearing agents should have a modifying action on the detrimental effects of steroids.

Surgical decompression of the femoral head been used widely and has produced favorable results in impending or early avascular necrosis [1,34,39]. With insufficient early detection of this disease, the treatment becomes impractical. Our study here reveals that prophylactic clofibrate treatment, started at the same time as the institution of steroids, can not only modify the ischemic phenomenon created by long-term steroid administration, but can also cause a dramatic increase in the femoral head blood flow. At the same time this treatment maintained the fat cell size and modified fatty accumulation and fat metabolism within the osteocytes of the steroid-treated rabbits; thus enhancing the chance of osteocyte survival. This treatment also has the effect of preserving normal femoral head pressure that could previously be maintained only through surgical decompression. More importantly, lipid clearing agents can modify an already manifested ischemic condition in the femoral head, as demonsrated by the gradual increase of blood flow, if started within 4 weeks of steroid treatment. We feel this should be beneficial in preventing the progression of ischemic effects induced in the femoral head by prolonged steroid administration.

We found that concomitant steroid plus clofibrate appeared to worsen liver necrosis in some of the steroid-treated rabbits. This resulted in a higher mortality rate and less resistance to systemic infection in the steroid plus clofibrate-treated rabbits. We feel this is an important side effect that is also being reported occasionally in human beings, and that it warrants further investigation before this particular agent is used clinically concomitantly with steroids.

References

1. Arlet J, Ficat P (1968) Diagnostic de l'osteonecrose femoro-capitale primitive au stade l(Stade preradiologique). Rev Chir Orthop 54:637–648
2. Boksenbaum M, Mendelson CG (1963) Aseptic necrosis of the femoral head associated with steroid therapy. JAMA Journal 184:262–265
3. Cosgriff SW, Diefenbach AF, Vogt William Jr (1950) Hypercoagulability of the blood associated with ACTH and cortisone therapy. Am J Med 9:752–756
4. Cruess, RL, Ross D, Crawshaw E (1975) The etiology of steroid-induced avascular necrosis of bone: A laboratory and clinical study. Clin Orthop 113:178–183
5. Cruess RL, Blennerhassett John, Macdonald FR, Maclean LD, Dosseter John (1968) Aseptic necrosis following renal transplantation. J Bone Joint Surg [Am] 50:1577–1590
6. Edstrom Gunnar (1961) destruction of hip joint in rheumatoid arthritis during long-term steroid therapy. Acta Rheum Scand 7:151–155
7. Fisher DE, Bickel WH (1971) Corticosteroid-induced avascular necrosis. A clinical study of seventy-seven patients. J Bone Joint Surg [Am] 53:859–873
8. Fisher DE, Bickel WH, Holley KE (1969) Histologic demonstration of fat emboli in aseptic necrosis associated with hypercortisonism. Mayo Clin Proc 44:252–259
9. Fisher DE, Bickel WH, Holley KE, Ellerson RD (1972) Corticosteroid-induced aseptic necrosis. II. experimental study. Clin Orthop 84:200–206
10. Freiberger RH, Swanson GE (1965) Aseptic necrosis of the femoral head after high dosage corticosteroid therapy. NY State J Med 65:800–804
11. Glimcher MJ, Kenzora JE (1979) The biology of osteonecrosis of the human femoral head and its clinical implications: III. Discussion of the etiology and genesis of the pathological sequelae: Comments on treatment. Clin Orthop 140:273–312
12. Gold EW, Fox OD, Weissfeld Steven, Curtiss PH (1978) Corticosteroid-induced avascular necrosis: An experimental study in rabbits. Clin Orthop 135:272–280
13. Harrington KD, Murray WR, Kountz SL, Belzer FO (1971) Avascular necrosis of bone after renal transplantation. J Bone Joint Surg [Am] 53:203–215
14. Helmann WG, Freiberger RH (1960) Avascular necrosis of the femoral and humeral heads after high dosage corticosteroid therapy. New Engl J Med 263:672–675
15. Hill RB Jr (1961) Fatal fat embolism from steroid-induced fatty liver. New Engl J Med 265:318–320
16. Hungerford DS (1975) Early diagnosis of ischemic necrosis of the femoral head. John Hopkins Med J 137:270–275
17. Hungerford DW, Zizic TM (1978) Alcoholism associated ischemic necrosis of the femoral head: Early diagnosis and treatment. Clin Orthop 130:144–153
18. Johnson LC (1964) Morphologic analysis in pathology: The kinetics of disease and general biology of bone. In: Frost HM (ed) Bone Biodynamics. Little, Brown, Boston, pp 543–654
19. Jones JP Jr, Engleman EP (1966) Osseous avascular necrosis associated with systemic abnormalities. Arthritis Rheum 9:728–736
20. Jones JP Jr, Sakovich L (1966) Fat embolism of bone. A roentgenographic and histological investigation with use of intra-arterial lipiodol in rabbits. J Bone Joint Surg [Am] 48:149–164
21. Jones JP, Engleman EP, Steinbach HL, Murray WR, Rambo ON (1965) Fat embolization as a

possible mechanism producing avascular necrosis (abstract). Arthritis Rheum 8:449

22. Kenzora JE, Steele RE, Yosipovitch ZH, Glimcher MJ (1978) Experimental osteonecrosis of the femoral head in adult rabbits. Clin Orthop 130:8–46

23. Kerboul M, Thomine J, Postel M, Merle D'Aubigne R (1974) The conservative surgical treatment of idiopathic aseptic necrosis of the femoral head. J Bone Joint Surg [Br] 56(2): 291–296

24. Moran TJ (1962) Cortisone-induced alterations in lipid metabolism. Morphologic and serologic observations in rabbits. Arch Pathol 73:300–312

25. Skanse B, Von Studnitz W, Skoog N (1959) The effect of corticotrophin and cortisone on serum lipids and lipoproteins. Acta Endocrinol 31: 442–450

26. Solomon L (1981) Idiopathic necrosis of the femoral head: Pathogenesis and treatment. Can J Surg 24:573–578

27. Sweetam DR, Mason RM, Murray RO (1960) Steroid arthropathy of the hip. Br Med J [Clin Res] 1:1392–1394

28. Wang GJ, Sweet DE, Reger SI, Thompson RC (1977) Fat cell changes as a mechanism of avascular necrosis of the femoral head in cortisone treated rabbits. J Bone Joint Surg [Am] 59:729–735

29. Gregg PJ, Walder DN (1980) Regional distribution of circulating microspheres in the femur of the rabbit. J Bone Joint Surg [Br] 62:(2):222–226

30. Lacombe P, Meric P, Seylaz J (1980) Validity of cerebral blood flow measurements obtained with quantitative tracer techniques. Brain Res Rev 2:105–169

31. Rudolph AM, Heymann MA (1967) The circulation of the fetus in utero. Methods for studying distribution of blood flow. Cardiac output and organ blood flow. Circ Res 21:163–184

32. Michelsen K (1967) Pressure relationships in the bone marrow vascular bed. Acta Physiol Scand 71:16–29

33. Michelsen K (1968) Hemodynamics of the bone marrow circulation. Acta Physiol Scand 73: 264–280

34. Ficat RP, Arlet, Jacques (1980) Ischemia and necroses of bone. Hungerford DS (ed) Williams and Wilkins, Baltimore

35. Chandler FA (1948) Coronary disease of the hip. J Int Coll Surg 11:34–36

36. Glimcher MJ, Kenzora JE (1979) The biology of osteonecrosis of the human femoral head and its clinical implications: 1. Tissue biology. Clin Orthop 138:284–309

37. Glimcher MJ, Kenzora JE (1979) The biology of osteonecrosis of the human femoral head and its clinical implications: II. The pathological changes in the femoral head as an organ and in the hip joint. Clin Orthop 139:283–312

38. Gourdou JF, Danet A, Guiraud R, Durroux R, Ficat P, Arlet J (1974) Necrose experimentale de lat tete femorale d'origine veineuse chez le chien (English abstract), Rev Rhum Mal Osteoartic 41:739

39. Larson RM (1938) Intramedullary pressure with particular reference to massive diaphyseal bone necrosis. Experimental observations. Ann Surg 108:127–140

40. McFarland PH, Frost HM (1961) A possible new cause for aseptic necrosis of the femoral head. Henry Ford Hosp Med Bull 9:115–122

41. Rutishauser E, Rohner A, Held D (1960) Experimentelle Untersuchungen über die Wirkung der Ischaemie auf den Knochen und das Mark, Virchows Arch [A] 333:101–118

42. Wang GJ, Lennox DW, Reger SI, Stamp WG, Hubbard SL (1981) Cortisone-induced intra-femoral head pressure change and its response to a drilling decompression method. Clin Orthop 159:274–278

43. Wilkes CJ, Visscher MB (1975) Some physiological aspects of bone marrow pressure. J Bone Joint Surg [Am] 57:49–57

44. Wang GJ, Hubbard SL, Reger SI, Miller FD, Stamp WG (1983) Femoral head blood flow in long-term steroid treatment (study of rabbit model) South Med J 76:12:1520–1532

45. Chandler HP, Reineck TF, eixson RL, Mc Carthy JD (1981) Total hip replacement in patients under thirty years old. J Bone Joint Surg [Am] 63:1426–1434

46. Bonfiglio Michael, Voke EM (1968) Aseptic necrosis of the femoral head and non-union of the femoral neck. Effect of treatment by drilling and bone grafting (Phemister technique). J Bone Joint Surg [Am] 50:48–66

47. Hungerford DS (1983) Treatment of ischemic necrosis of the femoral head. In: Evarts CM (ed) Surgery of the musculoskeletal system, vol 33. Churchill Livingstone, New York, pp 5–29

48. Marcus ND, Enneking WF, Massam RA (1973) The silent hip in idiopathic aseptic necrosis. Treatment by bone grafting. J Bone Joint Surg [Am] 55:1351–1366

49. Meyers MH, Jones, RE, Bucholz RW, Winger DR (1983) Fresh autogenous grafts and osteochondral allografts for the treatment of segmental collapse in osteonecrosis of the hip. Clin Orthop 174:107–112

Bacterial Adherence in Foreign Body Infection

David J. Schurman[1] and R. Lane Smith

Summary. Foreign body infection is a special clinical problem because with few exceptions standard treatment (debridement and antibiotics) normally effective for most bodily infections is ineffective. Prosthetic implants are common and infection is the second most common reason for failure. The reason that prosthetic infections fail to resolve with antibiotic therapy has remained a mystery, but new insights are beginning to penetrate this enigma. Antibiotics will not kill sensitive bacteria in a test tube when they are attached to an object in the test tube or the walls of the test tube. Evidence suggests that once attachment has taken place bacteria may proliferate in the presence of bactericidal antibiotic concentrations. The extracellular matrix of bacteria, glycocalyx, may in some instances, such as with *Staphylococcus epidermidis*, enhance survival of bacteria. Glycocalyx appears to promote rapid attachment to foreign bodies under some circumstances. Attachment itself seems to confer upon the bacteria the ability to survive normally lethal concentrations of antibiotics. Critical insights as to the mechanism for this invulnerability are likely to result from investigating genomic expression of the bacteria at the time of attachment.

Key words. Bacterial adherence — Foreign body infection — Glycocalyx — Staphylococcus — Antibiotics

Introduction

Modern surgery was introduced by Joseph Lister in the 1860s. Until that time, surgical infections were as common as 25%–50% in many series and many of these infections resulted in death. Prior to Lister's work the concept, and indeed, the word infection was well known and generally understood in terms of its occurrence and likely destructive capacity. It was Lord Lister's application of Louis Pasteur's discovery of the cause of putrefaction which allowed Lister for the first time to prove that human infection was caused by bacteria. These findings allowed the introduction of both antiseptic and aseptic techniques, which over the space of a year or two revolutionized surgical practice worldwide. The application of sterile technique and the use of antiseptic disinfectants, such as carbolic acid, reliably brought the infection rates down to 5%. This low rate of infection allowed the introduction of elective surgery on a practical basis and swiftly gave rise to modern surgery as we know it. Joseph Lister, himself, predominantly limited his practice to orthopedic surgery. He electively pinned hips and internally fixed a variety of other fractures. An infection rate of 5% formed a reasonable basis for elective surgery well into the 1960s. Most elective surgery dealt with soft tissues. Those situations where implants were used mostly involved temporary fixations, such as fracture fixation.

Prior to the advent of antibiotics, osteomyelitis was a very common problem and accounted for the majority of most orthopedic inpatients. Many of the worst consequences of osteomyelitis were brought under control by the application of surgical principles propounded by Winnet Orr in the 1930s. The introduction of antibiotics as they became available diminished the consequences of infection still further. The sulfa drugs were

[1] Division of Orthopedics R171, Stanford University School of Medicine, CA 94305, USA

introduced in the 1930s, penicillin in the early 1940s, and other antibiotics, thereafter. A 5% infection rate was still thought not unreasonable because most infections were transient in that they involved soft tissue structures which could, with good surgical and antibiotic care, heal themselves. Osteomyelitis was brought under control and was in many cases prevented by the early application of antibiotics by pediatricians and family physicians to almost any illness that presented with fever. Internal fixation for fractures was commonplace, but the infections that did occur were controlled by removing the fixation, appropriate debridement, and eventually the use of antibiotics.

With the introduction of total joint replacement by John Charnley, building on the work of earlier surgical implant procedures, such as the Smith-Peterson cup arthroplasty, the Judet brothers acrylic hemiarthroplasty, and the metal hemiarthroplasty introduced by Austin Moore and F.R. Thompson, 5% infection rates became increasingly intolerable. The consequences of having to remove the arthroplasty hardware to control infection led orthopedic surgeons to search for more certain means of reducing infection rates. Probably the most significant advances since Lister's principles in preventing infections were largely developed or implemented by orthopedic surgeons. These advances were the use of antibiotics prophylactically and the introduction of laminar flow clean air rooms. It should be remembered that when prophylactic antibiotics were introduced by orthopedic surgeons, infectious disease experts and most other physicians believed this to be folly. Today in major medical centers throughout the world, clean, elective surgical procedures which employ antibiotic prophylaxis and use clean air rooms have generally reduced infection rates to 1% or less.

The two most tenacious and relentless types of orthopedic infection are clearly those of osteomyelitis and foreign body infections. We now know that chronic osteomyelitis has much in common with foreign body infection. Osteomyelitis bone is dead bone without adequate microcirculation and without viable tissue. Dead bone, although autologous, behaves in many respects like a foreign body, especially with regard to cleansing the bacterial infection and colonization of the dead bone. The

reason that clinical success in treating foreign body infection has been so poor has remained a riddle throughout the twentieth century. It is only in recent years that this riddle has begun to untangle. Some of the mystery remains, but important inroads into a real understanding of the problem have been carved out recently.

One of the first clues as to the nature of foreign body infection was the fact that Staphylococcus epidermidis, normally a non-pathogen, or a minor transient colonizer of wounds, became recognized as the most common pathogen causing infection in foreign body infection, along with Staphylococcus aureus. Costerton, a Canadian microbiologist, developed great interest in the nature of bacterial growth on inanimate objects, such as occurs in the Alaskan pipelines. This interest was not just an intellectual curiosity but was stimulated by the fact that the bacterial growth in pipelines was a significant economic problem, inasmuch as it increased maintenance and decreased oil flowing through the pipelines. Costerton discovered that the bacteria which so readily attached to the walls of the pipes secreted an exoskeletal polysaccharide, often referred to as glycocalyx, biofilm, or slime. Costerton began investigating how bacteria stick [1,2] in situations involving human implants. Anthony Gristina [3,4] recognized the value of Costerton's work and applied it to orthopedic surgery. Gristina was among the first to recognize that Staphylococcus epidermidis was associated with a bacterial extracellular slime and he hypothesized that this slime was a major factor in the pathogenicity of Staphylococcus epidermidis in its relationship with foreign bodies.

Investigations in the 1980s, utilizing electron microscopy, showed a strong rationale for implicating bacterial slime as an important factor in foreign body infection. Scanning electron microscopy demonstrated that the appearance of osteomyelitic bone was similar to that of bone infected by foreign objects, with coherent microcolonies in a biofilm obscuring the surface of the bone [5].

Bacterial adherence is associated with a variety of interactive processes. These phases can be divided into a) transport of bacteria by diffusion or convective flow, b) initial contact and binding, c) attachment mediation by special anchoring structures, such as fibrils or polymers, and d) colonization characterized by newly formed cells proliferating and remaining together to form a biofilm [6]. A wide variety of clinical pathogens bind to a variety of matrix proteins, including laminin, collagen, fibronectin, vitronectin, and fibrin. The isolation and characterization of microbial receptors is underway [7].

Materials and Methods

Our own interest in bacterial attachment to foreign bodies provoked us to find quantitative methods of describe events. Methodology for looking at quantities of bacteria attaching to foreign objects was limited to microscopic examination of bacteria samples, or staining the biofilm substrate in situ. We were able to carry out a variety of experiments after simplifying the methodologies [8]. From a variety of dyes tested we found that Toluidine Blue Staining was most reliable and that Carnoy's solution was optimal for fixation of the slime. Once the surface bacteria were stained and fixed they could readily be solubilized in 0.2 M NaOH at 85°C for 1 h. Fifteen clinical strains of *Staphylococcus epidermidis* were evaluated and their biofilm production ranged continuously from a high to medium to low rate of stain (Figs. 1, 2). This direct, simple, and reproducible quantitative

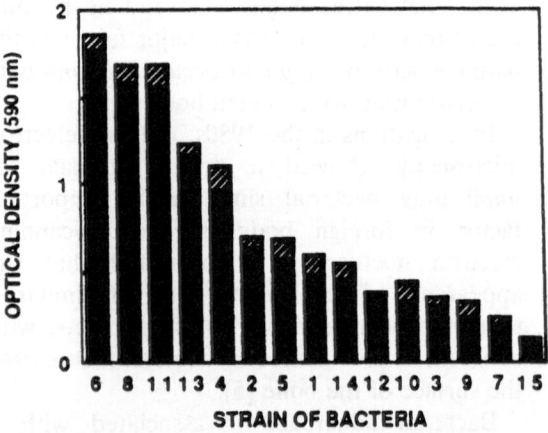

Fig. 1. Optical density of biofilm produced on glass culture tubes within a 24-h period. Experiments were performed in quadruplicate. The data show the means and the standard error of the mean. (From [8] with permission)

technique allowed us to investigate a series of interactions between bacteria and foreign bodies under in vitro circumstances.

An additional aid in the methodology of quantitative assessment of both the bacteria and the slime was the use of ^{3}H-thymidine. Through a series of experiments we were able to demonstrate that at least 81% of the marker was taken up by the bacterial DNA. Simultaneous use of ^{14}C-glucose and ^{3}H-thymidine allows one to determine the relative production of extracellular matrix per bacteria (Fig. 3). For *Staphylococcus epidermidis* . We were able to show that four times as much slime was produced per bacteria by a high slime producer than a low slime producer. Moreover, we were able to demonstrate that the production and accumulation of biofilm over time was a stable characteristic of different strains of *Staphylococcus epidermidis* [9].

Proline sutures of specific lengths were exposed to one of two types of *Staphylococcus epidermidis*. The first was a high producer of glycocalyx and the second a low producer of glycocalyx. These sutures were then placed in Triptycase soy broth in a glass test tube and each 24 h the suture was removed, washed three times and replaced in fresh broth for a total of 72 h. Utilizing our earlier methods, we were able to demonstrate quantitatively that the low producer of glycocalyx at the end of 24 h had one-tenth the number of bacteria on the surface of the suture as did the *Staphylococcus epidermidis* with high glycocalyx production. Over the 2nd and 3rd days, the high glycocalyx-producing *Staphylococcus epidermidis* grew at a geometric rate, as opposed to the low glycocalyx producing organism, which failed to show any increase in numbers of bacteria attached over that time period (Fig. 4). Thus it appears that slime production is responsible for increasing colonization of a foreign body by an order of magnitude initially, with continuing geometrical divergence thereafter.

In a series of additional experiments to characterize the rate of attachment of *Staphylococcus* to the suture, we found few or no organisms attached irreversibly to the suture in the first 5 h. Thereafter there was a geometric growth of bacteria, which remained firmly attached to the suture. This rate of growth continued at a constant rate for the next 3 days.

Fig. 2A,B. Transmission electron microscope pictures of two strains of *S. epidermidis* grown on cover slips for 24 h. Long measuring line = 0.5 μm, short line = 0.1 μm. Magnification, ×62 000. **A** High producer of biofilm; **B** low producer. (From [9] with permission)

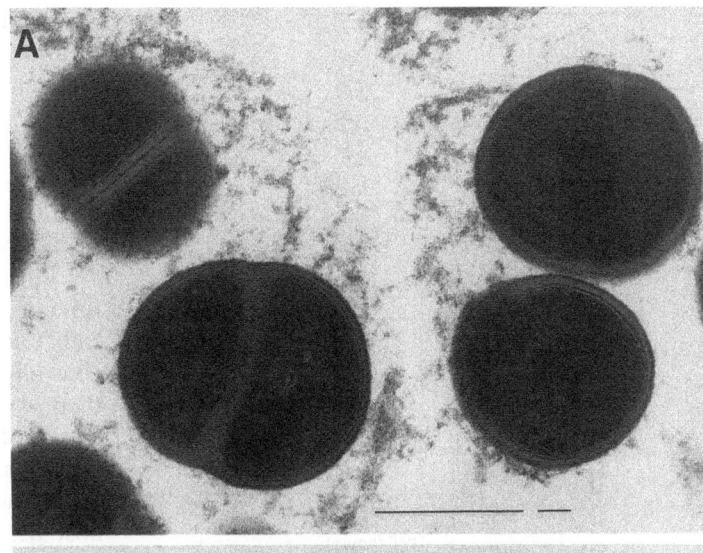

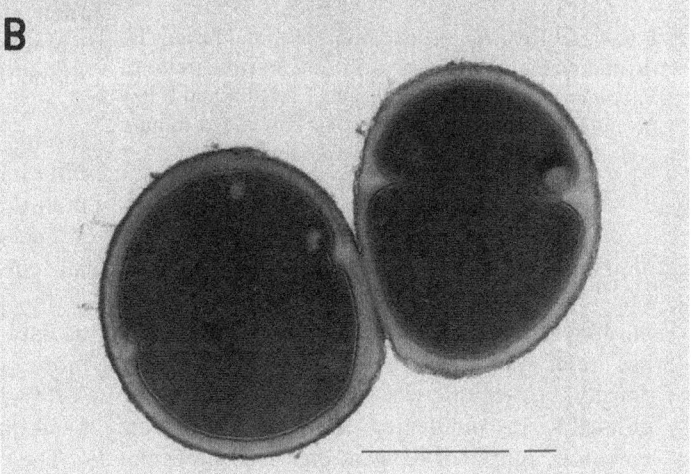

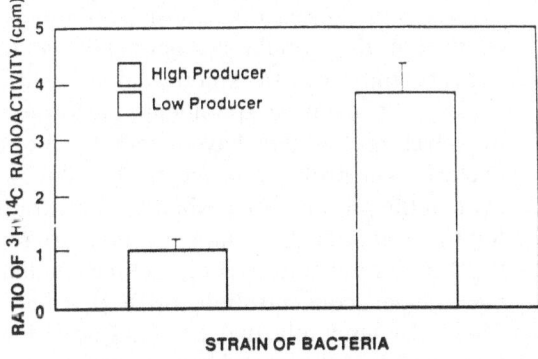

Fig. 3. Relative ratios of ³H-thymidine and ¹⁴C glucose incorporation in two strains (high vs low biofilm producer) of *S. epidermidis*. (From [9] with permission)

Bacterial Growth Rate

A summary of bacterial growth rates under different circumstances provides a few insights. Bacterial growth in culture broth under optimal circumstances proceeds at logarithmic rates until a maximum number is achieved, at which point bacterial growth ceases. At this point the bacteria remain fixed in number in what is called a stationary growth phase. These classic conditions relate to bacteria growing in nutrient broth under ideal temperature and oxygen conditions. The growth rate in broth is exponential, as compared to the geometric growth rate on foreign objects under optimal conditions. These differences in rates of growth are due in part to surface growth being somewhat limited by a two

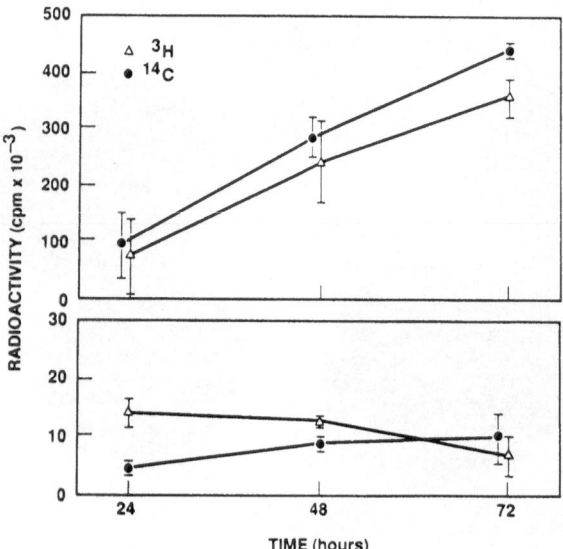

Fig. 4a,b. Relative incorporation of radiolabeled ³H-thymidine and ¹⁴C glucose over time in two strains of *S. epidermidis*. **a** High producer of biofilm and **b** low producer. Radioactivity represents counts per minute per sample. (From [9] with permission)

dimensional domain constraint. The reason that bacteria reach a stationary growth phase is multifactorial and highly complex. Historically it has been stated that with increasing bacterial density, growth rate ceases because of a buildup of local toxins and decreased access to adequate nutrition, supply of oxygen, etc. The molecular biology of this growth inhibition is not understood and the complexity of the situation will probably defy full explanation for some time. The growth rate of bacteria on foreign bodies has been studied very little.

Some bacteria have a low affinity for attachment to foreign bodies. The low affinity of attachment may also be associated with weak binding, such that the attachment that does occur may be readily reversible. Some bacteria empirically never reach a state of significant cell attachment to the foreign body and fail to proliferate with time. Those bacteria which readily adhere to foreign objects grow at a markedly diminished rate as compared to bacteria which are in free form in fluid unattached to foreign objects. Once cells of bacteria do attach to a foreign object in a stable fashion, their daughter cells may likewise form attachments with the foreign objects. After some

period the limited surface of the object is saturated. Now the daughter cells may either attach to one another, or break free and become unassociated with the foreign body. Bacteria associated with foreign bodies are typically referred to as sessile, and bacteria unassociated with foreign bodies are often referred to as planktonic.

Clinically, the rate of growth of bacteria on a foreign object is of very real concern. It is well known that infected objects may remain clinically quiescent for long periods and may then, without warning, flare up into acute processes of infection. During these flareups, the sessile bacteria on the foreign body partially break away and multiply independently in the host tissues and fluids. Under such conditions their growth rate once again increases and the whole spectrum of inflammatory reaction is re-incited.

As bacteria create an abscess away from the foreign body they once again become susceptible to antibiotic treatment much more readily than they do while they are in their sessile form attached to an implant. Most patients with intermittent symptomatic osteomyelitis learn that at the earliest phase of a recurrence they can usually abort episodic infection by taking antibiotics. The treatment is successful in curing the soft tissue infection but generally will not kill the bacteria attached to the foreign body.

The sensitivity of bacteria to antibiotics changes radically when they adhere to a foreign object. That is to say, the bacteria typically become quite insensitive to an antibiotic concentration that would normally kill them. It appears that growth kinetics alone will not explain this event. Experiments performed by ourselves and others have demonstrated that bacteria will proliferate, albeit at a slow rate, even in the presence of antibiotic concentrations ten times greater than amounts necessary to kill them in normal culture (i.e., 20 times minimum bactericidal concentration [MBC]) (Fig. 5). These studies imply that bacterial adhesion to foreign objects by itself elicits metabolic events in bacteria which make them insensitive to antibiotic concentrations well beyond the MBC. At this time this phenomenon remains unexplained.

Some bacterial genes are probably expressed differently according to whether bacteria are

Fig. 5. Bacterial adherence to proline suture material (stationary phase 1×10^9 STAPH EPI) and ^{3}H-thymidine uptake in the presence of $20 \times$ MBC antibiotic

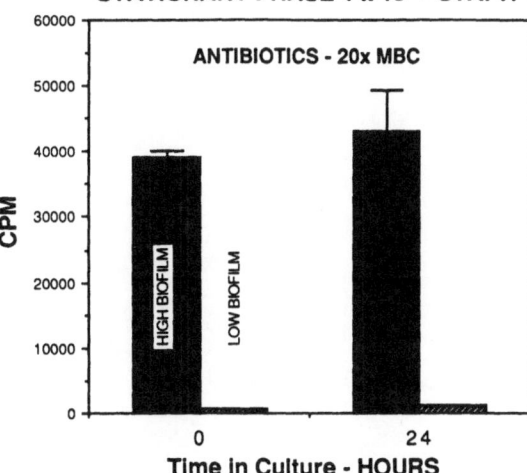

BACTERIAL ADHERENCE TO PROLENE SUTURE STATIONARY PHASE 1 x 10 ^{9} STAPH EPI

attached to an inanimate object or attached to other bacteria, or in suspension. Techniques are available currently which can identify specific genes which become expressed as the bacterial organism interacts with its environment. One would imagine that in the next several years specific genes and their products which govern bacterial adhesion and associated metabolic events will be isolated. These findings will bring a clearer insight into the governance of foreign body infection.

References

1. Costerton JC, Geesey GG, Cheng K-J (1978) How bacteria stick. Sci Am 238:86–95
2. Costerton JW, Irvin RT, Cheng KJ (1981) The bacterial glycocalyx in nature and disease. Annu Rev Microbiol 35:299–324
3. Gristina AG, Costerton J (1985) Bacterial adherence to biomaterials and tissue. J Bone Joint Surg [Am] 67:264–273
4. Gristina AG, Oga M, Webb LX, et al. (1985) Adherent bacterial colonization in the pathogenesis of osteomyelitis. Science 228:990–993
5. Pugsley MP, Sanders JR (1990) Infections of prosthetic joints. In Root RK, Trunkey DD, Sande MA (eds) New surgical and medical approaches in infectious diseases. Churchill Livingstone, New York, pp 229–244
6. Marshall KC (1985) Mechanisms of bacterial adhesion at solid water interfaces. In: Savage DC, Fletcher M (eds) Bacterial adhesion: Mechanisms and physiological significance. Plenum, New York, pp 133–161
7. Hook M, Switalski LM, Wadstrom T, Lindberg M (1989) Interactions of pathogenic microorganisms with fibronectin. In: Mosher D (ed) Fibronectin. Academic, New York pp 295–307
8. Tsai C, Schurman DJ, Smith RL (1989) Quantitation of glycocalyx production in coagulase negative *Staphylococcus*. J Orthop Res 6:666–670
9. Pett KV, Schurman DJ, Smith RL (1990) Quantitation and relative distribution of extracellular matrix in *Staphylococcus Epidermidis* biofilm. J Orthop Res 8:321–327

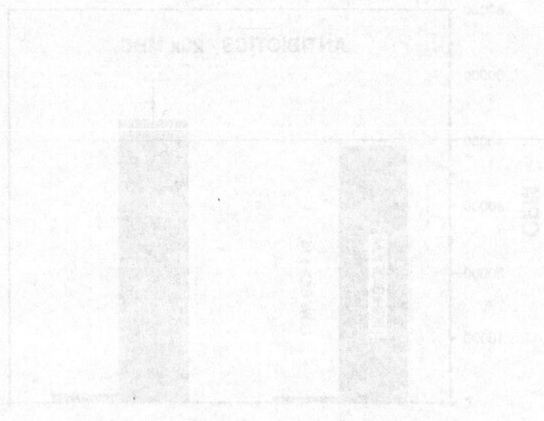

Part II. Joint Surgery and Its Problems

The Evolution of Hip Replacement

The title of my talk probably conjures up a picture of Charles Darwin, who took almost 40 years to tell his story of evolution. I have 40 minutes to tell mine. But I have the advantage of having seen virtually the whole evolution of joint replacement in my own lifetime. I'm sufficiently antique for that. And my account is a personal one, mostly involving people I knew.

The first artificial hip I knew about was put in by Philip Wiles of the Middlessex Hospital in 1936. Its design was based on that used for fracture fixation and if he'd had better materials it might have worked. But it didn't and he did only a handful. The first surgeon to do a substantial number of arthroplasties and to achieve even modest success was Smith-Petersen of Boston. He smoothed the rough arthritic surfaces of the joint and, to prevent them from sticking together, he interposed something between them. He tried celluloid, glass, and bakelite, but eventually he settled for vitallium.

Smith-Petersen described his famous vitallium cup arthroplasty to the Royal College of Surgeons of England in a Moynihan lecture in 1947. His results were reasonably good by the standards of those times. I think part of the reason for his success lay in his character. He was not only a supremely skilful surgeon, but was also a man of great empathy and kindliness; he was devoted to his patients, and they to him. But sometimes after his arthroplasties the femoral head became avascular, collapsed, and the pain recurred.

Working at much the same time in Oxford was Girdlestone, a completely different character. He was a deeply religious man. He prayed before every operating list. Naturally his enemies said this was essential prophylaxis. One can't help wondering if the biblical injunction "if thine eye offend thee pluck it out" inspired him to excise the head of the femur for a painful hip. This left the hip unstable, but quite often the patient lost his pain.

The next development came from Robert Judet of Paris. He was an ebullient, charming man with enormous surgical panache. Girdlestone's idea of cutting off the head appealed to him; but he and his brother Jean did something more. Having cut off the femoral head, they restored stability by putting in an acrylic one. I went to see them in the early 1950s and their results were spectacular. But, after a time, many of the prostheses broke. So people tried making them of metal, but then the stem broke, and eventually it was realized that the stem had to be protected by placing it inside the shaft of the femur. Austin Moore had devised such a prosthesis and used it to replace the femoral head after a fractured femoral neck. A few surgeons decided to try it for osteoarthritis and my colleagues and I published a series of 120, in which we had done just that. In our hands it gave better results than anything we had done before. But these results were still only moderate. As time went on, the prosthesis tended to burrow into the pelvis. Clearly the answer was to replace the acetabulum as well.

[1] Royal College of Surgeons, 35–43 Lincoln's Inn Fields, London WC2A 3PN, UK

The question was how to anchor it. One way might be to screw it into the pelvis; that's what Ring of Redhill did and still does.

His idea of using a screw was not new. As long ago as 1951, McKee produced an artificial hip derived from a lag screw. He only did a few cases and nearly all of them failed. But he was a very determined man and in 1956 he produced a second model. With this about half his cases were successful. But half were still failures and that was unacceptable.

At this point Charnley comes into the story. Sir John, half engineer, half surgeon, all genius. One day a patient with a Judet prosthesis told him that when he moved it squeaked. This triggered Charnley to study joint lubrication and he produced a model with a plastic acetabulum to reduce friction. What's more, he anchored both components with cement. McKee soon adopted cement also and then both he and Charnley began to have success rates of 90% or better.

That was in the early 1960s, and that's when I started doing total hips. The 60s — a decade of triumph for hip replacement; the patients were thrilled, and to surgeons it was a miracle. We saw complete cripples become virtually normal in next to no time; nothing in my surgical lifetime has been even remotely comparable. That was the 60s. What about the 70s? That was the decade of complications. Suddenly we were faced with a whole set of complications, some completely new to surgery. But these complications have turned out to be a vital part of the evolution of modern joint replacement, comparable with Darwinian evolution. In place of mutations supplying the raw material from which Nature selected the fittest to survive, we had complications from which surgeons selected the prostheses which survived longest.

I don't propose to discuss all the complications, just three. First infection, the complication we fear most and which may herald disaster. Once deep infection is established, if excising infected tissue and giving antibiotics don't clear it up, we may have to take out all the foreign material. Then, if we're brave, we can put in a new prosthesis immediately, using gentamicin-loaded cement. But we may prefer to play safe, to wait for everything to settle, leaving an excision arthroplasty, Girdlestone's operation. It's curious how this operation, which was virtually abandoned when replacement started, has come back into favor as the ultimate salvage operation.

But of course the best way of treating infection is not to get it. At one time Charnley had an infection rate of 9%. So he isolated the operating area, filtered the air and arranged its flow so that bacteria didn't fall into the wound. His infection rate dropped and dropped until it was well under 1%. But was it the ultraclean air which achieved this, or was it that he and his team had become very skillful? After all, they'd done thousands of hips. It was important to know, because health authorities had to decide whether hip replacement should be forbidden in conventional operation rooms. So the Medical Research Council (M.R.C.) set up a large-scale study, divided among a few hospitals, of which my own was one.

Our task was to do 8000 joint replacements between us. In my own unit, when we'd done our first 700, half with ultraclean air and half in a conventional set-up, the infection rate was slightly higher with ultra-clean air, though in both it was fairly low. But in the end ultra-clean air won. Not by much, and we now realize that, though its best to have ultra-clean air, other things are perhaps no less important — especially antibiotics, impervious clothing, and meticulous technique.

Antibiotics and technique everyone accepts. But the surgeon's clothing tends to be forgotten. Bacteria can get through the usual materials much too easily. There are, however, new materials which are so woven that bacteria cannot easily penetrate them and it would seem sensible to use these routinely during joint replacement.

Infection is one cause of loosening, but the commonest is probably poor application of the bone cement, though modern techniques which are much better are available. Another cause of loosening is trauma. We tend to forget that anyone who is active, and we've made these patients active, is liable at some time to fall over, and that also may lead to loosening.

But implants can loosen even without trauma, especially if the friction between the components is too great. That's one reason metal-on-metal prostheses were abandoned (another reason was that metal particles were abraded). We had to have low friction arthroplasties, such as metal on polyethylene. There's still some friction and metal products are absorbed;

they can be detected in the urine, for example. Fortunately this doesn't seem harmful. However, some metal products are not absorbed — could they do any harm? Well, local malignancy has been reported. This is extremely rare, but some of the new cementless prostheses have a roughened surface giving them a huge area of metal to bone contact. Perhaps we should think twice before putting these into very young patients. We always have to worry about implanting foreign materials.

Would biodegradables be safer? A surgeon in Burma used ivory for his hips. The host bone gradually replaced the ivory by creeping substitution. But elephants are not very common in the West and I can't see us using ivory. Another possibility is human material — there's no shortage of corpses. Most of the work on corpse bone has been done in the Soviet Union. In 1966 a Russian surgeon wrote a chapter about it in a book I was editing. He described how he took bone ends from corpses and put them into patients. If he stored the fresh corpse bone at −70°C for 25 days he seldom had any rejection, although he didn't use immunosuppressives. This material was satisfactory for replacing a tumor in a young person. But in this country we were operating on older people, and replacement of the corpse bone by the host bone takes several years and we couldn't expect elderly patients to remain off weight that long, which they would have to do, or the bone would crumble. So corpse bone was no good for most of our patients. And we went on using metal and polyethylene prostheses which we cemented into place.

We keep referring to cement and it was this substance, polymethyl methacrylate, which gave us in Britain a considerable lead over the United States in joint replacement. In the USA, anything implanted into the body has to be approved by the Food and Drug Administration. They needed a lot of reassurance that cement was safe before they would sanction its general use; and in the meantime we in Europe were gaining experience and using it quite safely.

The real problem with cement is not so much safety as the difficulty it causes when we need to revise a hip replacement. We have to dig out the cement that's deep down inside the femoral shaft; if it were only on the surface it would be so much easier. That's why double cups, which are

essentially surface replacements, were greeted with a fanfare of trumpets; but the complication rate was so high that they were soon virtually abandoned. However, there may be another answer. If we don't like digging out cement, why put it there in the first place? Cement may have been important in the early evolution of hip replacement, but now it might just be a vestigial remnant. With modern designs do we really need cement? And a recent twist in the evolutionary story is the development of porous-coated prostheses used without cement and anchored by what's called osseo-integration — bone ingrowth. Even more recent is the use of plasma-sprayed hydroxyapatite coating. Which also doesn't need cement and looks very promising. Joint replacement is still evolving. So it may be interesting to try looking into the future. I doubt whether, in 50 or 100 years time, we will still be inserting massive pieces of metal and plastic. It seems too unphysiological. Perhaps our successors will simply scrape off the damaged articular cartilage and rejuvenate the joint by applying a sticky paste of vigorous young chondrocytes: we're within sight of that already. After that it may not be long before somebody will be applying chondrocyte paste through an arthroscope.

But the molecular biologists might do better still — once they find the gene that switches on chondrogenesis. They could start with the double helix of DNA, uncoil the strands and separate them by high temperature or a strong alkali; that's routine. And they can break these strands into fragments with a restriction enzyme. They'll also take plasmids which have a fragment cut out of them, again by a restriction enzyme. Then the DNA fragment with the right gene will be mixed with the plasmid which has had a fragment cut out of it and DNA ligase will be added. The product will be recombinant bacteria, each of which contains the right fragment of human DNA, and these bacteria can be grown on ordinary agar.

This may sound fanciful, but molecular biologists can do all these things now, except for locating the gene for chondrogenesis. When they do that, perhaps the resulting material could be used to induce the formation of a new surface to the hip. And if all the other joint surfaces are renewed at the same time nobody will complain about that, will they? As long as they don't get a chondrosarcoma. So we may also need to find the gene that switches off chondrogenesis.

But before we are carried away too far into the future, let me finish by telling you the remarkable case of a woman whose x-ray was sent to me by a former registrar. She'd had a hip replacement some years earlier and now the x-ray looked appalling. There were broken screws, a fracture, loosening, penetration into the acetabulum — all sorts of complications. Of course there was an accompanying letter, and as I got to the bottom of the first page I read this, "Before you turn over, I would like you to guess the question this patient came to ask me". I tried. The first question I thought of was, "Where can I buy a strong wheelchair?". The second was, "Can you tell me if this was your first hip replacement or your second? — my lawyer wants to know". But when I turned over I found I was completely wrong. The question the patient had come to ask was this: "Doctor, when can you do my other hip — like this one!"

Hip Reconstruction Supplemented with Chiari Pelvic Osteotomy

Kazushi Hirohata, Tsukasa Matsubara, Tomio Shimizu, and Yasuhiro Saegusa[1]

Summary. Chiari's pelvic osteotomy combined with the reconstructive surgery such as CA, bipolar FHR and THR provided good long-term results in the treatment of coxarthrosis by creating a firm acetabulum. In order to facilitate the reconstructive surgery for the coxarthrosis secondary to CDH, the indication, surgical technique, and case presentation of supplementary Chiari's pelvic osteotomy was described.

Key words. Osteotomy — Ostoarthritis (hip) — Hip prosthesis — Acetabulum

Introduction

Congenital dislocation or subluxation of the hip is generally associated with acetabular dysplasia. Acetabular dysplasia is also observed in secondary coxarthrosis in adults. In the reconstruction of hips affected by coxarthrosis and acetabular dysplasia, pain-relief and stability of the affected hip should be obtained by improvement of its congruity and enlargement of the weight-bearing area.

In reconstructions of the hip such as cup arthroplasty (CA), femoral head replacement (FHR), and total hip replacement (THR), supplementary surgery is generally required for the acetabular dysplasia. In a previous report, Aufranc [1] reported also performing a vertical iliac wedge osteotomy in the CA. In order to provide bone stock for the acetabular re-

construction, Harris [2] has recently reported bone grafting using the resected femoral head, in THR, and this procedure has become widespread. We have supplemented Chiari's pelvic osteotomy in reconstructive surgery such as CA, FHR, and THR, since this procedure creates acetabulum which is biomechanically and biologically more stable than the above-mentioned shelf operation [3]. In this report, we describe the indications, operative procedures, and cases in which this procedure was utilized.

Selection of Cases

Indications for Cup Arthroplasty (CA)

Patients (20–45 years old) with severe acetabular dysplasia due to neglected congenital dislocation of the hip (CDH) are suitable candidates for this procedure. The highly dislocated femoral head is also able to be anatomically reduced to the primitive acetabulum.

Patients with osteoarthrosis secondary to subluxation of the hip with acetabular dysplasia who have severe pain and disability for ADL can be selected. In addition, a Sharp angle in frontal plane of over 55 degrees and a faux profile angle in the sagital plane of under 0 degrees are indications for this procedure.

Indications for Bipolar Femoral Head Replacement (Bipolar FHR)

Suitable candidates include patients (50–60 years old) with secondary coxarthrosis with acetabular dysplasia or a shallow acetabulum in

[1] Department of Orthopaedic Surgery, Kobe University School of Medicine, 7-chome, Kusunoki-cho, Chuo-ku, Kobe, 650 Japan

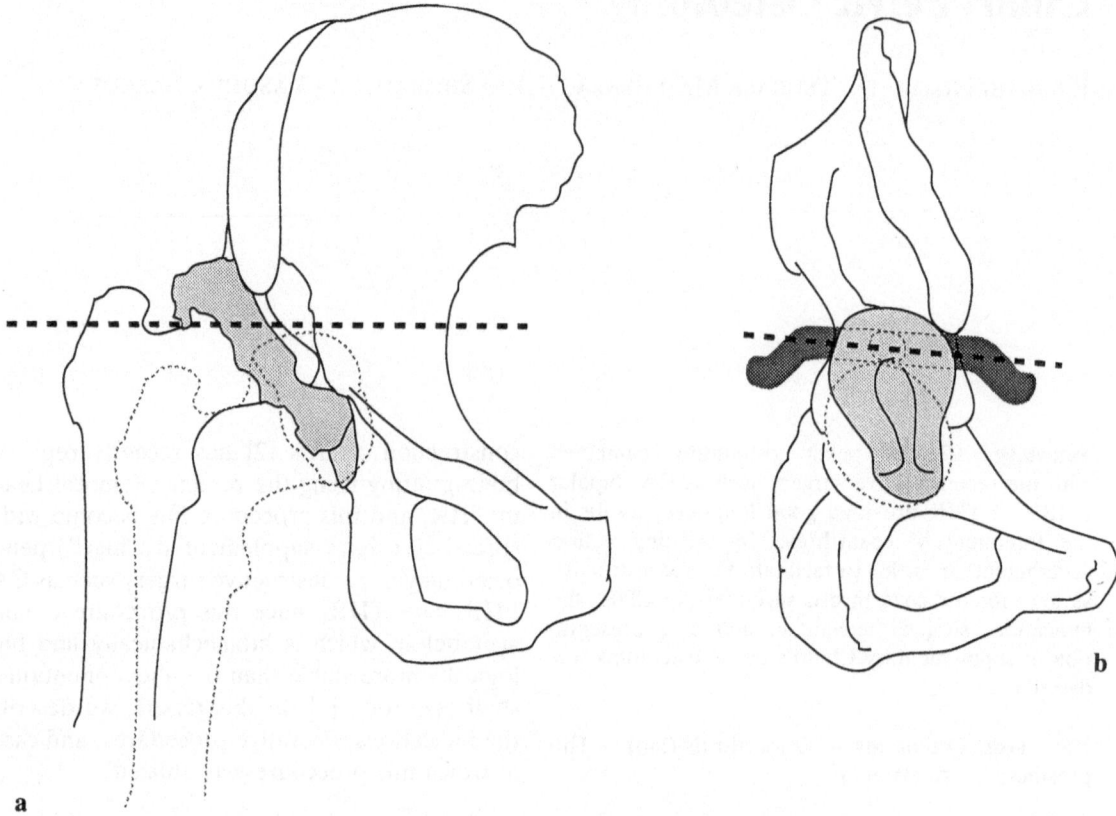

Fig. 1. Neglected CDH in an adult. **a** Anteroposterior view, and **b** lateral view. Osteotomy level is indicated by the *dotted lines* for the reduced femoral head. After osteotomy, the femoral head should be reduced into the primitive acetabulum

whom the subluxation of the femoral head has occurred with formation of marginal lipping and a double floor in the medial portion of the acetabulum. The Shenton line is broken and the acetabulum usually requires deep reaming.

Indication for Total Hip Replacement (THR)

Patients (50–70 years old) with an unstable type of hip dislocation with severe acetabular dysplasia or false acetabulum are suitable. Acetabuloplasty is required for firm fixation of the acetabular component, and equalization of leg discrepancy is needed. However, patients with severe osteoporosis must be excluded.

Surgical Procedure

The anterior approach of the hip is indicated for CA, and Watson-Jones' approach is generally for bipolar FHR or THR. After exposure of the hip, the capsule is completely resected. The tensor fasciae latae and gluteal muscles are detached at the outer portion of the iliac crest, and the abdominal and psoas are detached at the inner side of the iliac crest. The greater sciatic notch is subperiosteally exposed inside the iliac crest and the posterior portion of the ilium is also subperiostially exposed after resection of the limbus and joint capsule. One retractor is then inserted medially into the sciatic notch and the other is inserted laterally to cover the whole notch, to protect the sciatic nerve and vascular vessels. Pelvic osteotomy is then performed horizontally or ten degrees obliquely upward, using a Tuke saw at the level of the insertion of the rectus femoris (Fig. 1a,b). The proximal iliac bone is laterally shifted (approximately 40%–50% of its width) to reform the anterior and lateral portion of the dysplastic acetabulum. The proximal and distal portions of the ilium are trans-fixed by two K-wires. Reaming of the

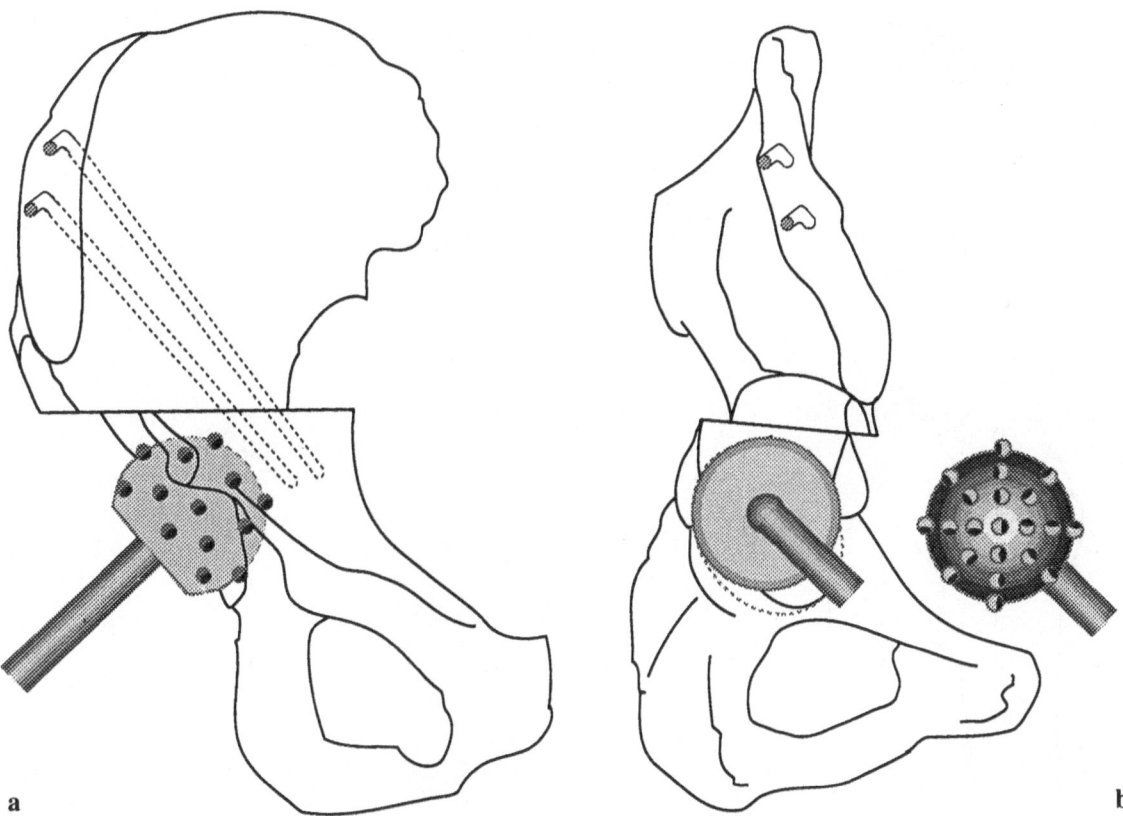

Fig. 2. Fixation of the osteotomized site — the primitive acetabulum is enlarged and deepened with a reamer; **a** anteroposterior view, **b** lateral view

primitive acetabulum is then performed, using a 44 to 50-mm diameter reamer, to create a new acetabulum with an appropriate diameter and depth for the cup, or femoral head, and the acetabular component (Fig. 2a,b). Since this pelvic osteotomy is done in one session using the same surgical approach, the additional time required is only approximately 10–20 minutes and additional bleeding is negligible.

Postoperative Care

Hip traction with the patient in a functional position is performed postoperatively for 3 weeks after CA and bipolar FHR, and in the following 3 weeks muscle strength exercises are given when the patient is in a supine position. A continuous passive motion device is used for this purpose. Depending on recovery of muscular strength, sitting in a wheel chair is permitted at 5–6 weeks after surgery. Weight bearing is permitted in gradations from partial to full, depending on recovery of muscle strength and the radiographic reappearance of joint space. Taking into consideration age, weight, muscle strength, and whether unilateral or bilateral replacement has been performed, the use of a cane is indicated for from 6 months to 1 year after surgery.

At Kobe University Hospital from 1975–1991, supplementary Chiari osteotomies were performed with CA (Fig. 3a), bipolar FHR (Fig. 3b), and THR in 84 hips in 81 cases (3 males, 78 females) with osteoarthrosis secondary to congenital dislocation of the hip. Patients' ages ranged from 17 to 54 years of age (average 35) for CA patients, 39–58 years (average 50.8) for bipolar FHR patients, and 52–66 years (average 58.0) for THR patients. There were no complications during surgery. Dissociation of the osteotomized ilium was observed in 2 patients during postoperative exercise, but bony fusion was established by casting for 4 weeks.

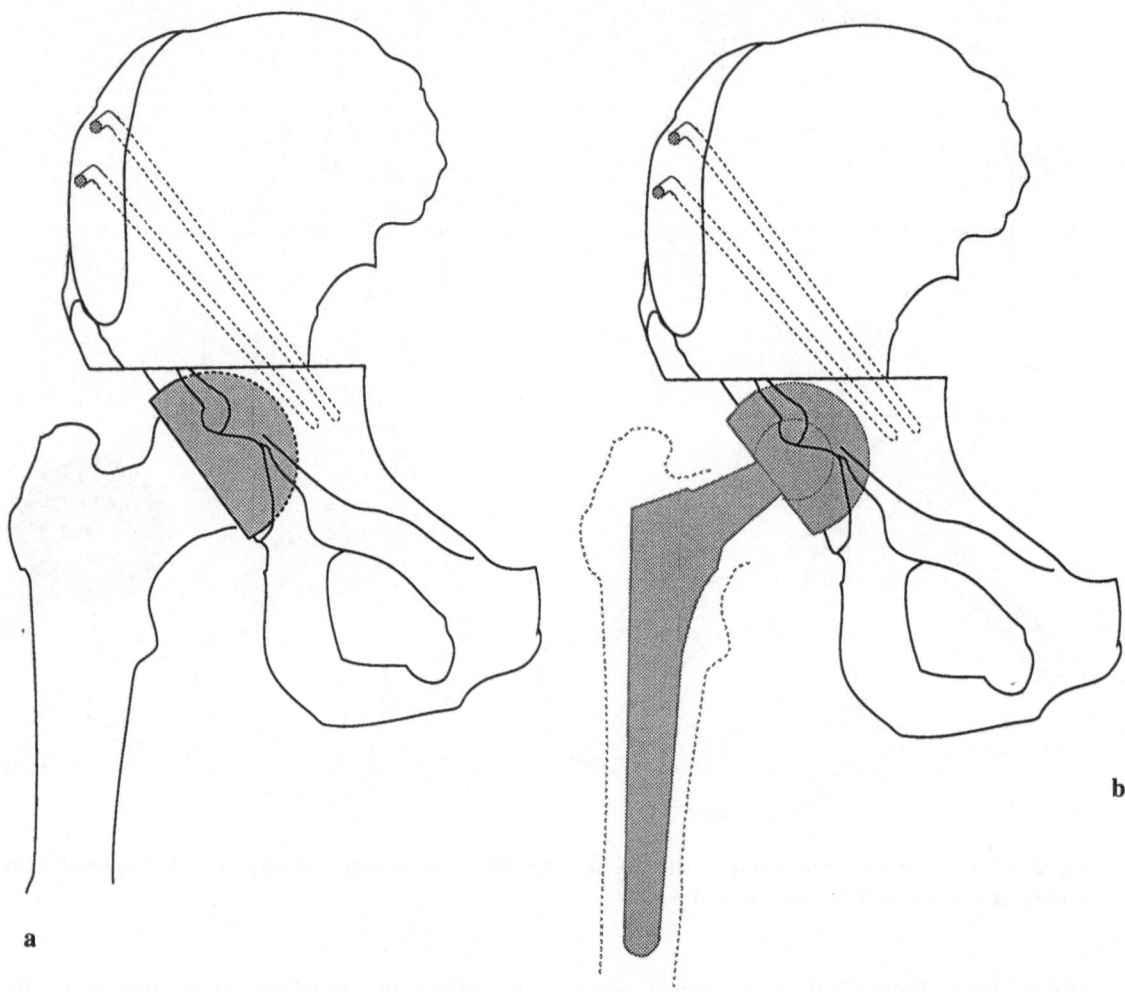

Fig. 3. a Supplemented Chiari's osteotomy for cup arthroplasty. **b** Supplemented Chiari's osteotomy for bipolar femoral head replacement arthroplasty

Case Reports

CA

Case 1 was a 45-year-old female with left osteoarthrosis secondary to CDH. The patient, although diagnosed with CDH, did not recieve any particular therapy. She complained of left hip pain after exercise at the age of 12 years, and this pain gradually increased. At hospitalization, when her condition was categorized according to the hip score of the Japanese Orthopaedic Association (JOA), she received a score of 10 points for pain, 15 points for gait, 16 points for ROM (flexion 90 degrees, abduction 10 degrees), and 20 points for ADL with a total score of 61. Chiari's osteotomy was performed

just above the primitive acetabulum, and the femoral head with the cup was reduced to the primitive acetabulum (Fig. 4a,b). Nine years later (Fig. 4c), although the patient has a slight gait disturbance and some slight restriction in ADL due to limited flexion, she has no pain and her JOA hip score has increased to 84 points.

Case 2 was a 43-year-old female with right osteoarthrosis secondary to CDH. The patient was not diagnosed with CDH during childhood. She had dull pain around the right hip after extended periods of walking, and this symptom gradually worsened. At hospitalization, her hip scores were: pain 20 points, gait 10 points, ROM 13 points (flexion 75 degrees, abduction 10 degrees), and ADL 16 points — a total of 59 points. Ten years after CA with Chiari's

Fig. 4. a Preoperative roentgenograph of CA in Case 1. Total hip score was 61 points. **b** Immediate postoperative roentgenograph. **c** Roentgenograph at 9-year follow-up. Total hip score was 84 points

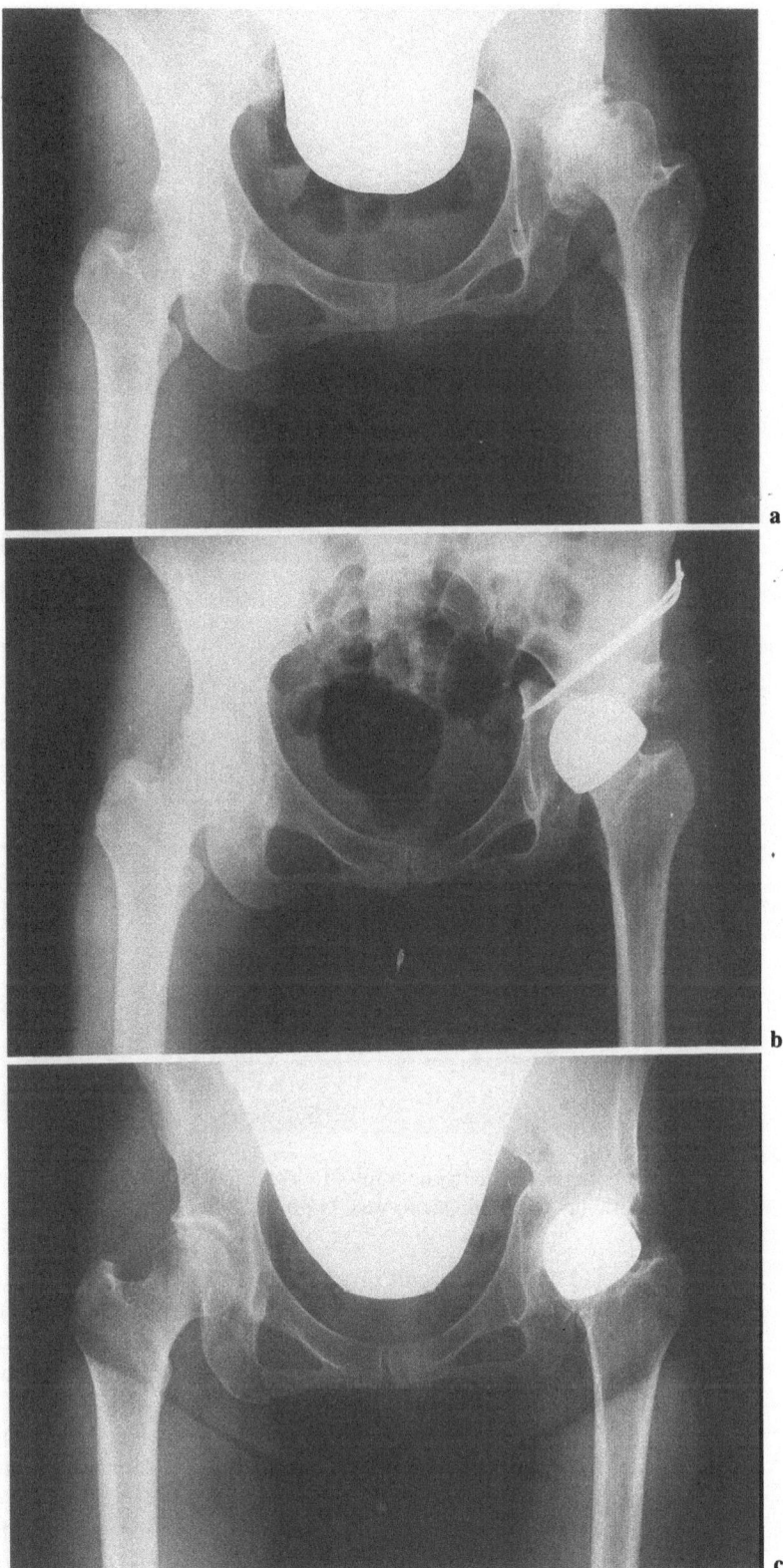

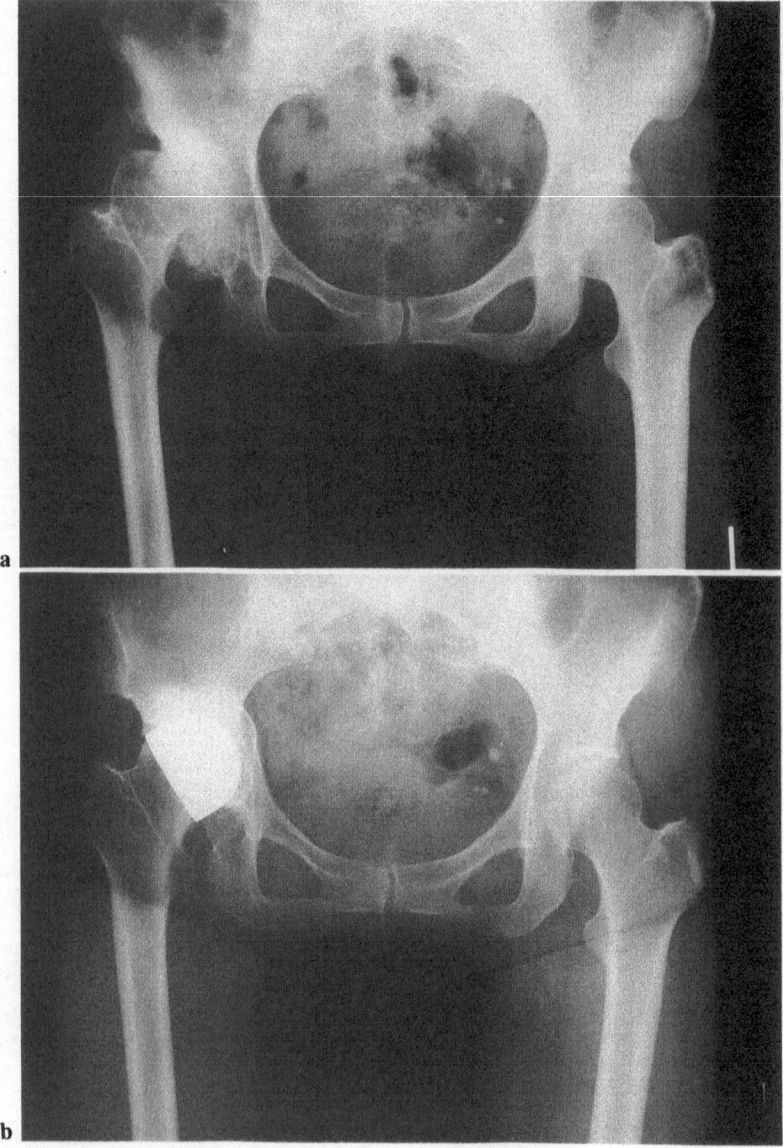

Fig. 5. a Preoperative roentgenograph of CA in Case 2. Total hip score was 59 points. **b** Roentgenograph at 10-year follow-up. Total hip score was 93 points

osteotomy, she has a slight gait disturbance but she has no pain, and the ROM of the hip is normal (JOA score 93 points) (Fig. 5a,b).

Bipolar FHR

Case 1 was a 57-year-old female with right hip osteoarthrosis secondary to CDH. The patient complained of right hip pain at the age of 52 years, and this pain gradually increased (Fig. 6a). At hospitalization she had a score of: pain 20 points, gait 10 points, ROM 13 points (flexion 85 degrees, abduction 10 degrees), and ADL 12 points — a total of 55 points. The patient also presented with a leg length discrepancy of 3 cm (lt > rt). The patient now has a total score of full marks, and the leg length discrepancy has been reduced to 5 mm (lt > rt) 5 years after bipolar FHR with Chiari's osteotomy (Fig. 6b,c).

Case 2 was a 45-year-old female with bilateral coxarthrosis. The patient had a past history of CDH and was treated by casting at the age of 1 year. She had left hip pain at 25 years of age. At hospitalization she presented with a score of:

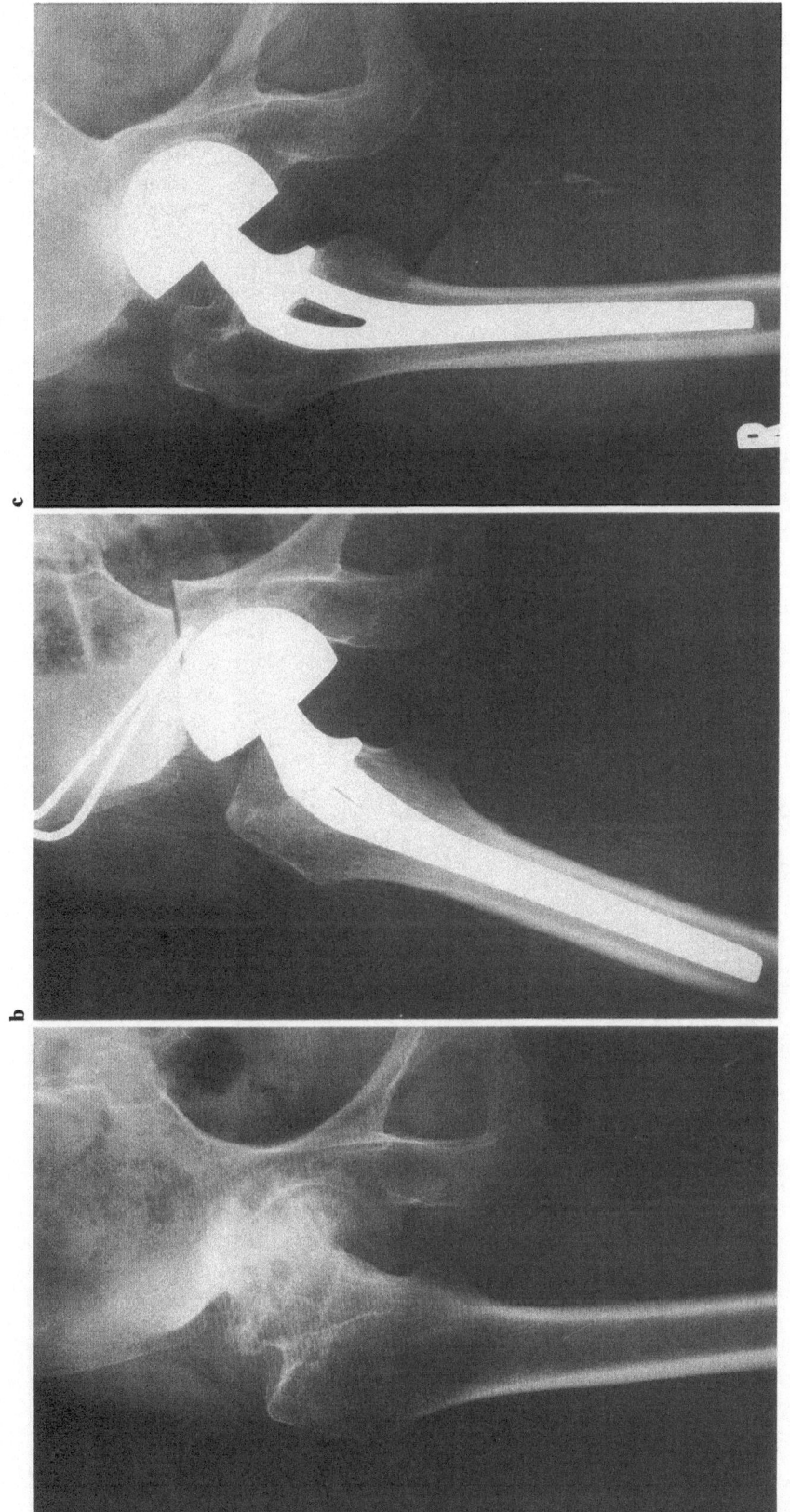

Fig. 6. a Preoperative roentgenograph of bipolar FHR in Case 1. **b** Immediate postoperative roentgenograph. **c** Roentgenograph 5 years after surgery reveals the reappearance joint space. The total hip score improved from 53 points to full marks

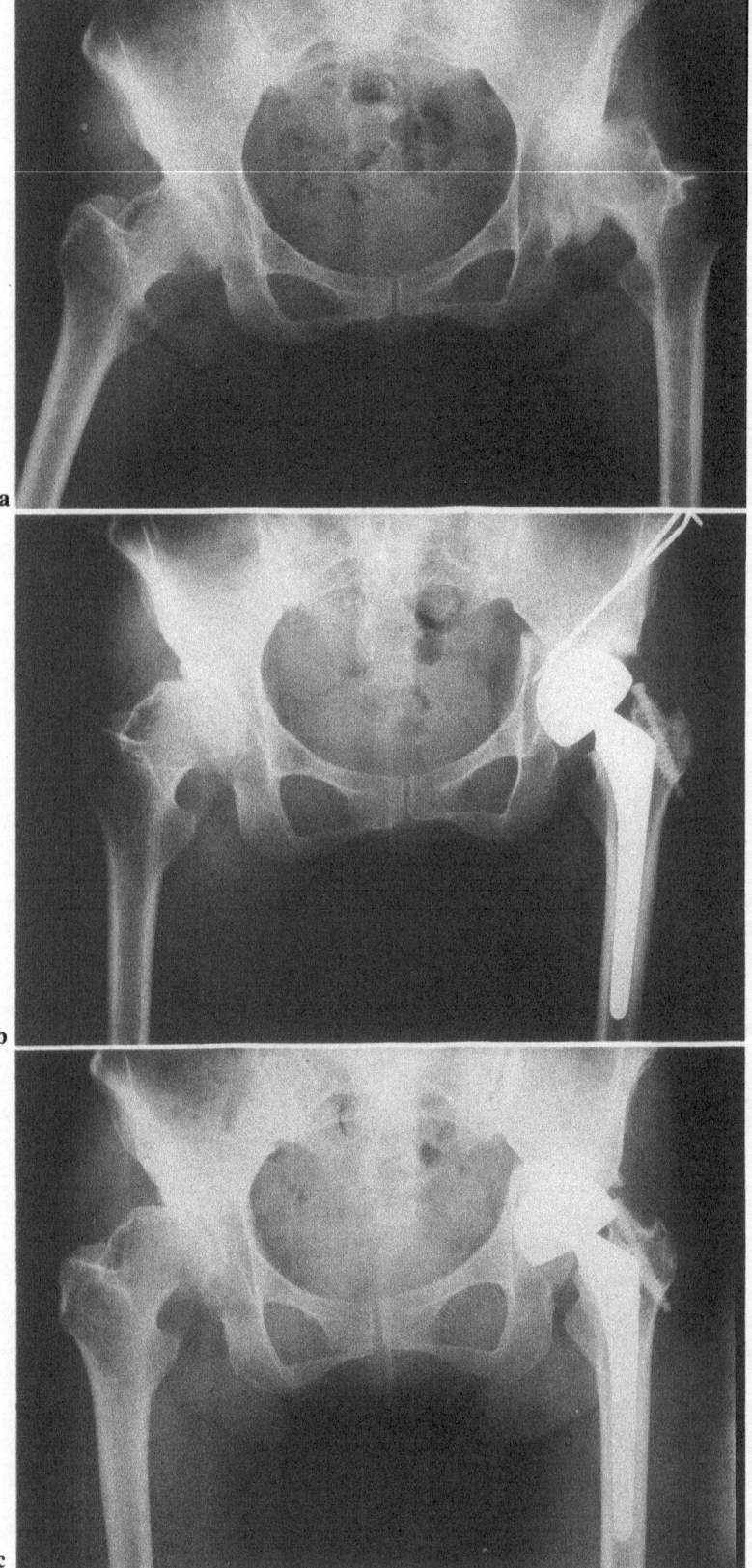

Fig. 7. a Preoperative roentgenograph of bipolar FHR in Case 2. **b** Immediate postoperative roentgenograph. Undue fracture of the major trochanter was fixed with a ceramic screw. **c** Roentgenograph at 3-year follow-up

Fig. 8. a Preoperative roentgenograph of THR in Case 1. **b** Immediate postoperative roentgenograph. **c** Postoperative roentgenograph 2 years after surgery. The preoperative total hip score improved and increased from 57 to 93 points

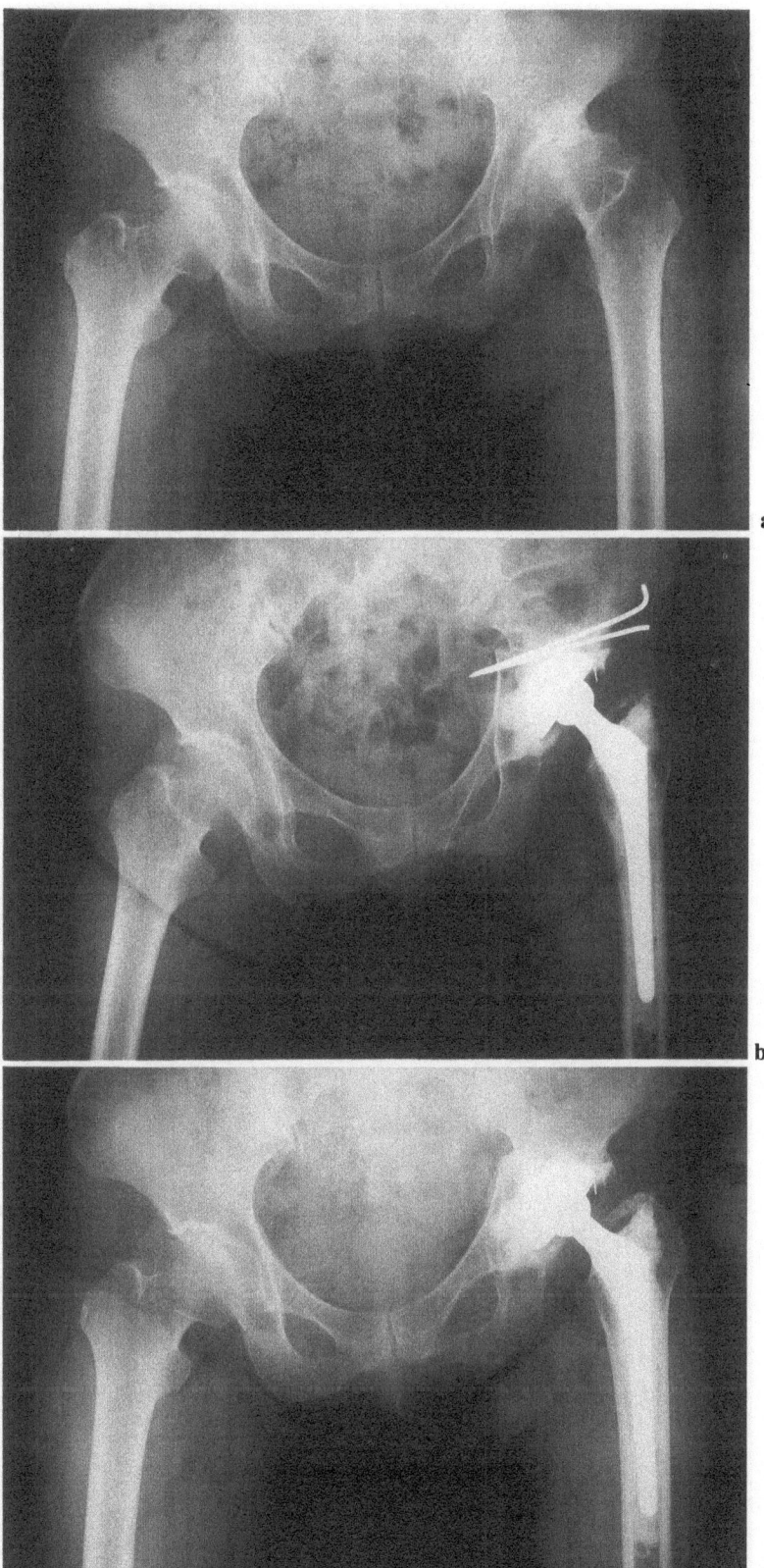

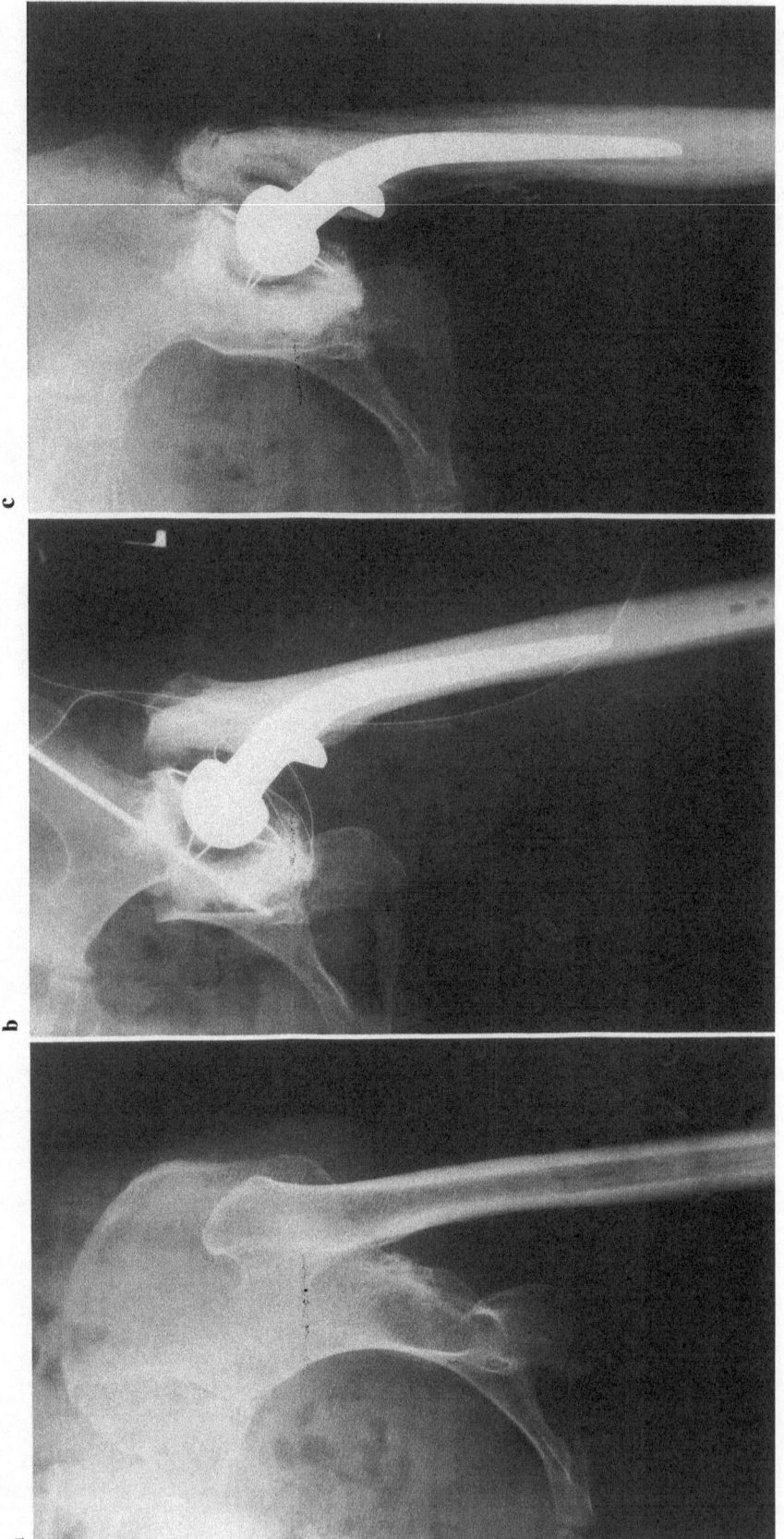

Fig. 9. a Preoperative roentgenograph of THR in Case 2. **b** Immediate postoperative roentgenograph. **c** Note the reduction of the femoral head in the primitive acetabulum. However, the total hip score increased from 60 to 65 points at the 10 year follow-up

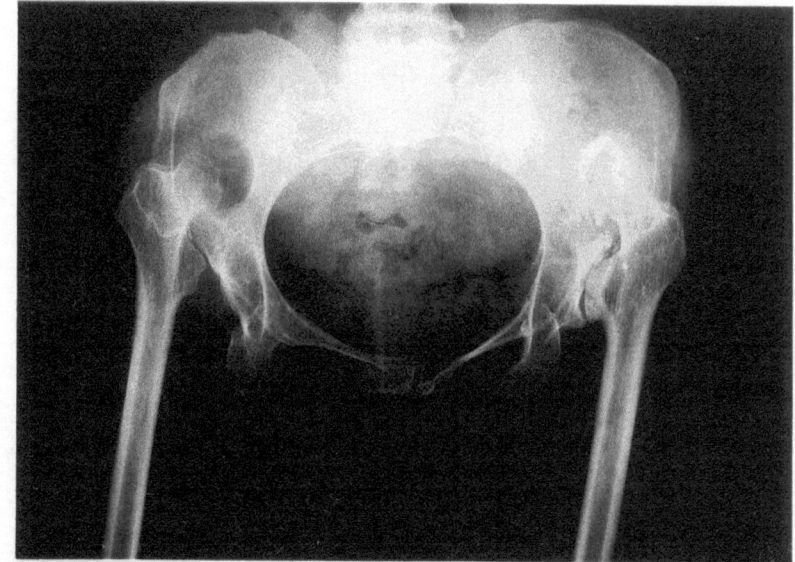

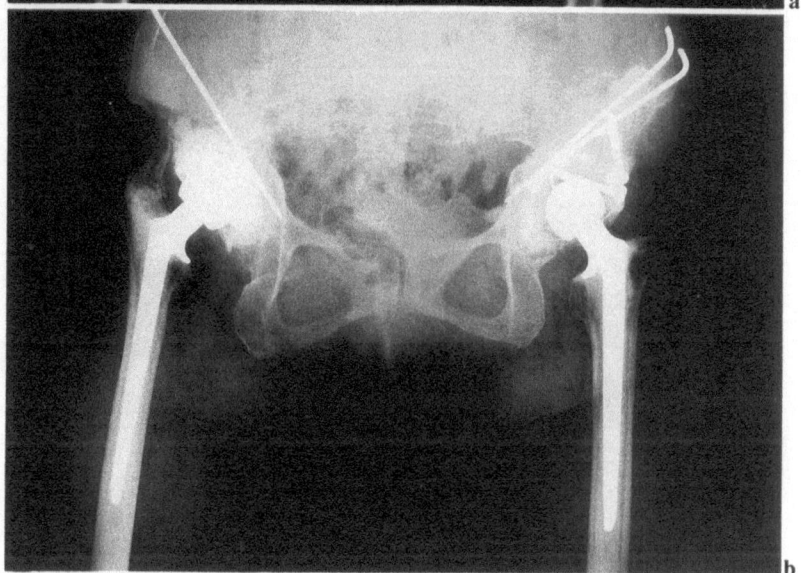

Fig. 10. a Preoperative roentgenograph of neglected bilateral CDH in an adult (THR, Case 3). **b** Roentgenograph 3 years after surgery on the left hip reveals satisfactory reduction. However, the postsurgery period is too short as yet to evaluate the result

pain 20 points, gait 15 points, ROM 11 points (flexion 60 degrees, adbuction 5 degrees), and ADL 11 points — a total of 57 points. The patient's score, as evaluated 3 years after bipolar FHR with Chiari's osteotomy, is 96 points and she has a slight restriction of abduction (Fig. 7a–c).

THR

Case 1 was a 62-year-old female with unilateral coxathrosis. The patient had neither a past history of CDH nor delayed development. Her complaint was of left hip pain which occurred when she was 57 years old. Her score at hos-

pitalization was: pain 10 points, gait 10 points, ROM 16 points (flexion 110 degrees, abduction 10 degrees), and ADL 11 points — a total of 57 points. Total replacement arthroplasty was supplemented with Chiari's pelvic osteotomy. The patient does not complain of hip pain, and there is no restriction of ROM 2 years after surgery (Fig. 8a–c).

Case 2 was a 52-year-old female with bilateral coxarthrosis who had been treated by casting following diagnosis of CDH. She complained of gait disturbance during childhood. She presented with hip pain during exercise at the age of 35. At hopitalization the patient's score was: pain 20 points, gait 5 points, ROM 18 points

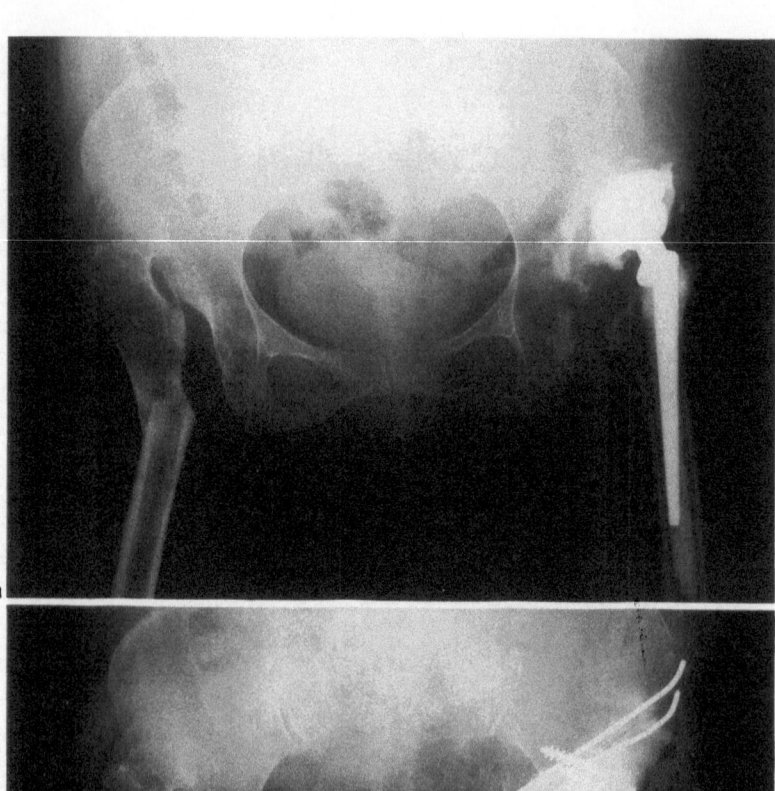

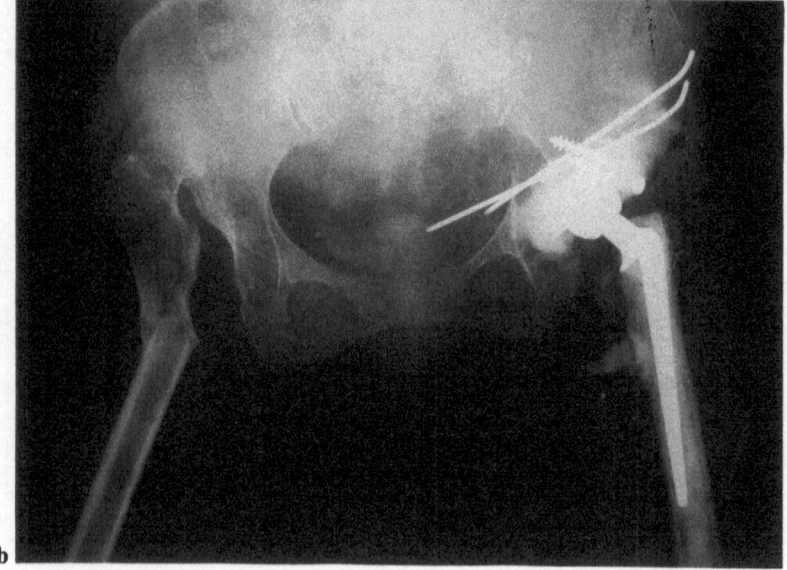

Fig. 11. a Roentgenograph of THR Case 4 before revision. b Roentgenograph after revision with supplementary Chiari's osteotomy. The short-term results are excellent

(flexion 90 degrees, abduction 20 degrees), and ADL 17 points — a total of 60 points. THR with Chiari's osteotomy was performed on the left hip. Ten years after surgery, the patient has no hip pain, but exhibits a slight gait disturbance and restriction of ROM, with a score of: pain 40 points, gait 10 points, ROM 10 points and ADL 5 points — a total of 65 points. Sinking of the femoral stem was observed radiographically, but there was no evidence of loosening of the acetabular component (Fig. 9a–c).

Case 3 was a 53-year-old female with bilateral coxarthrosis. She first walked shortly after first birthday. Gait abnormality was observed, and

she was diagnosed with CDH and treated by casting. She was not required to participate in physical education classes at school. She had slight hip pain which was treated only conservatively. She was hospitalized in 1986 because of severe right hip pain, and THR combined with Chiari's osteotomy was performed. The same procedure was performed on the left hip in 1988. Three years after the second surgical procedure, the patient walks with a cane. The short-term results of this latter operation appear to be highly satisfactory (Fig. 10a,b).

Case 4 was a 66-year-old female with bilateral coxarthrosis. The patient, although diagnosed with CDH, had not received any therapy. As her gait disturbance increased, and she was unable to walk long distances, she had an inter-trochanteric osteotomy in the right hip and an acetabuloplasty in the left hip at the age of 25. She was symptom-free until the age of 46, when bilateral hip pain appeared and increased. At the age of 66, the patient received a THR with an acetabular component fixed to the false acetabulum. As loosening of the acetabular component occurred 4 months postoperatively, and the gait disturbance increased because of pain, she was hospitalized at Kobe University Hospital. The radiograph taken at admission showed lateral upward dislocation of the acetabular component, together with the bone cement (Fig. 11a). This hip was revised with the performance of a THR with Chiari's pelvic osteotomy; the acetabular component was fixed in the primitive acetabulum (Fig. 11b). In addition, shortening of the femur was performed. Ten months after surgery the patient is now pain-free and performs gait exercises.

Discussion

Coxarthrosis with acetabular dysplasia and shallow acetabulum secondary to CDH has been treated by performing a shelf operation or acetabuloplasty. Reaming of the acetabulum and acetabuloplasty or vertical iliac osteotomy [1] have been combined with CA to gain an acetabulum with adequate depth and width. In 1984, we showed that in coxarthrosis with acetabular dysplasia, Chiari's osteotomy, when combined with cup athroplasty (CA), provided better clinical results [4], including improvement of ROM and ADL, rather than CA alone or CA with the Lance type of shelf operation. On the basis of this follow-up study, we have recommended that Chiari's pelvic osteotomy, in combination with femoral head replacement (FHR) and total hip replacement (THR) is indicated in patients with severe acetabular deficiency (Sharp angle >55 degrees; faux profile angle <0 degrees) and in those who have severe osteoarthrosis secondary to neglected CDH in adults [3].

Since Harris [2] reported THR combined with a shelf operation, using the resected femoral head, in coxarthrosis with severe acetabular dysplasia, this procedure has been the method of choice for many orthopedic surgeons [6]. Otto et al. [7] modified this procedure to promote fusion of the bone graft. When bone cement is used for the acetabular component, the time of remodeling and the fusion of the bone graft for the acetabuloplasty is uncertain. There is, therefore, risk of pseudoarthrosis or loosening of the transplanted bone graft. This is supported by a recent report of proximal migration of the femoral component after the performance of bipolar FHR combined with acetabuloplasty, using an autograft, in coxarthrosis with acetabular dysplasia [8]. We also had an experience with metallosis due to friction between the femoral component and the screw used for the fixation of the transplanted bone graft. Chiari's pelvic osteotomy provides biomechanical medialization of the center of the femoreal head, and makes it easy to reconstruct a firm acetabulum of appropriate depth and width. Furthermore, this procedure results in the full coverage of not only the latero-superior but also the anterior portion of the acetabulum by the translocation of the proximal ilium [2]. In bipolar FHR, as well as in CA, the acetabular cartilage is completely removed by reaming, but joint space reappears roentgenographically 3 months after surgery. This newly formed joint space consists of fibrous cartilage, and therefore protected weight bearing can be allowed in patients with a cane as soon as it appears. When sclerosis appears on the surface of the acetabulum, total weight bearing can be permitted as long as the patient has sufficient muscular strength. This usually occurs more than 6 months after surgery.

Hip reconstruction combined with Chiari's pelvic osteotomy, although it suffers from the drawback of the long time taken before weight-bearing or ambulation is possible (because of the reaming of cancellous bone), provides firm stability and long-term favorable results by enlarging the weight-bearing area.

References

1. Aufranc OE (1962) §IV General Surgical Technique; special points. In: Aufranc OE (ed) Constructive surgery of the Hip, Mosby, St Louis, pp 96–126

2. Chiari K (1955) Ergebnisse mit der Beckenosteotomie als Pfannendachplastik. Z Orthop 87: 14–26
3. Hirohata K, Shiba R, Shimizu T (1989) Follow-up results of Chiari pelvic osteotomy for patients with acetabular dysplasia. In: Hirohata K, Kurosaka M, Cooke TDV (eds) Joint Surgery Up to Date, Springer-Verlag, Tokyo, pp 35–49
4. Hirohata K, Shiba R, Ishida F, Sumi M (1984) Reevaluation of cup arthroplasty for coxarthrosis associated with acetabular dysplasia (in Japanese). J Jpn Orthop Ass 58:434–436
5. Harris WH, Crothers O, Oh I (1977) Total hip replacement and femoral head bone-grafting for severe acetabular deficiency in adults. J Bone Joint Surg [Am] 59:752–759
6. Kerboul N (1989) Totalprothesen-Implantation an der deformierten Hüfte am Beispiel der kongenitalen Hüftluxation. Orthopäde 18: 397–417
7. Otto KB, Baars GW, Nieder E (1989) Arthroplastische Therapie der kongenitalen Hüftgelenkdysplasie. Orthopäde 18:470–482
8. Hirohata K, Saegusa Y, Matsubara T, Shimizu T (1991) Hip Reconstruction for Coxarthrosis Supplemented with Chiari Pelvic Osteotomy. J of Joint Surg (in Japanese) 10:1209–1224

Management of the Infected Total Knee Replacement by Two-Stage Reimplantation

Alan H. Wilde[1] and John T. Ruth[2]

Key words. Reimplantation — Debridement — Cement spacer — Radiolucency — Mixed infections

Introduction

Infection following total knee arthroplasty can be a devastating complication resulting in a loss of knee motion and function and even in amputation. The incidence of knee infection following total knee arthroplasty has been reported to be from 2% in patients with osteoarthritis and 3% in patients with rheumatoid arthritis [1,2].

Treatment of the infected total knee arthroplasty has varied from aspiration of the knee and intravenous antibiotics, debridement of the knee either by open operation or by arthroscopy, with retention of the prosthesis along with intravenous antibiotics; debridement and removal of the infected knee prosthesis, and intravenous antibiotics; and arthrodesis of the knee, to two-stage reimplantation [3,4]. The purpose of this paper is to report our experience with two-stage reimplantation for the treatment of the infected total-knee arthroplasty.

As infection can remain dormant for prolonged periods, it is important to learn of longer-term experience with the treatment of septic total knee replacements by this method. The minimum follow-up in this series is 35 months with a maximum follow-up of 117 months.

Materials and Methods

Between May 1980 and October 1987, 21 two-stage reimplantations for the treatment of infected total knee arthroplasties in 21 patients were performed by the senior author at the Cleveland Clinic Hospital. One patient died of a myocardial infarction 6 weeks after the second-stage reimplantation total knee arthroplasty. All the remaining 20 patients were studied by interview either in person or by telephone and by physical and radiographic examination. The minimum follow-up was 35 months and the maximum was 117 months, the average follow-up being 52 months. There were 9 males and 12 females. The average age at the time of reimplantation was 69 years; the range was from 49 to 82 years. The preoperative diagnosis was osteoarthritis in 16 patients and rheumatoid arthritis in 5. The time between the index arthroplasty and the diagnosis and treatment of the infection in the total knee arthroplasty was less than 3 months in six patients, between 3 and 12 months in eight patients, and from 1 to 8 years in seven patients.

Treatment prior to two-stage reimplantation was with aspiration of the knee and intravenous antibiotics in four patients, debridement of the knee with retention of the prosthesis in two patients, arthroscopic debridement with intravenous antibiotics in two patients, and debridement and removal of the prosthesis with intravenous antibiotics in one patient.

The relationship between wound drainage greater than 6 days, hematoma drainage and wound separation, and the development of deep

[1] Case Western University, Cleveland, Ohio, USA
[2] Department of Orthopedic Surgery, The Cleveland Clinic Foundation, Cleveland, Ohio, USA

wound infection was also studied. Of 12 patients with infection that developed less than 1 year from the time of index arthroplasty, there was wound drainage in 6 days in four patients and wound separation in three patients.

The organisms that were cultured from the knee joint at the time of the first-stage debridement were *Staphylococcus* coagulase negative in nine patients, *Staphyloccus aureus* in two patients, *Streptococcus* group B in two, *Streptococcus bovis* in one, and *Enterococcus* in one patient. There also were mixed infections with *Staphylococcus aureus* and *Bacillus circulans* in one patient, *Staphylococcus* coagulase negative and *Enterococcus* in two, *Staphylococcus* coagulase negative and *Pseudomonas aeruginosa* in one, *Clostridium perfringens* and *Enterobacter cloacae* in one, and *Streptococcus* group B and *Propionobacterium* in one patient.

Intravenous antibiotic therapy was given after the first-stage debridement and removal of the prosthesis. The choice of antibiotics was based on culture and sensitivity results from three aerobic and anaerobic cultures taken from the cement membrane, synovium, and synovial fluid removed at the time of surgery. Intravenous antibiotics were given for an average of 5.2 weeks after the first stage debridement and removal of the prosthesis. The range of intravenous antibiotic treatment was from 3 to 12 weeks. The patients were evaluated pre- and postoperatively, utilizing a modification of the Hospital for Special Surgery Knee Score which evaluates pain, walking ability, stability of the knee, range of motion, alignment, ability to climb stairs, and use of ambulatory aids. Scores of 85–100 points are considered excellent, 70–84 good, 60–69 fair, and scores of less than 60 points were rated as poor results. The wounds of the operated knee were evaluated for redness, induration, drainage, and heat.

Preoperative Radiographic Evaluation

The preoperative roentgenograms of 14 patients were evaluated for radiolucencies of the bone/cement interface in the zones recommended by the Knee Society. The lucencies of all three components were measured on the antero-

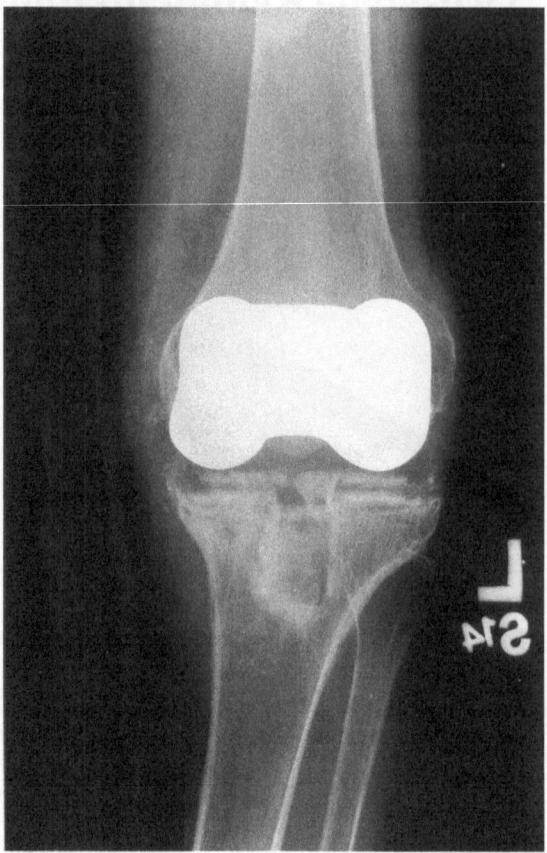

Fig. 1. Anteroposterior roentgenogram, showing wide radiolucencies around the tibial component of an infected total knee arthroplasty

posterior and lateral roentgenograms and were totaled. A radiolucency of 4 mm or less at the bone/cement interface was not considered significant, a radiolucency of 5–9 mm was felt to be questionable for loosening, and a radiolucency of 10 mm or more suggested possible impending loosening. There were nine patients with total radiolucencies of 10 mm or more; this value was as much as 26 mm in some cases. One patient had a total radiolucency of 8 mm. Three patients had total radiolucencies of less than 4 mm. There was one patient who had had a medial hemiarthroplasty who had a 2 mm radiolucency completely around the tibial component on the anteroposterior and lateral roentgenogram associated with subsidence. On the femoral side, there was only 1 mm radiolucency in zone 4 posteriorly (Fig. 1).

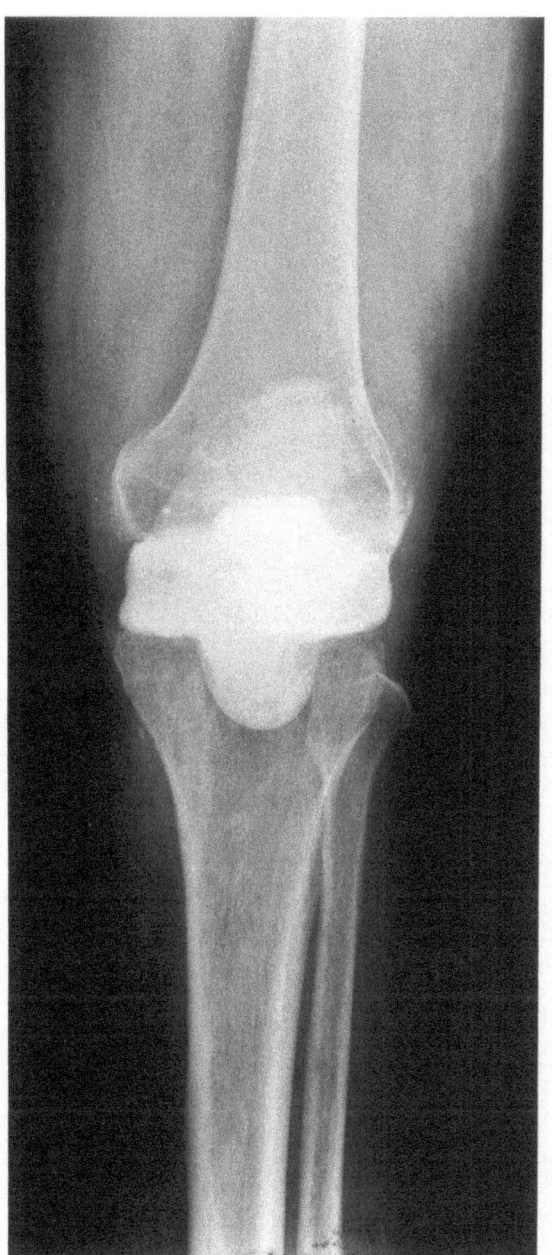 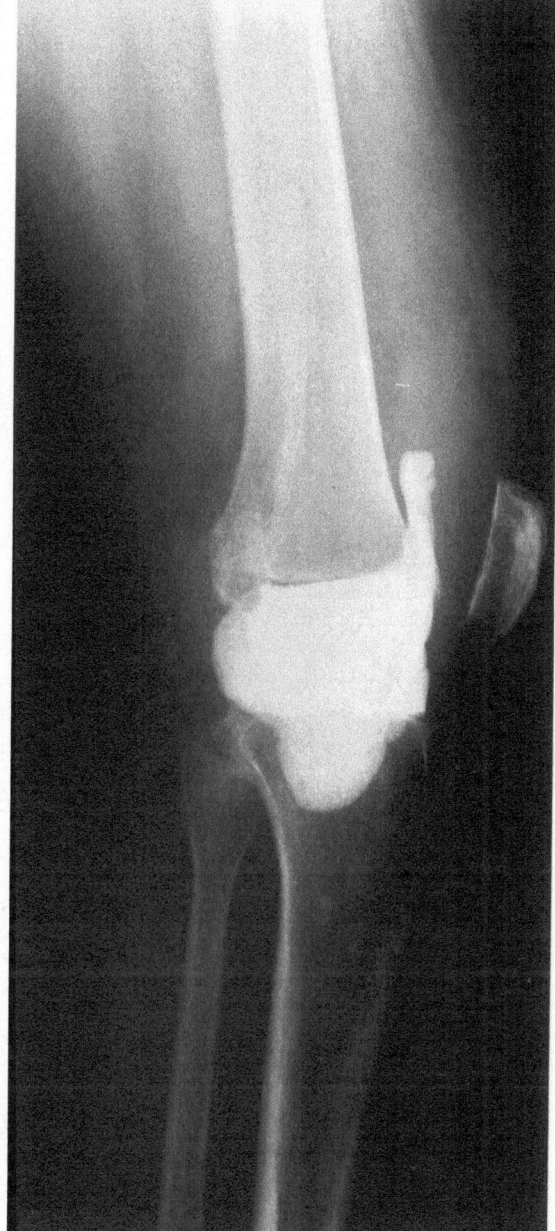

Fig. 2. Anteroposterior roentgenogram of the knee, showing the antibiotic/cement spacer

Fig. 3. Lateral roentgenogram of the knee, demonstrating the antibiotic/cement spacer. Note the extension of the cement spacer onto the anterior aspect of the femur to maintain the suprapatellar pouch

First-Stage Operation

The first stage of the operative management is debridement of sinus tracts and synovium. The prosthesis, cement membrane, and cement are removed. One or 2 mm of the bony surfaces of the femur, patella, and tibia are debrided with a power saw. The synovium, cement membrane, and synovial fluid are submitted for three aerobic and anaerobic cultures and sensitivities. The bone surfaces of the joint are thoroughly lavaged. Postoperatively, the knee was immobi-

Table 1. Results of two-stage reimplantation for infected total knee replacement

Case	Diagnosis	Type of prosthesis	Organism	Interval to infection	Antibiotics in spacer/cement at revision	Interval to reimplantation (in weeks)	Revision prosthesis	Outcome	Follow up knee score/rom (Length of follow-up)
1. F.C.	OA	Total Condylar	Staph. Coag. Neg.	4 years	Cefazolin/Cefazolin	12	Insall-Burstein	Con't. Inf. Revised elsewhere	48/5–90° (50 months)
2. A.G.	OA	Guepar	Staph. Coag. Neg.	3 months	No Spacer/Tobramycin	104	Total Condylar III	Success	93/0–90° (36 months)
3. M.J.	OA	Insall-Burstein	P. aeruginosa and Staph. Coag. Neg.	2 months	Tobramycin/Tobramycin	6	Total Condylar III	Success	80/5–105° (46 months)
4. W.K.	OA	Townley	B. circulans and Staph. Coag. Pos.	1 month	Tobramycin/Gentamicin	3	Total Condylar III	Success	88/10–100° (48 months)
5. W.L.	OA	Guepar	Staph. Coag. Neg.	8 years	Gentamicin/Gentamicin	6	PCA revision	Success	67/25–60° (76 months)
6. G.M.	RA	Total Condylar	Staph. Coag. Neg.	7 months	Cefazolin/Unknown	6	Total Condylar III	Success	89/0–120° (56 months)
7. S.N.	OA	Insall-Burstein	Staph. Coag. Neg.	6 months	Vancomycin/Gentamicin	5	Total Condylar III	Success	93/0–90° (35 months)
8. J.O.	OA	Unicondylar	Staph. Coag. Neg.	2 months	Tobramycin/Tobramycin	4	Total Condylar III Post. Stab. Insall-Burstein	Success	86/10–70° (50 months)
9. M.S.	RA	Attenborough	Strep. Bovis	22 months	No Spacer/Oxacillin	12	Custom Rot. Hinge	Success	65/0–100° (117 months)
10. S.W.	RA	Total Condylar	Strep. Group B	3 years	Tobramycin/Cefazolin	4	Total Condylar III	Success	73/15–105° (63 months)
11. A.M.	RA	Geometric	Strep. Group B	58 months	No Spacer/Vancomycin	3	Total Condylar III	Success	Expired 5 years postop (51 months f/u)
12. E.M.	OA	Insall-Burstein	Enterococcus and Staph. Coag. Neg.	2 months	Tobramycin/Gentamicin	8	Insall-Burstein	Success	96/105° (72 months)

	Diagnosis	Prosthesis	Organism	Interval	Antibiotics	No.	New Prosthesis	Outcome	ROM (follow-up)
13. J.B.	Acromegaly with OA	Total Condylar III	*Enterococcus*	8 months	Tobramycin/Gentamicin	6	Total Condylar III	Success	68/0–80° (45 months)
14. D.D.	RA	Total Condylar III	*Staph. Coag. Neg.*	20 months	No Spacer/No Antibiotics	6	Total Condylar	Failure Fusion	
15. R.B.	OA	Post. Stab. Insall-Burstein	*C. perfringens Enterobacter Cloacae*	9 days	No Spacer/Cefazolin	3	Post. Stab. Insall-Burstein	Failure Fusion	
16. L.P.	OA	Post. Stab. Insall-Burstein	*B. Strep. Propriono Bacteria*	34 months	Tobramycin/Tobramycin	5	Total Condylar III	Success	96/0–105° (36 months)
17. B.S.	OA	Post. Stab. Insall-Burstein	*Staph Coag. Neg.*	7 months	Tobramycin	4	Total Condylar III	Success	(35 months)
18. R.L.	OA	Post. Stab. Insall-Burstein	*Staph Coag. Neg.*	3 months	Vancomycin/Vancomycin	5	Total Condylar III	Success	98/0–115° (35 months)
19. H.T.	OA	Post. Stab. Insall-Burstein	*Staph Coag. Neg. and Enterococcus*	11 months	Tobramycin/Tobramycin	4	Total Condylar III	Success	Phone (42 months)
20. C.D.	OA	Unknown	*Staph aureus*	22 months	Cefazolin/Cefazolin	14	Post. Stab. Insall-Burstein	Died	6 weeks postop MI
21. F.C.	OA	Post. Stab. Insall-Burstein	*Staph aureus*	4 weeks	Tobramycin/Tobramycin	4	Total Condylar III	Failure Fusion	

OA, osteoarthritis; RA, rheumatoid arthritis; Con't. Inf., continued infection; Post, Stab., Posterior stabilized

lized by an antibiotic-impregnated cement spacer (Figs. 2, 3) in 16 patients. An external fixator was utilized in two patients. No immobilization was used in three patients (Table 1).

Second-Stage Operation

The interval between the first-stage and the second-stage operations ranged from 3 weeks to as long as 104 weeks. The average was 10.6 weeks, the median was 5 weeks. The patient with *Clostridium perfringens* and *Enterobacter cloacae*, which developed from hematogenous seeding of the total knee prosthesis from an ascending cholangitis was reimplanted at 3 weeks. The one patient who had a second-stage operation at 104 weeks had had a first-stage operation performed at another hospital.

The second stage operation consisted of another debridement of the synovium and the cement membrane and removal of the cement spacer. Specimens of the synovium and cement membrane were submitted for three aerobic and anaerobic cultures. An additional 1–2 mm of bone from the femur, patella, and tibia were removed with a power saw. The bony surfaces and joint were thoroughly lavaged. A new prosthesis was implanted, mixing powdered antibiotic with the methylmethacrylate in powder form prior to the application of the monomer. The antibiotics used in the cement were selected according to the preoperative culture and sensitivity reports.

The types of components used at the time of reimplantation were the Total Condylar III prosthesis in 10 patients, posterior stabilized Insall-Burstein prosthesis in 5, PCA revision prosthesis in 1, Kinematic rotating hinge in 1, and the constrained Condylar prosthesis in 1 patient (Table 1). All of the reimplantations were performed in horizontal flow laminar airflow operating rooms. The operating team all wore helmet aspirator systems. Intravenous antibiotics were instituted from the start of induction of anesthesia and were continued for less than 1 week in 10 patients, from 1 to 4 weeks in four patients, and for 4 weeks in four patients. Intravenous antibiotics were given for 4 weeks in two patients with positive cultures from the time of reimplantation and two patients with rheumatoid arthritis.

Oral antibiotics were used for 3 weeks or less in three patients. Two of these patients had positive cultures at the time of reimplantation. The third patient had rheumatoid arthritis and prolonged drainage from the knee wound. Oral antibiotics were given for 6 weeks in one patient who had a positive culture at the time of reimplantation, for 4 months in one patient who had coagulase-negative *Staphylococcus* culture at the time of reimplantation, for 8 months in a patient with rheumatoid arthritis, and for longer than 12 months in three patients with rheumatoid arthritis.

There were seven patients who had positive cultures at the time of reimplantation. One patient had *Clostridium perfringens* from a hematogenous spreading from ascending cholangitis into his total knee replacement. After reimplantation, *Enterobacter cloacae* was cultured which ultimately led to a knee fusion. In another patient, the original infecting organism was cultured in one of three cultures at the time of reimplantation. This patient received IV antibiotics for 1 week following reimplantation, followed by 4 months of oral antibiotics. Five years after reimplantation, reinfection occurred with the original infecting organism. The remaining five patients have been free of infection at the time of follow-up.

Complications

Wound dehiscence occurred in three patients, which required debridement and closure of the wound. There was one intraoperative fracture of the lateral femoral condyle that was treated by internal fixation by screws. In another patient, a supracondylar fracture occurred 3 weeks postoperatively, which was treated successfully in a long-leg cast.

Deep vein thromboses were detected on postoperative venograms in four patients. There were also high probability lung scans in two patients, strongly indicating pulmonary emboli. All these patients received anticoagulation with heparin and Coumadin. Venography and lung scans have been performed routinely on all of our patients undergoing replacements of the hip and knee since January 1984.

There were seven patients with hematomas that drained for longer than 6 days. There

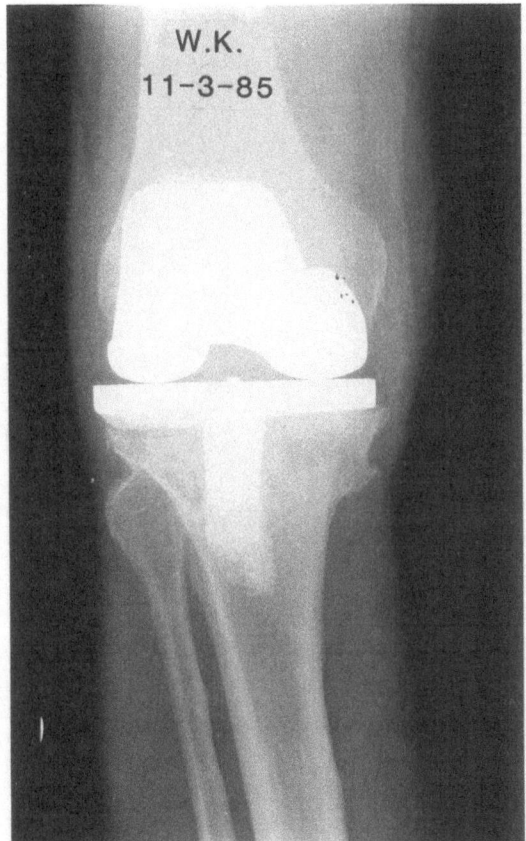

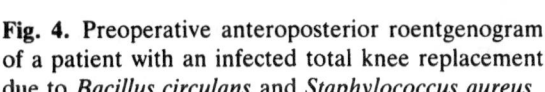

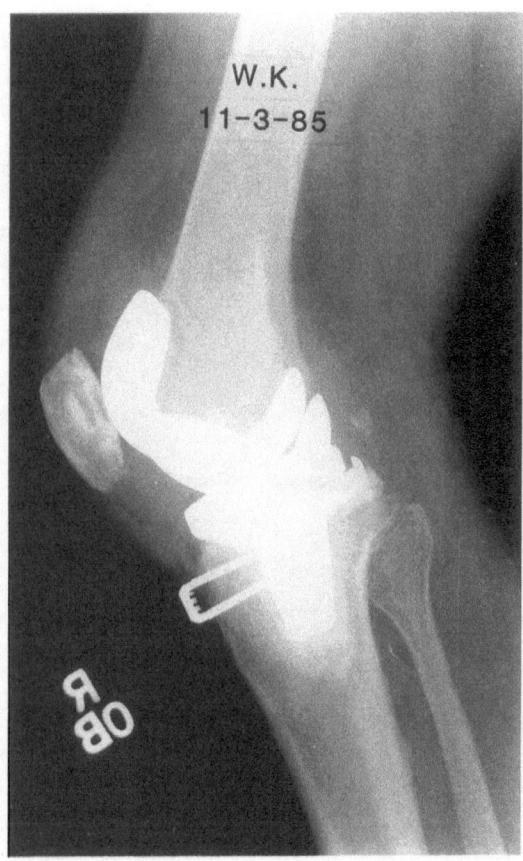

Fig. 4. Preoperative anteroposterior roentgenogram of a patient with an infected total knee replacement due to *Bacillus circulans* and *Staphylococcus aureus*

Fig. 5. Lateral roentgenogram of the patient shown in Fig. 4

was one recurrent patellar subluxation, which required an open lateral release and advancement of vastus medialis. There was one patellar fracture, which occurred 23 months postoperatively, which was treated by patellectomy due to comminution of the fracture. Finally, there was one death 6 weeks postoperatively, from myocardial infarction in a patient with preexisting arteriosclerotic heart disease.

Results

All the patients were evaluated, either by personal examination and roentgenograms or by telephone, except for the one patient who died with a myocardial infarction 6 weeks postoperatively. Follow-up was 100% on the group that could be studied. Time of follow-up averaged 52

months. The range was from 35 months to 117 months.

Of the 20 patients who could be studied, 16 were clinically free of infections. Three had undergone removal of the prosthesis and knee fusion, and one patient had continued infection with the original infecting organism 5 years after reimplantation. The rate of success with regard to infection at the time of follow-up was 80% (Figs. 4–7).

Postoperative knee scores were obtained in 14 patients. The average postoperative Hospital for Special Surgery knee score was 80 points. The range was from 48 to 98 points. The results were excellent in 41%, good in 11.7%, fair in 23.5%, and poor in 23.5%. The four poor results included three knee fusions and the one patient with continued infection in the operative knee.

The postoperative range of motion in flexion averaged 98 degrees with a range of 60–120

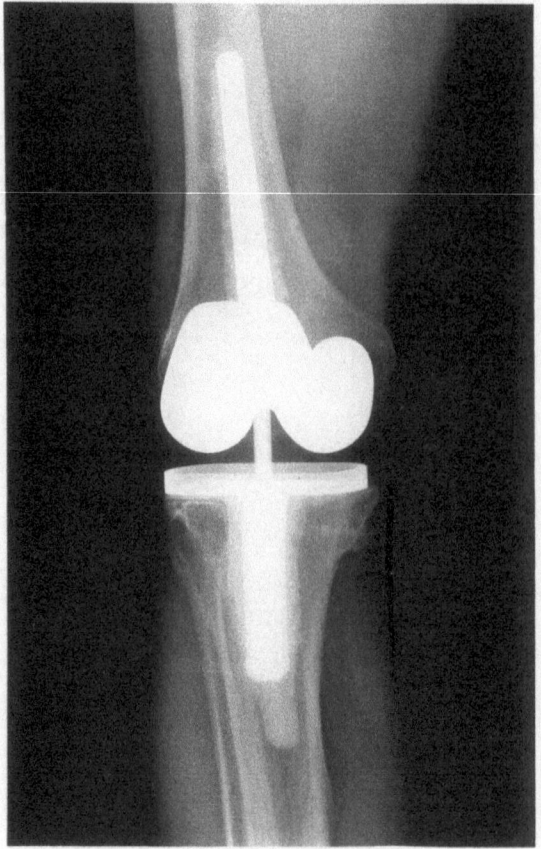

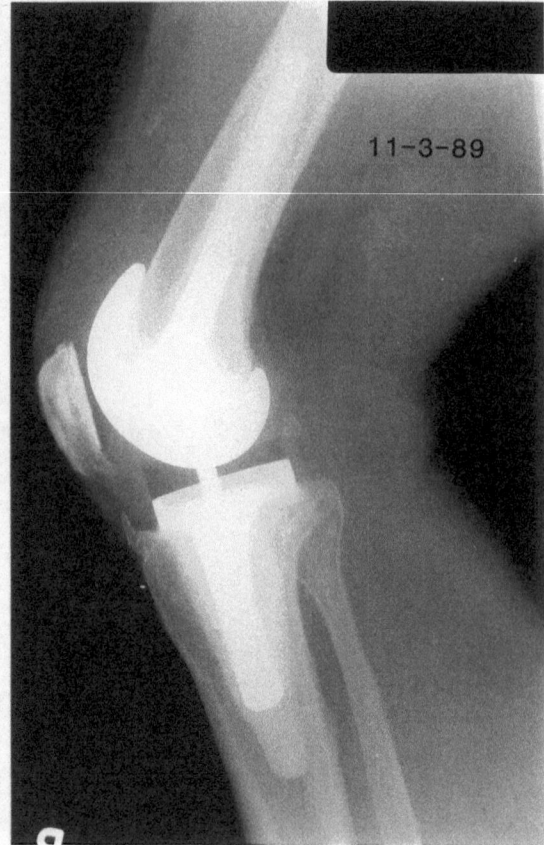

Fig. 6. Anteroposterior roentgenogram of the patient shown in Figs. 4 and 5; 4 years after a two-stage reimplantation

Fig. 7. Lateral roentgenogram of the patient shown in Fig. 6

degrees. The average postoperative extension was 4 degrees, with a range of 0–25 degrees.

There were two patients who underwent patellectomy. The knee scores on the two individuals were 65 points and 80 points. There were four patients who did not have replacement of the patellar articular surface due to insufficient bone remaining. Their knee scores were 67, 73, 89, and 96 points. The range of motion in the two patients who had had patellectomy was 5–105 degrees and 0–100 degrees. The ranges of motion in those patients who did not have a patellar component were 25–60 degrees, 0–120 degrees, 15–105 degrees, and 0–105 degrees.

Radiolucencies at the bone/cement interface were characterized, using the zones recommended by the Knee Society. The radiolucencies for femoral, tibial, and patellar components were totaled. Eighteen patients had postopera-

tive roentgenograms. There were six with total radiolucencies of 4 mm or less, eight with total radiolucencies of 5–9 mm, and four with radiolucencies greater than 10 mm. Of those with radiolucencies greater than 10 mm, the radiolucencies totaled, 13, 14, 15, and 19 mm.

Removal of the knee prosthesis and fusion were performed on three patients for continued infection. All three patients obtained a fusion. One patient developed ascending cholangitis due to *Clostridium perfringens*, which was cultured from the gall bladder and subsequently from the patient's knee replacement. The knee replacement was removed and intravenous antibiotics were given. The knee wound was packed open and was redebrided 2 days later. A reimplantation was performed after 3 weeks of intravenous penicillin treatment. After the reimplantation, *Enterobacter cloacae* was cultured, and the wound continued to drain. The prosthesis was removed, and the knee was fused. There has been no drainage from the wound since that time. A second patient with rheumatoid arthritis developed an infection in the knee due to *Staphylococcus* coagulase negative. The prosthesis was removed, and intravenous antibiotics were given for 5½ weeks postoperatively. After reimplantation, this patient had chronic intermittent drainage due to *Candida albicans* for a period of 2½ years. Ultimately, the knee prosthesis was removed, and the knee successfully fused. There was no recurrence of infection 30 months following fusion. The third patient developed an infection due to *Staphylococcus aureus*. After removal of the prosthesis, intravenous antibiotics were given for 4½ weeks before reimplantation. One month after reimplantation the wound began draining again due to *Staphylococcus aureus*. The prosthesis was removed, and the knee fused. Two years after the fusion with an intramedulary rod, an abscess of the knee was drained, and 3 months later, after the wound had healed, the intramedullary rod was removed.

Discussion

Two-stage reimplantation for the treatment of the infected total knee replacement, using intravenous antibiotics for an average of 5.2 weeks, and an antibiotic-impregnated cement spacer for mobilization of the knee has been shown to be successful in 80% of the patients, who were apparently free of infection for an average of 52 months or 4.3 years. This information confirms our earlier report, which also showed a success rate of 80% after an average follow-up of 33 months or 2.9 years [5].

The use of antibiotics with cement beads has been previously reported in the treatment of the infected total knee replacement. Ten of 11 knees were treated successfully with this method [6]. Gentamicin has also been utilized in cement for the treatment of one case of a knee replacement infected with *Staphylococcus aureus* [7]. Antibiotics have been used as well in the treatment of the infected total hip replacement [7,8]. The cement spacer has several advantages. It provides stability and makes an external fixator or a cast unnecessary. It provides comfort and convenience for the patient. It can be left in

place for prolonged periods if necessary while the patient is waiting for the second-stage reimplantation. It maintains the length of the collateral ligaments and the suprapatellar pouch. It makes the second-stage exposure easier. It decreases operating room time when compared with the use of an external fixator. It also provides a vehicle for the delivery of antibiotics.

The infected total knee replacement has been salvaged in 11 of 11 knees without the use of an antibiotic cement spacer. The follow-up averaged 33 months in that series [9]. The hospital length of stay averaged 12 weeks for those patients, however. Other methods for the treatment of the infected total knee replacement have included debridement with component removal and 48 hours of suction irrigation with satisfactory functional results in nine of 11 knees [10] and in 12 of 12 knees [11]. The time interval between the first and second stages in Insall's series [9] was 6 weeks. Short time intervals between the first and second stages do not appear to be as successful. In the papers authored by Rand, when the knees were reimplanted 2 weeks or less after the first-stage debridement removal of the components was satisfactory in only 35% of cases [12,13].

Not all antibiotics can be used in bone cement. Cefazolin, Clindamycin, Erythromycin, Gentamicin, Oxacillin, Penicillin G, Tobramycin, and Vancomycin have been shown to be suitable for use in bone cement [14–23]. When powdered antibiotic is mixed with powered polymethylmethacrylate, there has not been shown to be any significant decrease in the compressive or tensile strengths of the cement [20,21].

The type of bone cement used does seem to influence the rate of diffusion and the length of time of diffusion of the antibiotics from the bone cement. Palacos has been shown to be superior to Simplex bone cement in that regard [15,20]. It has also been shown that toxic levels of Gentamicin do not appear in the serum after instillation of the antibiotic and bone cement. The concentrations of Penicillin and Gentamicin were greater at the bone/cement interface than in the serum [8].

Two of the failures in our series occurred with *Clostridium perfringens* and *Candida albicans*. These cases have been reported previously [4,24]. There has been another case reported of a failure to clear a total knee replacement of infection with *Candida albicans* after multiple attempts of debridement [25].

The finding of a positive culture at the time of the second-stage procedure did not imply failure in this series. Of seven patients with positive cultures after the reimplantation of the total knee replacement, only two resulted in continued infection. Therefore, 71.5% of the patients in whom there was a positive organism present at the second-stage procedure were apparently free of infection at the time of follow-up. Obviously a longer period of follow-up is desirable in all of these cases before one can be certain that they are truly free of infection. It is well known that infection can remain dormant in bones and joints for prolonged periods.

Patellar components could not be reinserted at the time of reimplantation in four patients, due to inadequate bone being available. In this instance, the patella was shaped in order to glide in the patellar groove of the femoral component. This may be preferable to a patellectomy, but we lack specific data to support this concept.

Currently we aspirate the knee at weekly intervals following the first-stage debridement and removal of the prosthesis. If the knee is sterile, then reimplantation can be performed at 4 weeks after the first-stage procedure if the patient's condition and nutrition permits. If the aspiration reveals persistent infection, a second debridement and insertion of a new antibiotic spacer is performed. Intravenous antibiotics are continued for a longer period prior to reimplantation. Proper nutritional support of patients throughout the course of their treatment is important, and reimplantation may need to be delayed until the serum albumin is about 3.5 g and the total lymphocyte count is above 1500. If infection recurs following the second-stage reimplantation, there are the treatment options of removal of the prosthesis and knee fusion or another attempt at two-stage reimplantation. Patients with a history of repeated infections, or those who are immunologically compromised, or those with difficult organisms to treat (such as *Candida albicans* and *Clostridium perfringens*) or those who have antibiotic-resistant organisms should most likely be considered for knee fusion.

References

1. Grogan TJ, Dorey F, Rollins J, Amstutz HC (1977) Deep sepsis following total knee arthroplasty. J Bone Joint Surg [Br] 59:197
2. Knutsen K, Lindstrand R, Lingren L (1986) Survival of knee arthroplasties — A nationwide multicentre investigation of 8000 Cases. J Bone Joint Surg [Br] 68:795
3. Bliss DG, McBride GG (1985) Infected total knee arthroplasties. Clin Orthop 199:207
4. Levine M, Rehm SJ, Wilde AH (1988) Infection by *Candida albicans* of a total knee arthroplasty. Clin Orthop 226:735
5. Wilde AH, Ruth JT (1988) Two-stage reimplantation for infected total knee arthroplasties. Clin Orthop 236:23
6. Borden LS, Gearen PF (1987) Infected total knee arthroplasty. J Arthrop 2(1):27
7. Hovelius L, Josefsson G (1979) An alternative method for exchange operation of infected arthroplasty. Acta Orthop Scand 50:93
8. Carlsson AS, Josefsson G, Lindberg L (1973) Revision with Gentamycin-impregnated cement for deep infections in total hip arthroplasties. J Bone Joint Surg [Am] 60:1059
9. Insall JB, Thompson FM, Brause BD (1983) Two-stage reimplantation for the salvage of infected total knee arthroplasty. J Bone Joint Surg [Am] 65:1087
10. Walker RH, Schurman DJ (1984) Management of infected total knee arthroplasties. Clin Orthop 186:81
11. Brause BD (1982) Infected total knee replacement — diagnostic, therapeutic, and prophylactic considerations. Orthop Clin North Am 13(1):245
12. Rand JA, Bryan RS, Morrey BF, Westholm F (1986) Management of infected total knee arthroplasty. Clin Orthop 205:75
13. Rand JA, Bryan RS (1983) Reimplantation for the salvage of an infected total knee arthroplasty. J Bone Joint Surg [Am] 65:1081
14. Chapman MW, Hadley WK (1976) The effect of polymethyl-methacrylate and antibiotic combinations on bacterial viability. J Bone Joint Surg [Am] 58:76
15. Elson RA, Jephcott AE, McGechie DB (1977) Antibiotic-loaded acrylic cement. J Bone Joint Surg [Br] 59:220
16. Hill J, Klenerman L, Trustey S, Harrow RB (1977) Diffusion of antibiotics from acrylic bone-cement in vitro. J Bone Joint Surg [Br] 59:197
17. Hott SF, Fitzgerald RH, Kelley PJ (1981) The depot administration of penicillin G and

gentamicin in acrylic bone cement. J Bone Joint Surg [Am] 63:793

18. Hughes S, Field CA, Kennedy MRK, Dash CH (1979) Cephalosporins in bone cement. J Bone Joint Surg [Br] 61:96
19. Lawson KJ, Marks KE, Rehm SJ, Brems J (1990) Vancomycin versus tobramycin elution from polymethylmethacrylate cement: An invitro study. Orthopaedics 13:521–524
20. Marks KE, Nelson CL, Lautenschlager EP (1976) Antibiotic-impregnated acrylic bone cement. J Bone Joint Surg [Am] 58:358
21. Murray WR (1984) Use of antibiotic-containing bone cement. Clin Orthop 190:89

22. Schurman DJ, Trindale C, Hirshman P, Moser K, Kajiyama P, Stevens P (1978) Antibiotic-acrylic bone cement composites. J Bone Joint Surg [Am] 60:978
23. Wahlig H, Dingeldein E (1980) Antibiotics and bone cements. Acta Orthop Scand 51:49
24. Wilde AH, Sweeney RS, Borden LS (1988) Hematogenously acquired infection of a total knee arthroplasty by *Clostridium perfringes*. Clin Orthop 229:228
25. Goodman JS, Seibert DG, Reahl GE, Glecklev RW (1983) Fungal infection or prosthetic joints: A report of two cases. J Rheumatol 10:494

Excimer Laser in Joint Surgery: Experimental Basis and Clinical Experience

W. Puhl and R. Fischer[1]

Summary. In our hospital XeCl laser has been used in joint surgery and especially in treatment of osteoarthrosis since 1989. To judge the effect caused by laser we radiated fresh human cartilage with constant power density and varying pulse rates. The tissue damage next to the cutting crater was examined by lightmicroscopy and by SEM. There was a good ablation rate with little tissue damage and no laser-specific histological changes.

From our clinical experience we report the results of 25 patients treated with new fiber systems. In those cases we obtained smooth and stable cartilage surfaces combined with a good ablation rate. Postoperative results were comparable to those achieved by mechanical shavers. This makes XeCl laser to our laser of choice in joint surgery.

Key words. Excimer laser — Joint surgery — Articular cartilage — Thermal effects

Introduction

At the beginning of the 1960s, laser was introduced into various fields of medicine. In 1961 Campbell [1] was the first to use laser equipment in ophthalmology. Goldman [2] started at about the same time using laser in dermatology.

In joint surgery, laser offered little advantage as long as energy transmitting systems small enough for arthroscopic use were missing. Only the development of a small mirror system for transmitting the energy from CO_2 lasers enabled the use of the CO_2 laser in joint surgery, begun by Whipple [3]. In 1981, Glick [4] achieved laser meniscectomies, using a new fiber system with a small diameter. Wavelengths in the far UV portion made it difficult to find adequate fibers for energy transfer in excimer lasers. Only in 1987 were special quartz fibers suitable for those wavelengths developed to maintain sufficient energy transfer for the XeCl excimer laser.

Interaction between laser energy and tissue takes place if photon energy is transmitted from the laser to molecular structures. In most lasers used in joint surgery, such as the CO_2 laser (9600–10 600 nm) the Nd:YAG laser (1064 nm) and the Ho:YAG laser (2100 nm) the transmitted energy leads to heating of the radiated tissue. Inside the tissue low power densities (below 150 W/cm^2) cause necrosis and higher power levels lead to vaporization of intracellular water. Power densities between 10^4 and 10^6 W/cm^2 are required for the excision and cutting of tissues. Next to the cutting crater there is always an area that is changed by heat transmission. The extent of tissue damage depends, among other things, on laser wavelength, working conditions (contact or non-contact appliance, pulse rate), and tissue precooling.

Excimer lasers emit light in the UV portion of the light spectrum (e.g., KrF 248 nm, XeCl 308 nm, XeF 351 nm). Due to these wavelengths, most of the energy is absorbed in the tissues in the first few 10 μms. Thus power densities reaching between 10^9 and 10^{11} W/cm^2 lead to disintegration of molecular structures. In comparison to the photothermal ablation of the above-mentioned lasers there is almost no thermal damage tissue when precise cutting is achieved.

[1] Orthopedic Clinic, University of Ulm, Germany

Our general intention in joint surgery is to carry out cutting and ablation that is as exact as possible with as little damage to the surrounding healthy tissue as possible. In osteoarthrosis, in particular, we try to remove all affected osteoarthrotic cartilage by both smoothing the surface and leaving healthy chondral areas undamaged.

Materials and Methods

In November 1989 we installed a 308 nm XeCl excimer laser (Max 10 Fa. Arthrex, Munich FRG) in our hospital, using it mainly in arthroscopic treatment of knees, shoulders, and ankles, but especially in knee surgery, due to the numbers of knees treated here.

In an experimental setup we used hyaline joint cartilage obtained in joint replacements and fibrocartilage obtained by meniscectomies. All tissue samples were kept in normal saline solution and radiated within 24 hours postoperatively. To compare our results with similar experiments we used air as the laser-tissue interface. The samples were radiated with the fiber at a distance of 1 mm with a rectangular beam application, using a round-shaped fiber with a diameter of 0.9 mm (AR-9020 Fa. Arthrex, Munich FRG). The specimens were radiated with 30 mJ per pulse using various pulse rates and a pulse duration of 70 ns.

Half of the specimens were stained with hematoxilin-eosin, PAS, or Goldner and were examined by light microscopy. The rest were examined by scanning electrone microscope (SEM). Regarding knee joint surgery, from August 1990 (when we received new fibers with a better transmission rate) to February 1991, we treated 25 patients. The laser was used 10 times for debridement of cartilage in chondromalacia II or III, according to Outerbridge [5], at the femoral condyles, 8 times in chondromalacia II or III retropatellar, 6 times for partial or complete meniscal resection, 10 times to remove plicae and 2 times for arthroscopic synovectomies. Chondromalacia in small areas was treated by laser alone; in defects of large extent we used a mechanical shaver, first smoothing the edges and surface and afterward using the laser. All patients had a follow-up while staying in the hospital (usually 6–8 days) and afterward when they were seen in our outpatient department.

Results

The cartilage specimens were fixed, stained, and examined by light microscopy. There was an obvious relationship between pulse rate and depth of ablation. The walls of all craters appeared smooth with no evidence of carbonization. The transitorial zone surrounding the craters showed uniform structural changes. The diameter of this zone increased with the pulse rate. There was no obvious border between this

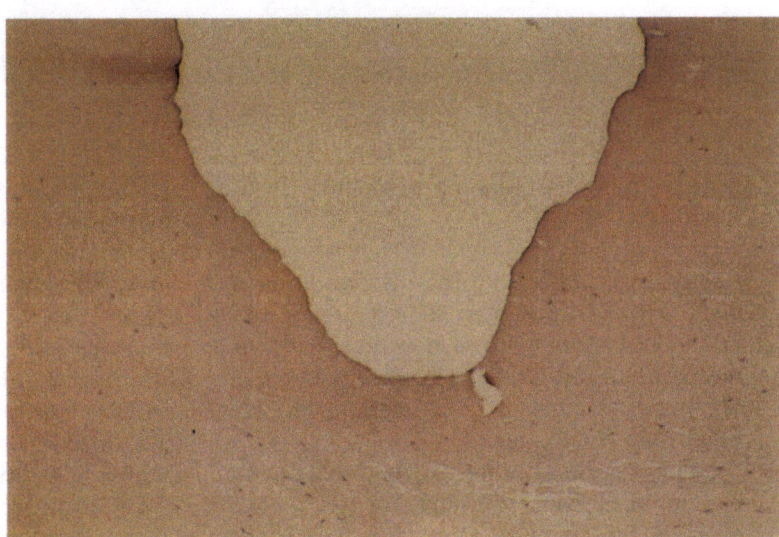

Fig. 1. Laser cut light microscopy. (HE stained)

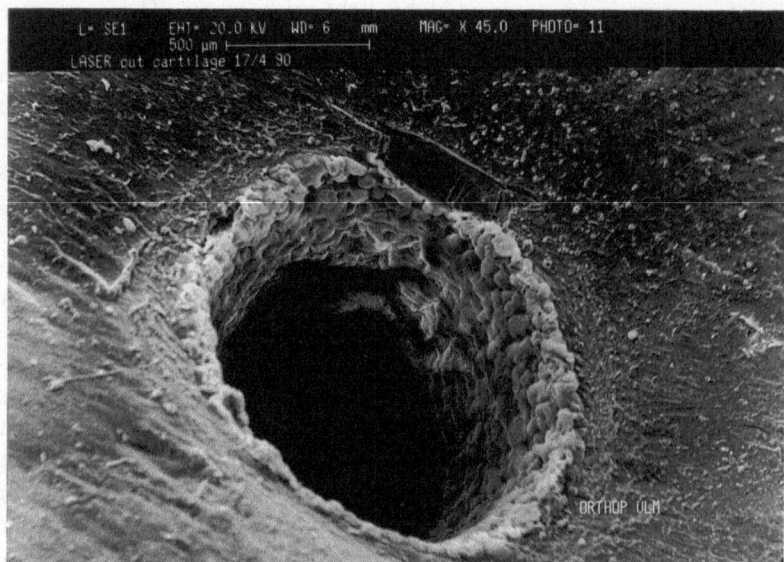

Fig. 2. Laser cut scanning electron microscopic (SEM) examination

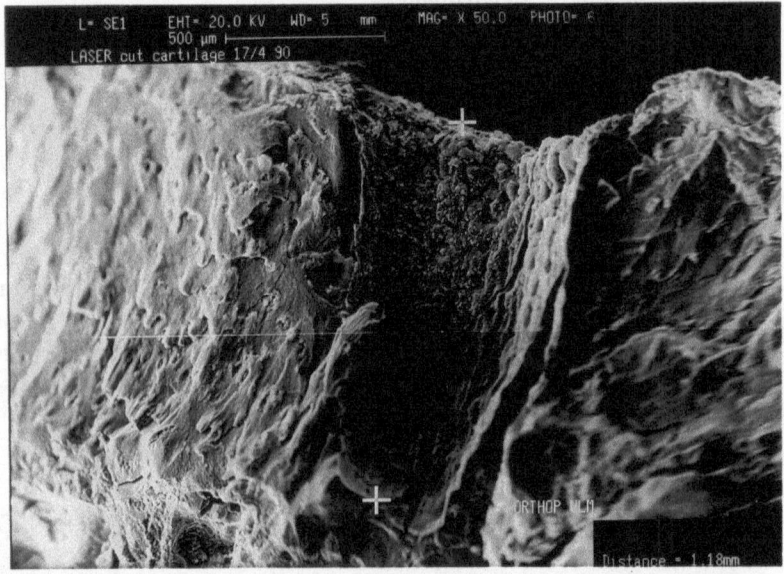

Fig. 3. Laser cut SEM examination

zone and the surrounding apparently healthy tissue (Fig. 1).

SEM indicated a small area with uniform structure beneath the sharply visible crater edge. Further away from the crater, the tissue gradually lost its uniform structure, with some matrix becoming visible. This area changed into apparently normal cartilage without any clear borderline (Figs. 2 and 3).

Neither in the light microscopic examinations nor in SEM could we find any laser-specific changes.

Comparing the XeCl laser to mechanical shaver instruments in joint surgery, we found a lower ablation rate but much better results in smoothing the surface of the cartilage, using an excimer laser. While the surface after shaver use appeared rather bumpy on examination, the cartilage treated with the excimer laser showed a smooth surface. The formerly soft chondromalacic cartilage showed a hardened, almost sealed, surface.

The postoperative results of our patients treated with laser arthroscopic surgery were not significantly different from those of patients treated with shaver instruments alone. Post-operative intensity of pain, joint effusion, and range of movement were approximately the same in both groups. There was no difference in results, not only for the patients treated between August 1990 and February 1991, but also for those patients treated with the XeCl laser between November 1989 and August 1990 (when examined on follow-up).

Our experience in using the XeCl excimer laser in arthroscopic operations is that it is possible to achieve an ablation rate as effective and almost as good as that obtaining when mechanical shavers are used.

The main problem in the beginning was that the transmission of energy was insufficient, due to the fibers (AR-9020 Fa. Arthrex, Munich FRG) used. Fibers could only transmit barely enough energy for cartilage ablation. After frequent use and resterilization, the transmission rate decreased, leading to a power density below 10^9 W/cm^2, thus minimizing the ablation rate while increasing thermal damage. Furthermore, treatment of chondromalacia at the retropatellar surface or the femoral condyles was difficult to achieve with handpieces working only in a forward position. A rectangular beam application is necessary for optimal photon absorption.

Since August 1989, we have been using new fiber systems (AR-9010 Fa. Arthrex, Munich FRG) with which a better energy transmission is possible. There are also fibers (AR-9040 Fa. Arthrex, Munich FRG) available with a tip curved in a 30° angle for better energy application to the retropatellar and condylar cartilage. Using these fiber systems, we found the ablation rate much increased, almost reaching that of mechanical shaver instruments, leaving a smooth and hardened cartilage surface.

However, with frequent use of the fibers, we also found a significant decrease in transmission.

Discussion

Lasers used in joint surgery are the CO_2 laser, as a representative of gas lasers, the Nd:YAG and HO:YAG lasers which use a solid active medium, and the XeCl laser, an excimer laser that produces photons via excited dimers.

One generally accepted advantage of lasers in arthroscopic operations is that lasers, due to the small diameter of the fibers and handpieces, can work in the enclosed and narrow parts of the joints (e.g., in resection of the posterior part of the meniscus) with no damage to the surrounding cartilage. However, there is much discussion about the "best laser" to be used in joint surgery.

We favor the XeCl excimer laser for the following reasons.

Excimer Laser Works Via Photoablation with Almost No Thermal Damage of Surrounding Tissue

This effect was described initially by Srinivasin [6] as "ablative photodecomposition".

In our experiment, cartilage damage could be seen only in an area of few μms next to the cutting crater. The cutting depth correlates with the power density and pulse rate of the laser.

Hohlbach [7] and Kroitzsch [8], who examined the effect of XeCl laser on human cartilage in vitro, also found similar results.

In comparing our present in vitro results to the effects of excimer laser in joint surgery we have to take into account the fact that we used air as the laser-tissue interface, knowing that photoablation is improved while thermal damage is reduced in a fluid medium [9]. In arthroscopic operations we use Ringerlactate as the laser-tissue interface.

Furthermore, we cannot judge whether the chondrocytes next to the transitorial zone that appeared unchanged in our histologic slides would still be vital in an in vivo experiment.

In comparing several lasers in vitro Siebert [10] demonstrated that there was only a small area of obviously damaged tissue following XeCl laser use, while Nd:YAG and Ho:YAG lasers produced high thermal damage. Trauner [11], examining tissue damage after the application of CO_2 and Ho:YAG lasers, found an even larger area of thermal damage after Ho:YAG radiation.

Adopting pulse rate to the thermal relaxation time constant Grossweiner [12], using a Nd:YAG laser, and Siebert [13], using a Ho:YAG laser, were able to decrease tissue damage but could not achieve the results achieved with the excimer laser.

Excimer Laser Enables Us to Ablate Almost All Single Tissue Layers, Resulting in an Almost Smooth Surface. Joint Surgery Can Thus be Performed Really Gently

This smooth surface can be seen in macroscopic as well as in microscopic examinations. In trying to smooth the surfaces of osteoarthrotic human cartilage in vitro, Siebert [10] found good results when using the XeCl laser. None of the other lasers tested had similar results.

Up To Now There Are No Known Side Effects of XeCl Laser Use

Until now we have treated about 100 patients, using the XeCl laser. We have had no complications so far.

Raunest [14], who treated 70 patients with chondromalacia stage II or III according to Outerbridge [5] with either a XeCl laser or with mechanical instruments had significantly superior results in the group treated with the laser. Although he did not state how many of the patients in each group had chondromalacia stage III, and although he used a modification of a score developed for postoperative follow-up of knee instability in his follow-up of patients with arthrosis, the results are quite interesting.

In the postoperative control of our patients we could not confirm such results as we had comparable results in both groups. Of course, prospective randomized examinations are necessary to judge whether there are any significant differences in the follow-up of patients treated with laser and patients treated with mechanical instruments.

One cannot tell for certain that there is no risk of mutagenicity from the use of excimer laser radiation, but, up to now, there has been no known case of malignant disease following excimer laser radiation. Examinations performed by Kochevar [15] and Peak [16] have demonstrated that there is only a small risk of mutagenicity from the use of 308 nm XeCl laser radiation.

The Main Disadvantage of the XeCl Laser in Comparison to Mechanical Instruments is a Lower Ablation Rate

There are still problems to be solved concerning the transmission of the quartz fibers. Frequent use of the fiber reduces the transmission rate, leading to a power density below $10^9 \, W/cm^2$ at the tissue surface, thus reducing ablation rate while increasing thermal damage. Several groups are now attempting to improve the transmission rate to increase the percentage of available laser energy at the tissue surface. The first encouraging results using tapered fibers support the hope that there might be better fiber systems available in the next few years.

In spite of these difficulties, we find the XeCl excimer laser to be the least damaging laser for cartilage treatment available today. Our in vitro examinations as well as those of others would confirm this. However, up to now one can only estimate the extent of chondrocyte damage in vivo. In examining the healing conditions of laser defects in vivo, Schultz [17] and Hardie [18], using Nd:YAG lasers, and Borovoy [19], using a CO_2 laser, found a greater extent of cartilage damage than that expected from in vitro results. Therefore our results need further proof by way of in vivo examination.

In laser synovectomy, where there is also the necessity of a good coagulation effect, the XeCl laser might be of less interest. In such cases one might prefer the Ho:YAG laser or the CO_2 laser. But since treating osteoarthrotic cartilage demands the least damage of healthy chondrocytes possible, in those cases we will continue to prefer the XeCl laser to other lasers now available.

References

1. Campbell CJ, Rittler MC, Koester CJ (1963) The optical laser as a retinal coagulator; an evaluation. Trans Am Acad Ophthalmol Otolaryngol 67:58–67
2. Goldmann L, Blancy DJ, Kindel DJ Jr (1963) Pathology of the effect of the laser beam on the skin. Nature 197:912–14
3. Whipple TL, Caspari RB, Meyers JF (1982) Arthroscopic meniscectomy by CO_2 laser vaporization in a gas medium. Orthop Trans 6:136–42
4. Glick J (1981) YAG Laser meniscectomy. Presented at the Triannual Meeting of the International Arthroscopy Association of North America, Rio de Janeiro, Brazil, August 1981
5. Outerbridge RE (1964) Further studies of the

etiology of chondromalacia patellae. J Bone Joint Surg [Br] 46:179–90

6. Srinivasin R (1986) Ablation of polymers and biological tissues by ultraviolet lasers. Science 234:559–65

7. Hohlbach G, Möller KO, Schramm U, Baretton G (1989) Experimentelle Ergebnisse der Knorpelabrasio mit einem Excimer-Laser. Histologische und elektronenmi-kroskopische Untersuchungen. Z Orthop 127:216–21

8. Kroitzsch U, Laufer G, Egkher E, Wollenek G, Horvath R (1989) Experimental photoablation of meniscus cartilage by excimer laser energy. Arch Orthop Trauma Surg 108:44–48

9. Kolbe T, Hibst R, Steiner, R (1990) Untersuchungen zu Parametern der Excimer-Laser-Angioplastie in Bezug auf Effizienz und Gewebeschäden. In: Steiner R (Hrsg) Verhandlungsbericht der Deutschen Gesellschaft für Lasermedizin e.V. 5. Jahrestagung 28.–30.9.1989. EBM-Verlag, München, pp 36–47

10. Siebert WE, Kohn D, Wirth CJ (1990) Histologische und rasterelektronenmikroskopische Veränderungen an Knorpeloberflächen nach Bearbeitung mit verschiedenen Lasern im Vergleich zu mechanischen Instrumenten. In: Steiner R (Hrsg) Verhandlungsbericht der Deutschen Gesellschaft für Lasermedizin e.V. 5. Jahrestagung 28.–30.9.1989. EBM-Verlag, München, pp 334–42

11. Trauner K, Nishioka N, Patel D (1990) Pulsed Ho:YAG laser ablation of fibrocartilage and articular cartilage. Am J Sports Med 18(3): 316–20

12. Grossweiner LI, Al-Karmi AM (1988) Tissue heating with pulsed Nd-YAG laser. SPIE 908: 145–50

13. Siebert WE, Wirth CJ (1990) Der Laser an der Schwelle zur klinischen Anwendung in der Orthopädie. Laser Brief 18:3–4

14. Raunest J, Löhnert J (1990) Arthroscopic cartilage debridement by excimer laser in chondromalacia of the knee joint. Arch Orthop Trauma Surg 109:155–59

15. Kochevar IE (1989) Cytotoxicity and mutagenicity of excimer laser radiation. Lasers Surg Med 9: 440–45

16. Peak MJ, Peak JG, Moehring MP, Webb RB (1984) Ultraviolet light action spectra for DNA dimer induction lethality, and mutagenesis in E. coli with emphasis on the UVB region. Photochem Photobiol 40:613–20

17. Schultz RJ, Krishnamurthy S, Thelmo W, Rodriguez JE, Harvey G (1985) Effects of varying intensities of laser energy on articular tissue. Lasers Surg Med 5:577–88

18. Hardie EM, Carlson CS, Richardson DC (1989) Effects of Nd:YAG laser energy on articular cartilage healing in the dog. Lasers Surg Med 9:595–601

19. Borovoy M, Zirkin RM, Elson LM, Borovoy MA (1989) Healing of laser-induced defects of articular cartilage: preliminary studies. J Foot Surg 28(2):95–99

Implant Debris from Total Joint Arthroplasties: Studies on the Mechanisms Responsible, the Amounts of Debris Generated, and the Implications in Loosening and Infection

Timothy Wright[1]

Summary. The release of metallic and polymeric debris to the tissues and fluids surrounding total joint replacement components is a significant problem with serious implications affecting the longevity of the arthroplasty. Measurements of metallic debris levels suggests that of the common implant metals, titanium alloy generates more debris, though this conclusion is based on levels measured in tissues collected at revision from around implants which had already failed. Similar measurements performed on synovial fluid samples obtained from aspiration of both well-fixed and loose implants support this finding. However, the debris levels were much lower in the fluid samples from around the well-fixed implants, suggesting that much of the metallic debris around failed joint replacements is a result of rather than a cause of the mechanical loosening itself. Based on the abundance of polymeric debris generated in the joint and on the wide range of shape and size of the debris, polymeric debris may play a more important role in eliciting a deleterious biological reaction than metallic debris. Techniques for clinically improving the situation exist, including improving component design to minimize the stresses associated with damage to the polyethylene articulating surface.

Key words. Joint arthroplasty — Polyethylene — Implant debris — Surface damage — Metal levels

Introduction

Despite the dramatic decrease in the incidence of sepsis following total joint arthroplasty, infection remains a serious complication. Bio-
materials play a role in the etiology of infection by adversely affecting the host response and by providing a surface on which pathogens can dwell, secluded from circulating immune factors and antibiotics [1,2]. Though the effect on the host defense mechanism is dependent, along with other factors, on the type of biomaterial, experimental evidence shows that most of the implant materials commonly used in total joint replacements can adversely influence the incidence of infection [3]. Furthermore, the tissue response is more pronounced in articulating implants, such as total joint replacements, than in stable implants, presumably due to the added particulate debris generated from wear of the joint surfaces [1].

It also appears that implant loosening, a more prevalent complication than infection, is influenced by the presence of particulate forms of biomaterials. There is growing evidence that bone resorption, with the subsequent loss of fixation of the implant, is a direct result of the biological reaction to large amounts of debris [4,5]. Cells activated by the presence of particulate debris release cytokines, which in turn, can elicit bone resorption [6].

To understand the problem of debris-related complications and to design joint components which will last longer, a comprehensive approach has been taken. The mechanisms by which debris can be generated from the articulating surface have been determined by observing damage on retrieved components and by measuring the levels of implant debris from tissues and fluids collected from around total joint arthroplasties.

[1] Department of Biomechanics, The Hospital for Special Surgery (affiliated with New York Hospital and Cornell University Medical College) New York, NY 10021 USA

To further examine the specific problem of ultra high molecular weight polyethylene debris, stresses which cause surface damage as a result of contact with the opposing metallic component were investigated. Surface damage due to wear can generate excessive amounts of polyethylene debris. Examining the stresses occurring on and within polyethylene components provides insight into the damage mechanisms. Stress analysis can also be used to establish the effects of changes in design variables that control the resistance of the component to surface damage.

Observations on Retrieved Prostheses

Observations performed on retrieved polyethylene total joint components have been used to identify damage modes responsible for the release of particulate debris [7–9]. The two most severe damage modes, pitting and delamination, are caused by fracture of the polyethylene at a depth of 1–2mm below the articulating surface. These two damage modes result in the release of large amounts of debris. The amount of damage observed on retrieved components increased significantly with patient weight, with the length of time the component was implanted, and (for patellar components) with the range of motion achieved post-operatively [8–10]. Furthermore, damage was related to the design of the articulating surfaces, with more nonconforming surfaces experiencing greater damage [10]. The correlations with weight and time reveal that the damage is dependent on both the applied load and the number of loading cycles, supporting the hypothesis that fracture is the primary mechanism. The correlation with range of motion demonstrates that damage will be greater as greater function is restored to the patient.

Observations on retrieved components have also been used to identify damage modes occurring on metallic components. Articulating surfaces of titanium alloy implants were found to be moderately scratched, even after short implantation times (2–3 years or less) [11]. This differs from the articulating surfaces of the other two common implant metals (cobalt alloy and stainless steel) that generally remained polished while implanted. The stem portions of hip implants from all three alloys were often found to be abraded, presumably due to articulation against the surrounding cement mantle as the implant loosened.

Observations on Retrieved Tissues

Observations have also been made on periarticular tissues collected from around total joint implants during revision surgery. Atomic absorption spectrophotometry [12] has been used to identify and measure the metallic content in tissues obtained from around titanium alloy [11], cobalt-chromium alloy [13], and stainless steel components. The major alloying elements were determined, together with barium [14], a major constituent of acrylic bone cement.

For example, cobalt, chromium, nickel, and molybdenum levels were measured in periarticular tissue from 22 individuals who underwent revision hip surgery for failed cemented total joint replacements in which the femoral component had been fabricated from cobalt alloy. The average duration of implantation was 9.8 years (range 1 month to 18 years). The reason for removal was aseptic loosening in 16 cases, and infection in 6 cases. Total tissue content of the four elements ranged from 2.7 to 250 µg of, metal per g of dried tissue (with a mean total tissue content of 39 µg/g); however, within each case, the tissue metal content varied more widely. The total tissue metal content in cases revised for infection was higher than the metal content in cases revised for aseptic loosening (Table 1).

Ratios of the individual constituent elements generally reflected the cobalt chromium alloy composition, suggesting that metal debris was present predominantly as wear particles. Only for tissues with very low metal content did departures of these ratios indicate the presence of ionic corrosion products.

Histological examination of the tissues from these cases revealed primarily fibrosis, histiocytic reaction, hemorrhage, and necrosis. Polyethylene and cement particles were prevalent in a majority of the sections examined, while metallic particles were seen only in tissues from the infected hips. The polyethylene debris varied over a wide range of shape and size and was found both within cells and in the extracellular material.

Table 1. Mean tissue metal content and durations of implantation for three groups of patients with cobalt alloy hip prostheses [13]

Infected (n = 6)		Aseptic Loose cup and stem (n = 12)		Aseptic Loose cup (n = 4)	
Metal content (μg/g)	Duration (months)	Metal content (μg/g)	Duration (months)	Metal content (μg/g)	Duration (months)
5.6	13	6.7	112	2.7	94
6.2	29	8.6	34	7.1	148
25.0	153	9.0	124	10.8	184
25.8	12	13.7	191	12.2	74
124.8	211	14.7	186		
250.0	160	16.4	126		
		17.0	203		
		18.5	124		
		37.6	88		
		67.2	117		
		70.1	155		
		97.8	130		
Mean ± SD	Mean ± SD	Mean ± SD	Mean ± SD	Mean ± SD	Mean ± SD
72.9 ± 97.5	96 ± 88	32.2 ± 30.0	132 ± 47	8.2 ± 4.3	125 ± 50

The mean barium content determined from the tissues in these cases was 1374 μg/g (range 151–6300 μg/g). Assuming that bone cement is 10% (w/w) $BaSO_4$ and that the barium does not leach preferentially from the cement, this value corresponds to 23 μg of cement per g of dried tissue. No correlation was found between barium content and content of the metallic alloying elements. Metal content did not differ significantly between tissue from one anatomical site compared to tissue from another site around the joint. But tissues from the cement-bone interface had a barium content significantly higher than the barium content measured in tissues from the capsule.

The extremely low metal content measured in cement-bone interfacial tissues and the few metallic particles seen histologically suggest that metallic particles may have been less important in inflammatory reaction and loosening than cement or polyethylene particles. Furthermore, much of the metallic debris may have been generated over that short period of time after significant loosening had occurred. This would explain the lack of correlation between average tissue metal content or histological findings and duration of implantation. Since accumulating evidence implicates debris particles in the generation of foreign body tissue reaction and the accompanying bone destruction, the smaller amounts of metal and wide range of values suggest a greater importance of cement and polyethylene than of metallic debris as a cause of the loosening of cemented prostheses.

Debris Levels in Synovial Fluid

To further test the conclusion concerning metallic debris, a prospective study was performed to measure the synovial fluid content of prosthesis metals and barium in well-fixed and loose total hip arthroplasties [15]. Synovial fluid was collected from 37 hips that had well-fixed implant components and 44 hips that had components that were loose, requiring revision surgery. Approximately equal numbers of implants made from the three common alloys were included and the number of well-fixed and loose implants was about equal for each type of material.

The content of prosthesis elements measured was substantially higher in synovial fluid from hips with loose implants than from hips with well-fixed implants, with particularly high levels noted for loose titanium alloy implants (Table 2). There was, however, considerable overlap in content between well-fixed and loose implants. The metal content in synovial fluid was considerably higher than reported values for blood or serum, suggesting that the synovial mem-

Table 2. Metal content in synovial fluid from hips with well-fixed and loose stainless steel, cobalt alloy, and titanium alloy prostheses [15]

	Well-fixed	Loose
Element	(n = 11)	Stainless steel (n = 13)
Chromium	6 (1–16)	17 (1–137)
Nickel	7 (0.1–35)	20 (2–162)
	(n = 19)	Cobalt alloy (n = 23)
Cobalt	2 (0.4–6)	21 (0.2–152)
Chromium	6 (0.2–16)	19 (0.8–238)
Nickel	9 (0.2–34)	12 (0.2–52)
	(n = 7)	Titanium alloy (n = 8)
Titanium	5 (0.1–13)	109 (13–194)
Vanadium	Not detectable	0.4 (Not detectable – 2)

Entries are mean values with range in parentheses

brane acts as a barrier to prevent dissolved metals from diffusing out of the joint fluid.

The amount of cement debris in the fluids from around well-fixed implants was apparently much lower than that from around loose implants. The mean barium content in the well-fixed implants was 19 µg/l of fluid (range 1–51 µg/l) versus 302 µg/l (range 30–1900 µg/l) in the loose implants. This finding suggests that much of the cement debris was generated as a result of further mechanical damage to the cement mantle after mechanical loosening had initiated such damage.

Damage Mechanisms for Polyethylene Implants

To investigate the mechanisms responsible for the damage modes observed on retrieved polyethylene implants, we began by determining the stresses occurring on and within these components as a result of contact with the opposing metallic component. We used experimental methods [16,17], approximate elasticity solutions [18], axisymmetric finite elements analyses [19], and fully three-dimensional finite element analyses [20]. The experimental analyses of contact stresses in total knee tibial components showed a strong influence of both geometry and material. The measured contact stresses were higher for more nonconforming components and for components fabricated from carbon fiber-reinforced, rather than plain, polyethylene.

Unlike the experimental methods, the theoretical structural analyses made it possible to vary design parameters independently and to determine stresses within the polyethylene, as well as on the surface. These analyses were used, therefore, to assess the risk of surface damage in specific contemporary total knee and total hip replacements and to determine the effects of altering the designs of these implants.

Contact between nonconforming articulating surfaces in total knee components resulted in significantly higher contact stresses on the polyethylene surface than in the case of contact between articulating surfaces in total hip components. This is consistent with the observations of surface damage on retrieved polyethylene components, which demonstrated that the less conforming tibial components from total condylar type total knee replacements experienced greater damage than acetabular components from total hip replacements.

Although contact stresses are higher in tibial components, they occur at the center of the contact area, where the principal stresses tangent to the surface are also compressive. This results in a large component of hydrostatic compression. These stresses should not be expected to cause damage modes, such as pitting and delamination, that are more prevalent in these components than in acetabular components.

These observations can be explained, however, by comparing the values of the principal and shear stresses for the specific knee and hip component geometries [20]. The range of the maximum principal stress was much greater for the knee component than the hip components. The maximum shear stress occurred beneath the surface for the knee component, but at the surface for the hip components. This was true even though the magnitudes of the maximum shear stress were similar for both the knee and hip components.

The effects of the large compressive and tensile maximum principal stresses are compounded in the knee replacement because the contact area can change size and orientation and move with respect to the tibial component during articulation. Therefore, points on the tibial component surface will be subjected to cyclic stresses which vary between tension and compression. These cyclic stresses are consistent with the initiation and propagation of surface cracks in a direction which is initially perpendicular to the surface. Points on the surface of polyethylene hip joint components are also likely to be subjected to cyclic stresses, but the range of the stresses is much smaller.

The subsurface location of the maximum shear stress in the tibial component may also explain the surface damage seen on retrieved implants. The maximum shear stress occurs at a depth of 1–2 mm, which is about equal to the depth of the pits and delamination observed in retrieved implants. The location of the largest value of maximum shear stress is consistent, therefore, with the initiation of subsurface cracks or with the change in the direction of cracks that are initiated at the surface and propagated perpendicular to the surface under the influence of the maximum principal stresses.

Many contemporary total knee designs have articulating surfaces much less conforming than those of the total condylar type knee implant used in the stress analyses just described [20]. This is particularly true of some cruciate-sparing designs that have nearly flat tibial surfaces, supposedly to allow sufficient joint laxity for the posterior cruciate ligament to function properly. Since the stresses associated with surface damage all increase with decreasing conformity, stresses in these less conforming joint designs would be expected to be greater.

Experimental studies of contact stresses [17] support this assumption, as do recent observations on retrieved PCA type tibial components removed because of excessive wear after only 4–5 years of service [21]. These components showed large areas of delamination [22], much more severe than that observed on more conforming Insall/Burstein total condylar components [6].

The studies of polyethylene components provide design criteria for minimizing the stresses associated with surface damage [20]. In particular, minimum polyethylene thicknesses for knee and hip components should be used. Maintaining a minimum of 6 mm thickness for acetabular components and 8 mm for total condylar type tibial components will minimize these stresses. Also, a compromise must be sought between alteration of the design of the articulating surfaces to improve the con-

formity and the potential adverse effect on joint kinematics [20].

Other factors may increase the stresses due to contact forces. The physical properties of several retrieved polyethylene hip and knee implants were investigated [23,24]. Based on measured density changes, the elastic modulus of polyethylene apparently increased during the time the implant was in vivo. The increase in elastic modulus was not uniform through the thickness of the component, but varied with depth from the articulating surface. The maximum increase in modulus occurred at the surface of acetabular components and at a depth of about 1 mm in tibial components. Since the stresses due to contact increase with increased modulus, in vivo degradation will result in increased stress magnitudes which further increase the risk of surface damage and subsequent debris generation [23].

Acknowledgments. This work has been a collaborative effort of researchers at The Hospital for Special Surgery, including Foster Betts PhD, Donald Bartel PhD, Eduardo Salvati MD, Clare Rimnac PhD, Manjula Bansal MD, and William Brien MD. The support of the National Institutes of Health (Grants AR01737 and AR38905), the Robert Patterson Fund, and the Clark Foundation is gratefully acknowledged.

References

1. Gristina AG, Kolkin J (1983) Total joint replacement and sepsis. J Bone Joint Surg 65-A: 128–134
2. Salvati EA (1990) Infected total hip replacement. In: Evarts C (ed) Surgery of the musculoskeletal system. Churchill Livingstone, New York, pp 4475–4495
3. Petty W, Spanier S, Shuster JJ, Silverthorne C (1985) The influence of skeletal implants on incidence of infection. J Bone Joint Surg 67-A: 1236–1244
4. Mirra JM, Marder RA, Amstutz HC (1982) The pathology of failed total joint arthroplasty. Clin Orthop 170:175–183
5. Howie DW, Vernon-Roberts B, Oakeshott R, Manthey B (1988) A rat model of resorption of bone at the cement-bone interface in the presence of polyethylene wear particles. J Bone Joint Surg 70-A:257–263
6. Galante JO, Lemons J, Spector M, Wilson PD Jr, Wright TM (To be published) The biologic effects of implant materials. J Orthop Res

7. Wright TM, Rimnac CM, Faris PM, Bansal M (1988) Analysis of surface damage occurring in carbon fiber-reinforced and plain polyethylene tibial components from posterior stabilized type total knee replacement. J Bone Joint Surg 70-A: 1312–1319

8. Hood RW, Wright TM, Burstein AH (1983) Retrieval analysis of total knee prostheses: a method and its application to forty-eight total condylar prostheses. J Biomed Mater Res 17: 829–842

9. Figgie MP, Wright TM, Santner T, Fisher D, Forbes A (1989) Performance of dome-shaped patellar components in total knee arthroplasty. Trans 35th Ortho Res Soc 14:531

10. Wright TM, Burstein AH, Bartel DL (1985) Retrieval analysis of total joint replacement components. In: Fraker A, Griffin C (eds) Corrosion and degradation of implant materials. American Society for Testing Materials, Philadelphia, pp 415–428

11. Agins HJ, Alcock NW, Bansal M, Salvati EA, Wilson PD Jr, Pellicci PM, Bullough PG (1988) Metallic wear in failed titanium-alloy total hip replacements. J Bone Joint Surg 70-A:347–356

12. Betts F, Yau A (1989) Graphite furnace atomic absorption spectrometric determination of chromium, nickel, cobalt, molybdenum and manganese in tissues containing particles of a cobalt-chrome alloy. Anal Chem 61:1235–1238

13. Betts F, Wright TM, Salvati E, Boskey A, Bansal M (to be published) Metal analysis and histological grading of periarticular tissues from cobalt alloy total hip revision arthroplasties. Clin Orthop

14. Betts F, Wright TM, Salvati E, Boskey A (1990) Barium content of tissues from revision total hip arthroplasties. Trans 36th Ortho Res Soc 15:457

15. Brien WW, Salvati EA, Betts F, Bullough PG, Wright TM, Buly R, Garvin K (to be published) Metal levels in cemented total hip arthroplasty: a comparison of well-fixed and loose implants. Clin Orthop

16. Wright TM, Fukubayashi T, Burstein AH (1981) The effect of carbon fiber reinforcement on contact area, contact pressure and time dependent deformation in polyethylene tibial components. J Biomed Mater Res 15:719–730

17. Hood RW, Wright TM, Fukubayashi T, Burstein AH (1981) Contact area and pressure distribution in contemporary total knee designs. In: Van Buskirk WC, Woo SL-Y (eds) 1981 Biomechanics Symposium. American Society of Mechanical Engineers, New York, pp 233–236

18. Wright TM, Bartel DL (1986) The problem of surface damage in polyethylene total knee components. Clin Orthop 205:67–74

19. Bartel DL, Wright TM, Edwards D (1983) The effect of metal backing on stresses in polyethylene. In: Hungerford DS (ed) The hip. CV Mosby, St Louis, pp 229–239

20. Bartel DL, Bicknell VL, Wright TM (1986) The effect of conformity, thickness, and material on stresses in UHMWPE components for total joint replacement. J Bone Joint Surg 68-A:1041–1051

21. Tsao AK, Mintz LJ, McCrae CM, Stulberg SD, Wright TM (to be published) Severe polyethylene failure in PCA total knee arthroplasties. J Bone Joint Surg

22. Wright TM, Rimnac CM, Stulberg SD, Mintz L, Tsao AK, Klein RW, McCrae C (to be published) Wear of polyethylene in total joint replacements: observations from retrieved PCA knee implants. Clin Orthop

23. Elbert KE, Kurth M, Bartel DL, Eyerer P, Rimnac CM, Wright TM (1988) In vivo changes in material properties of polyethylene and their effects on stresses associated with surface damage of polyethylene components. Trans 34th Ortho Res Soc 13:53

24. Eyerer P, Ke YC (1984) Property changes of UHMW polyethylene hip cup endoprostheses during implantation. J Biomed Mater Res 18: 1137–1151

Part III. Miscellaneous Conditions in Orthopaedics

How Should We Treat Fractures?

A. Graham Apley[1]

The title of this talk is "How should we treat fractures?", but really the important question is "How should we treat people?" — people who happen to have broken bones. If, for example, a person breaks their leg, all they want at the end of treatment is that the leg should be long enough to reach the ground, face the way they're going, and enable them to sit, stand, walk, and run. Which was not difficult till Röntgen came along. But ever since he invented x-rays, that's what most surgeons treat instead of treating people. What's more, surgeons assume that their help is needed in getting a fracture to join; that they must put it in plaster, or plate it, or something. But fractures join without surgeons needing to immobilize them.

An anthropologist named Schultz dug up the bones of 118 wild apes and found evidence of 65 fractures. And they had all joined — except in one situation. The only place he found non-union was in the neck of the femur, where we still get non-union today. Clearly, most fractures in apes join without being immobilized. And it's no different in humans. Take the clavicle. It nearly always joins, though most of us treat a fractured clavicle simply with slings, which don't immobilize it at all. Short of plating, which is unnecessary, we can't immobilize a clavicle, but it still joins.

Of course most fractures join, whether they are immobilized or not; otherwise land animals could not have evolved. The interesting question is why — why do they join? This used to puzzle

[1] Royal College of Surgeons 35-43 Lincoln's Inn Fields London WC2A 3PN, UK

me until one day when I suddenly realized why they join. Fractures join . . . because the bone is broken. I know this sounds childish. If you want to sound scientific, you can call it a feedback mechanism, which it is. Movement at the fracture site — a site which is unacceptable to Nature — provokes callus, which prevents that movement. A typical feedback mechanism — though all it means is that fractures join because the bone is broken. McKibbin has verified this experimentally. He has shown that movement leads to callus, but if the fracture is held rigidly no callus forms. Clinically we knew this already. If a fractured femur is fixed with a very tight fitting nail there's no movement and no callus. But if the nail is loose, there is movement and callus forms.

So why treat fractures at all? Well, partly because they're painful, and partly to avoid malunion. So, if a fracture is displaced, we reduce it and then hold it to stop it hurting and to prevent redisplacement. But we only want to hold the fracture, the joints should be kept moving. Here we have a conflict. We're trying to hold something, and yet to move something nearby. We have two ways of resolving this conflict. With a fractured femur, for example, we can hold the reduction by traction and keep the knee moving while the fracture joins. Or we can hold it with a nail, again keeping the knee moving till the fracture joins. But there's a difference. With fixation the patient can go home much sooner — unless something goes wrong. It may get infected and then the patient might be in hospital for months and end up with a stiff knee. So we have a second conflict: speed versus safety. If we try to hurry, we take risks.

It is this dual conflict — hold vs move and speed vs safety — which I believe is at the heart of all fracture treatment. I call it the fracture quartet and these factors — hold, move, speed, and safety — are the ones we should consider when comparing our methods of treatment such as plaster, traction, and metal fixation.

With plaster the weak member of the quartet is "move" — the joints tend to get stiff. The broken bone bleeds, the blood clots, and if the limb is kept still in plaster everything sticks together. Especially if, like Lorenz Bohler in Vienna and Watson-Jones in England, we insist that the joints above and below the fracture must both be included in the plaster. But, as we've seen, fractures join whether they're immobilized or not. So why include the joints?

With a fractured shaft of humerus, for example, perhaps a sling is enough. Then the patient can exercise the joints. And, because gravity holds the bone straight, the fracture should join in good position. But there's a snag. A sling may be satisfactory while the patient is standing up, but when the patient lies in bed or sits in an armchair the fracture angulates and that's painful. So its much kinder and more sensible to support the arm, in a cast-brace, leaving the shoulder and elbow free.

Sarmiento, the modern exponent of bracing, reported a series of 85 humeral shaft fractures treated in this way, and the only one which failed to join was through a secondary deposit. Functional bracing is an important technique and the principle is simple. A fractured shaft can't shorten or angulate much unless the soft tissues can expand. They can't expand if they're encircled by plaster or a plastic, so the fracture can't displace significantly; and the joints are free to move.

That was a fractured shaft. But with an articular fracture any kind of splint is bound to include the joint. And if we keep a fracture into a joint splinted, stiffness is inevitable. Salter showed why. He damaged the articular surface of rabbits' knees. If he kept them in plaster, they got adhesions and stiffness. If he kept them moving they healed and were fine.

Clearly what articular fractures need is movement. One way of achieving this is by internal fixation of the fracture, and in the hands of one of the great master surgeons the results are excellent. But what are the results when fixation is done not by a great master, but by an ordinary average surgeon? And we should always remember that most surgeons are average — that's what the word average means. The average surgeon is an average surgeon. Roberts in 1968 published the results of a large series of tibial plateau fractures treated by a number of different surgeons — some experienced, some not, so they constituted an average. And internal fixation didn't do very well, nor did plaster. Traction — skeletal traction through the upper tibia, came out best. And in 1983 Hayes presented a similar series; again traction came out best.

With traction, knee movements can begin early, as soon as the patient is comfortable enough to bend the knee on the bed. They can begin even earlier if the patient lets the knee bend through the bed passively, and then extends it actively. You can't do that on most hospital beds. So at my hospital we designed special beds and on these they move much better. We found that they sometimes moved so vigorously that they developed pin track sepsis. This was because friction was excessive and the pin rotated in the tibia. So we devised special swivels with ball bearings. These have almost no friction and now we have no problem with skeletal traction.

Using traction like that, 90% of our tibial plateau fractures have done well. Of course with internal fixation the great masters also get a 90% success rate. There's more than one way of treating a fracture. But traction is easier and safer than fixation, and you don't have to be a great master to get good results.

That was traction without a splint. Most people would say you couldn't treat a fractured femoral shaft in that way. You couldn't hold it well enough for it to join in good position. "Hold" would be the weak member, unless you used a splint — a Thomas splint. This splint was designed and made by Hugh Owen Thomas, the father of orthopedics. But he was a cantankerous individual and it is quite likely that his splint would have died with him but for his nephew, Robert Jones, who was not only a great surgeon, but was also loved by everyone. Now, in the First World War, gunshot fractures of the femur had a mortality of 80% — 80%! When Robert Jones became director of military orthopedics he introduced his uncle's splint and cut the mortality to 20%.

The Thomas splint was fine for transport, but used for definitive treatment it led to stiffness of the knee. So people modified it to permit knee movement. There were many modifications, but I think the best was the one devised by my old chief, George Perkins. He was a genius and this showed in the way he modified the splint — he simply threw it away. Because, he said, it wasn't the splint that mattered, it was the traction.

Does simple traction work? Well, Buxton in 1981 published a series of 54 consecutive femoral shaft fractures all treated by traction without a splint. And they all joined — non-union can occur with this method but is rare, and any mal-union is usually slight. So clearly "Hold" is *not* the weak member of the quartet. But there is a weak member: "Speed". Buxton's patients were in hospital for 12–16 weeks. Most people nowadays get them up much sooner, by applying a cast-brace as soon as the fracture is sticky, at 4–6 weeks. This method is safe and it works.

If we want to get the patient home quicker still we can, of course, fix the fracture with an intramedullary nail. Kuntscher made these popular during the Second World War. The German army depended on mobility and speed, with large numbers of motorbikes. So they had many fractured femurs and tibias. The quickest way of dealing with these was nailing, and if this meant taking risks — well, war is a risky business.

Nailing brings me to our third method of treatment, metal fixation. There are two main kinds. External fixation has improved enormously in the last 10 years. It is particularly useful for open fractures with a lot of soft tissue damage. Soft tissues heal better if the broken bone is held still. And once the soft tissues are healing the patient can be up and about while the fracture is uniting — though union may take a long time and, with very rigid fixation, it takes a very long time — because it's so rigid and callus doesn't form.

But if we want to fix a closed fracture, many surgeons prefer to use internal fixation. There's still a weak member of the quartet: safety. It's not safe — at least it's not always safe. Modern technology and antibiotics have made internal fixation much safer than it used to be. And about 25 years ago a group of Swiss surgeons founded AO, the Association for Osteosynthesis. They made fixation a science — precision engineering.

But AO doesn't stand for "Always Operate". It's all very well if a fit young man with a fracture is taken from the ski slopes to some wonderful new hospital, with all the equipment in the world. And if one of the great master surgeons is waiting to operate on him himself. But it's not like that everywhere. The patient may be scraped off a muddy road and taken to some little hospital with poor equipment, and there waiting for him is a young registrar, who's read about internal fixation and who's just waiting to have a try at it. Well, if this registrar fixes the fracture, we musn't be surprised if sometimes it ends up a mess. It is quite true that internal fixation can give excellent results, but it can also give terrible results.

The secret is to know how to do it and, even more important, when. The indications are difficult to formulate, because there are so many variables — the patient, the injury, the surgeon, the assistants, the equipment, the operating room — everything. I've found it best to teach that the indications are like a staircase. On the bottom step is the inexperienced surgeon with limited equipment; he or she should use internal fixation only when the alternatives (traction or plaster) are even more dangerous than unskilled surgery — as they may be with the elderly, for example. As the skill and equipment of the surgeon and the team increase, so the indications also may increase.

How do residents acquire their skill? Well, first they learn it by reading, by assisting, and by attending courses. Then they need practice. We used to practise on patients. But today we have plastic bones; residents can and should practise on dead bones — in a workshop. But they should practise *all* the methods of fracture treatment, not only fixation. Bracing is often done badly and skeletal traction very badly.

Only when surgeons have mastered all the methods of treatment can they treat any fracture — and only then can they answer our original question: "How should we treat fractures?". And that, as far as fractures are concerned, is the Craft of Surgery. But "How should we treat people?"; that's much more difficult. That needs experience, judgment, kindness, and compassion — human qualities. That's the Art of Surgery — it needs time and humanity.

Bone Graft Substitutes in Fracture Management: Basic Science and Clinical Results

ROBERT W. BUCHOLZ[1]

Summary. The experimental and clinical results of several osteoconductive, porous calcium phosphate ceramic materials were studied. Interporous hydroxyapatite, derived from a South Pacific coral, has proven to be as effective as autogenous cancellous bone for the filling of traumatic metaphyseal defects. Collagraft, a composite of hydroxyapatite/tricalcium phosphate ceramic, bovine dermal collagen, and autogenous bone marrow aspirate, is effective in the filling of comminuted cortical defects. These materials are biocompatible, bioinert, and osteoconductive. When used in conjunction with rigid internal fixation, they are as effective as autogenous graft, with the possible exception of their use in segmental diaphyseal fractures. The major complication with these materials has been slow bone remodeling and a slightly higher refracture rate. Definition of their role in the routine filling of traumatic bony defects awaits further experimental and clinical studies.

Key words. Bone graft substitute — hydroxyapatite — tricalcium phosphate — composite

Introduction

A variety of porous calcium phosphate biomaterials has been studied over the last 15 years as bone graft substitutes. These osteoconductive implants share certain properties which make them promising as substitutes for standard bone autografts and allografts. In addition to having pore dimensions and configurations which mimic those of either cancellous or cortical bone, these ceramic materials are, to a variable degree, bioinert and bioabsorbable. Bone has an affinity to regenerate on the surfaces of these ceramic materials, and the rate of new bone formation appears to be equivalent to that in conventional bone grafts. The two major bone graft substitutes which have been investigated to date are a biologically-derived block form of hydroxyapatite called interporous hydroxyapatite and a composite of calcium phosphate ceramic with bovine dermal collagen called Collagraft.

Interporous Hydroxyapatite

Although hydroxyapatite implants have been fabricated from several different scleractinian reef-building corals, most research has focused on the block hydroxyapatite from a coral genus named *Goniopora*. The exoskeleton of *Goniopora* coral has longitudinal channels of 500 to 600 μm in diameter with interconnecting fenestrations averaging 260 μm in diameter. The average wall (trabecular) thickness is 130 μm. These pore dimensions of the exoskeleton are continuous and interconnected throughout the coral.

The hydroxyapatite implant from this coral exoskeleton is formed by a simple hydrothermal exchange reaction which converts the calcium carbonate structure of the coral into pure hydroxyapatite [1,2]. During this chemical conversion, the unique microarchitecture of the coral exoskeleton is maintained, but all of the organic material is removed. The resultant brittle hydroxyapatite implant, called inter-

[1] Department of Orthopedic Surgery, University of Texas, Southwestern Medical School Dallas, TX 75235-8883, USA

Fig. 1. a Cross section and **b** longitudinal section of interporous hydroxyapatite derived from *Goniopora* coral. (original magnification ×3)

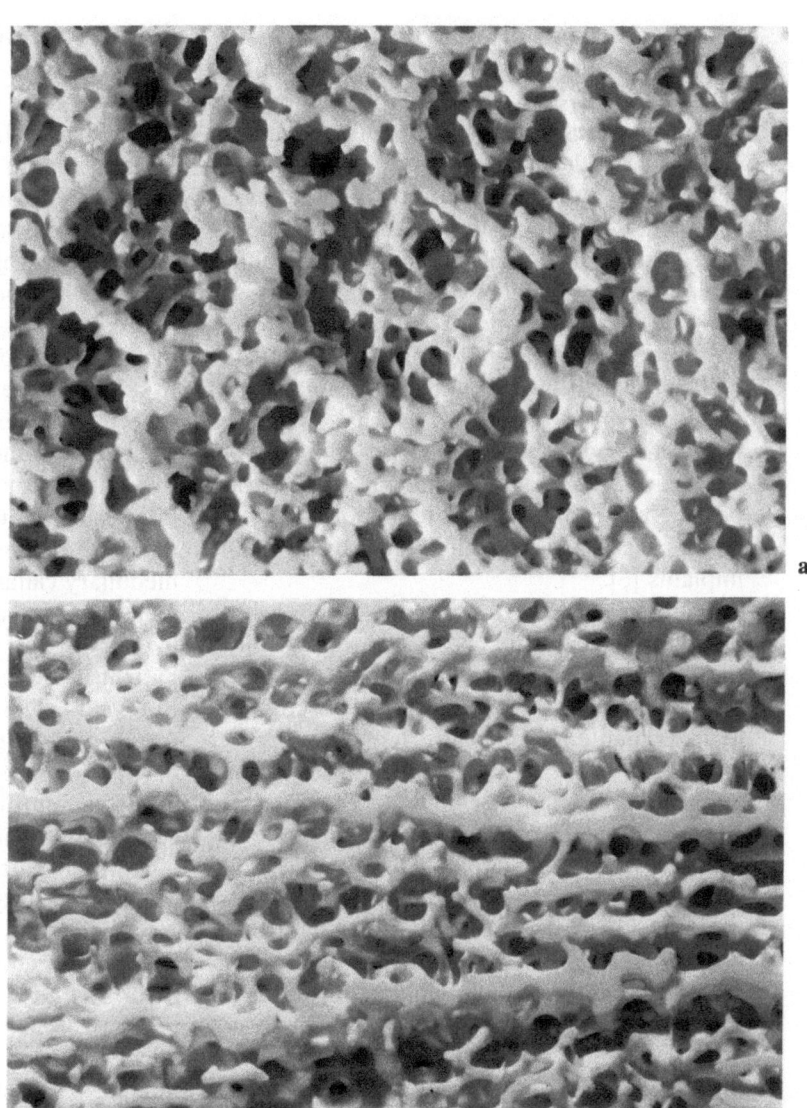

porous hydroxyapatite, has pore dimensions which closely match those of human cancellous bone (Fig. 1).

Basic Research with Interporous Hydroxyapatite

Several animal models have been used to test the efficacy of interporous hydroxyapatite in the filling of long bone defects. In a proximal tibial metaphyseal model in dogs, a 1cm^3 defect along the anterior lateral aspect of the proximal metaphysis was made bilaterally. On one side, a block of interporous hydroxyapatite was contoured to the defect, and on the contralateral side, a similar sized cortical cancellous graft from the iliac crest was used. Radiographic and histomorphometric techniques were used to assess the amount of bone regeneration in the bilateral defects at 2, 4, 6, and 12 months. On the hydroxyapatite side, the specimens contained compact (cortical) bone along the external surface of the implant in the area of the cortical window. The interior of the hydroxyapatite in the area of the medullary canal was filled with trabecular bone. The volume fractions of soft tissue, bone, and hydroxyapatite were approximately 52%, 13%, and 35%, respectively. The total amount of bone regeneration into the hydroxyapatite implants at the various study intervals was comparable to that in the contralateral autograft specimens. Histologically, the regenerated bone stained well with Alizarin and showed multiple osteoid seams. In none of the specimens was there a fibrous membrane between the regenerated bone and the underlying hydroxyapatite surface. The cellular elements within the implants were consistent with what was seen in normal bone with regard to simultaneous apposition, maintenance, and turnover of new bone. No inflammatory or immunologically reactive cells were noted within the hydroxyapatite implants [3].

While the amount of regenerated bone within the hydroxyapatite appeared to be equivalent to that within the autograft, determination of the mechanical properties of the regenerated bone/hydroxyapatite composite required further animal studies [4]. Mechanical testing of the implant alone demonstrated that its compressive strength ranged from 412N/cm^2 with the compressive load applied parallel to the channel axes, to 84N/cm^2 with the load applied perpendicular to the channel axes. However, similar mechanical testing of *Goniopora* implants 6 months after implantation demonstrated ultimate strengths up to 3500N/cm^2. This increase in strength of the implant over time with bone regeneration into its pores parallels what is seen in cancellous autografts inserted for similar periods of time. The increased strength of both cancellous graft and *Goniopora* grafts in a tibial metaphyseal defect in dogs was attributed to the onlay of new bone on the trabeculae of graft or hydroxyapatite. While the strength of the bone/hydroxyapatite composite may change over time with bone remodeling, it appears that there is no significant difference, after approximately 3 months, in the mechanical properties of the hydroxyapatite compared to those of cancellous bone. It was concluded that while the hydroxyapatite implant is quite brittle and weak at the time of implantation, the mechanical properties of the implant, with rapid bone regeneration into the implant pores, quickly approach those of autogenous cancellous grafts.

Clinical Studies

Approval from the Food and Drug Administration for human investigation with interporous hydroxyapatite in traumatic defects of long bones was obtained in 1982. The protocol for its use included both metaphyseal and diaphyseal bony defects, although the majority of patients enrolled had periarticular fractures with metaphyseal defects. The material was provided in block form and was fashioned intraoperatively to fill any size of metaphyseal or diaphyseal defect. The majority of the fractures were treated by standard techniques of open reduction and internal fixation with rigid immobilization of the major fracture fragments. Any bone defects in either the trabecular bone of the medullary canal or the cortex of the bone were measured, and an appropriate sized block of the hydroxyapatite was contoured and inserted. All patients were followed at regular intervals for up to 8 years. The results were assessed according to clinical function and radiographic appearance of the fracture. While no concurrent control group was enrolled in the study, the results were compared to historical controls at two of the institutions participating in the study.

The clinical and radiographic results in over 150 patients with long term follow-up have been analyzed. No adverse reactions to the hydroxyapatite have been apparent. The time to union, functional outcome, and rate of complications have been similar in the study and in control populations. Serial radiographs have shown no evidence of a radiolucent line around the hydroxyapatite suggesting a fibrous interface between the hydroxyapatite and the surrounding bone. No fragmentation of the hydroxyapatite was apparent in any case where stable fixation of the fracture was achieved. Radiographs up to 8 years following implantation, however, have shown little evidence of biodegradation of the hydroxyapatite. The porous architecture of the hydroxyapatite was still clearly visible on long-term radiographs.

Included within the larger series of 150 patients was a smaller pilot study population with tibial plateau fractures. Forty patients with closed tibial plateau fractures and associated metaphyseal defects treated between 1981 and 1985 were randomized into either an autogenous bone graft control group or an interporous

Fig. 2. a Anteroposterior and lateral radiographs of a split-compression type of lateral plateau fracture. **b** Postoperative radiographs demonstrate an anatomic reduction with buttressing of the osteochondral fragments with a large block of radiodense hydroxyapatite

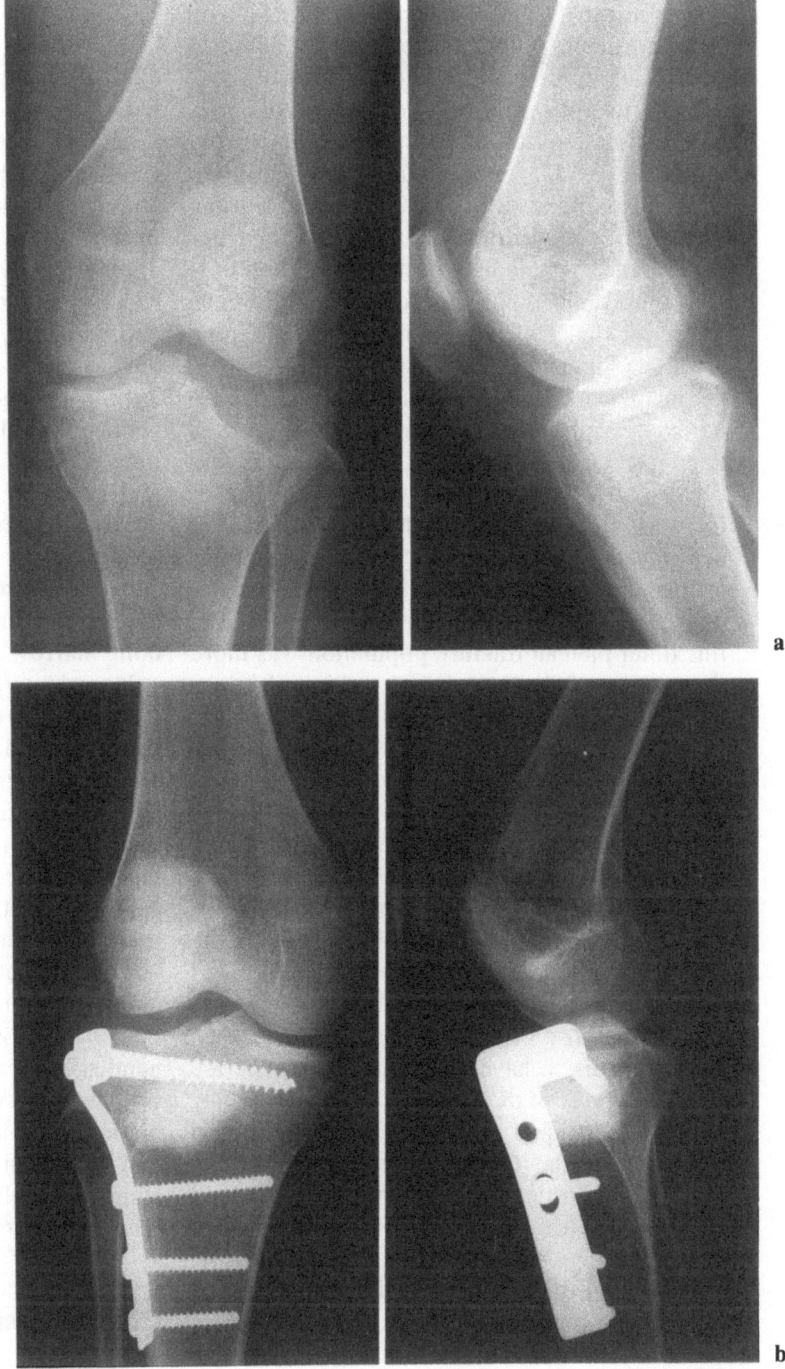

hydroxyapatite group. The purpose of this specific study was to assess the results with the hydroxyapatite implant compared to autogenous controls in a specific fracture pattern with all variables controlled. The demographic data on the study ($n = 20$) and control ($n = 20$) groups were comparable, as was the degree of comminution, the fracture patterns, and the amount of fracture displacement. At final follow-up examination (15.4 months after surgery for the autograft controls and 34.5 months after surgery for the hydroxyapatite implant patients), the results in the two groups were comparable. The time to fracture union, as measured by obliteration of all major fracture lines, averaged 2.5–3 months in both groups. The amount of articular depression at follow-up was equal in the two groups. Eleven autograft cases and 15 hydroxyapatite cases had no progressive settling of the articular surfaces, as judged by comparison of the immediate postoperative and final follow-up radiographs. There was no difference in the incidence of post-traumatic degenerative arthritis. Similarly, there was no difference in the incidence of complications, including painful hardware, infection, soft tissue problems, and knee instability. From this randomized study on tibial plateau fractures, it was concluded that for this specific fracture, the block form of hydroxyapatite was as effective as corticocancellous autograft for the filling of any metaphyseal defects. (Fig. 2) The clinical outcome in this tibial plateau fracture population was more dependent on the severity of the initial injury and the presence of any postoperative complications than it was on the use of either autograft or hydroxyapatite to fill the fracture defects [5].

It is concluded from these experimental and clinical studies that: (1) interporous hydroxyapatite is biocompatible, but does not biodegrade at an appreciable rate, (2) while the material itself is quite brittle, once regenerated bone fills its pores, its mechanical properties are similar to those of autogenous bone graft, (3) bone appears to have an affinity to regenerate on the surfaces of the hydroxyapatite, especially within the unique pore size and configuration provided by the *Goniopora* material, (4) the material is most effective when it is surrounded by viable cancellous or cortical bone, and (5) its clinical use should be limited to traumatic metaphyseal defects until further experimental and clinical data are available. The major concern with the material has been with its effect on bone remodeling. There have been three cases of refracture following use of the hydroxyapatite in a diaphyseal location. Because of its potentially adverse effect on bone remodeling, porous hydroxyapatite (in shaft fractures of long bones) is probably contraindicated. Its proper place in the management of long bone fractures will not be definitively defined until further experimental and clinical research is performed.

Collagraft Bone Graft Substitute

Collagraft is a composite of granular hydroxyapatite-tricalcium phosphate, bovine dermal collagen, and autogenous bone marrow aspirate. The porous calcium phosphate ceramic consists of granules approximately 0.5–1.0 mm in diameter. The granules are composed of approximately 65% hydroxyapatite and 35% tricalcium phosphate, with a pore volume of approximately 70%. The fibrillar collagen is 95% Type 1 collagen with small amounts of Type 3 collagen, and is similar to the fibrillar collagen used for dermal injections. At the time of application, 2.5 gm vials of the ceramic and 2.5 ml of fibrillar collagen are mixed. Immediately prior to insertion, 2 cc of autogenous bone marrow aspirated from the iliac crest is added to the composite. For larger sized defects, greater amounts of the ceramic, collagen, and bone marrow aspirate can be added.

Experimental work has focused on the use of Collagraft in diaphyseal defects of long bones [6]. In an ulnar defect model of the dog, Collagraft was found to be nearly as effective as autogenous cancellous bone, as measured by time to union and strength of the regenerated bone. Further studies have shown it to be clearly superior to either the ceramic granules alone or the bovine collagen alone.

The concept for this composite is that the ceramic and collagen provide an osteoconductive matrix for bone regeneration, while the autogenous bone marrow provides osteoprogenitor cells and growth factors to stimulate bone formation. Because of its potential osteoinductive and osteogenic properties, Collagraft has been clinically applied in more demanding fractures than has the *Goniopora* hydroxyapatite.

Clinical Results

Starting in September 1986, a multicenter prospective randomized study comparing Collagraft to autogenous cancellous bone graft has been conducted under the auspices of the Food and Drug Administration. Two hundred and sixty-seven patients with traumatic defects of long bones have been enrolled to date. These include 128 patients receiving cancellous autograft and 139 patients receiving Collagraft.

Only adult patients between the ages of 18 and 70 with a fracture of the humerus, radius, ulna, femur or tibia were enrolled. Any fracture older than 30 days was excluded. Similarly, any open fracture of grade 3B or 3C and pathologic fractures were excluded.

All study patients were randomized by computer-generated random block order into test and control groups. All patients were prospectively followed by physical examinations, serial radiographs, and reporting of all adverse events and complications. An independent radiologist performed the blinded, non-biased evaluation of the radiographs.

Analysis of the data at the 6- and 12-month follow-up visits showed the results in the control and study populations were equivalent. The mean operative time for the Collagraft group was approximately 30 min shorter than that for the autograft group. The radiographic scores judging union and bone regeneration showed no statistical difference between the Collagraft and autograft groups. There were 12 (7.5%) wound healing complications in the Collagraft group and 20 (13.3%) in the autogenous control group, including complications at the iliac crest donor site. The Collagraft group included 9 fracture site infections, while the control group had 13. There were six cases of loss of fixation and seven cases of delayed union and nonunion in the Collagraft group for an overall fracture healing complication rate of 8.1%. The overall rate of fracture healing complications in the control group was 6%, including two cases of loss of fixation and seven cases of delayed union and nonunion. There have been three refractures in the Collagraft group and one refracture in the control group. Overall, there was no statistically significant difference in the clinical or radiographic results between the control and study populations [7].

Discussion

After nearly 15 years of experimental and human investigation, certain conclusions regarding ceramic bone graft substitute materials can be made. First, these calcium phosphate biomaterials appear to be bioinert without inciting any immunological or inflammatory reaction. Bone appears to have an affinity to grow on the surfaces of these materials, especially those composed primarily of hydroxyapatite. Primary lamellar bone regenerates on the surface of the implants without any preliminary fibrous or cartilaginous stage of tissue ingrowth. Second, these materials are mechanically brittle and weak. When subjected to the normal loading of long bones, they tend to fragment, thus losing their osteoconductive properties. Any use in a fracture setting, therefore, necessitates rigid internal or external fixation of the bone to prevent such loading during the early stages of fracture repair. Third, when used in a block form, these materials function as well as, if not better than, morsellized autogenous graft for the maintenance of position of articular fragments. They have an excellent spacer effect, while at the same time providing a matrix for bone regeneration. Fourth, the usefulness of these materials for acute diaphyseal fractures is limited. Even with the addition of collagen and autogenous bone marrow aspirate, the rapidity and amount of callus is less than what is seen with standard autogenous cancellous graft. While no difference in the clinical or radiographic results is evident in diaphyseal fractures with mild degrees of comminution, segmental defects of long bones represent a more demanding indication for the material and their efficacy in this setting is as yet unproven. Fifth, these materials are especially helpful in the avoidance of bone graft donor site morbidity [8]. As with bone bank allograft, these materials eliminate such problems as chronic pain, wound complications, and skeletal defects, which often accompany iliac crest and other donor site harvesting of bone graft.

The major disadvantage of these ceramic materials is their potentially adverse effect on bone remodeling. The hydroxyapatite phase of the ceramic is bioabsorbed at a very slow (nonappreciable) rate. Radiographs at 8 years following implantation do not appear to be appreciably different from immediate postoperative radiographs with regard to the density or quantity of ceramic. Despite the feasibility of aligning the longitudinal pores of the ceramic in line with the weight bearing forces of the long bone, the composite of ceramic and regenerated bone is biomechanically inferior to normal corticocancellous bone. In areas of high stress concentration, such as the shaft of a long bone, the presence of the hydroxyapatite jeopardizes the strength of the bone and may predispose to recurrent fracture. Although there has been no statistically significant difference in the rate of refracture to date, longer term follow-up studies will be necessary.

References

1. Weber JN, White EW (1973) Carbonate materials as precursors to new ceramic and polymer materials for biomedical applications. Min Sci Eng 5:151
2. Roy DM, Linnehan SK (1974) Hydroxyapatite formed by coral skeletal carbonate by hydrothermal exchange. Nature 247:220
3. Holmes RE, Bucholz RW, Mooney V (1986) Porous hydroxyapatite as a bone graft substitute in metaphyseal defects. J Bone Joint Surg 68A: 904–911
4. Holmes RE, Mooney V, Bucholz RW (1984) A coralline hydroxyapatite bone graft substitute: Preliminary report. Clin Orthop 188:252–262
5. Bucholz RW, Carlton A, Holmes RE (1989) Interporous hydroxyapatite as a bone graft substitute in tibial plateau fractures. Clin Orthop 240:53–62
6. Moore DC, Chapman MW, Marske D (1987) The evaluation of a biphasic calcium phosphate ceramic for use in grafting long bone defects. J Orthop Res 5:356–365
7. Cornell CN, Lane JM, Chapman MW, et al. (1991) Multicenter trial of Collagraft as bone graft substitute. J Orthop Trauma 5:1–8
8. Younger EM, Chapman MV (1989) Morbidity at bone graft donor sites. J Orthop Trauma 3: 192–195

Embryology of Human Meniscus

HANS K. UHTHOFF and JUN KUMAGAI[1]

Summary. The development of the menisci was studied in knees of 94 human embryos and fetuses. As early as the 7th week of gestation, menisci can be observed as triangular cell condensations. Around the 10th week, blood vessels appear at the periphery of the menisci. Later on they penetrate into the outer third of the menisci. Only in the anterior and posterior horns can vessels be seen in the tip of the menisci. We found no evidence that menisci evolve through a discoid stage nor did we find a single discoid meniscus. During the prenatal period, the matrix of the menisci consists of collagen; no fibrocartilage could be detected.

Key words. Human meniscus — Embryology — Blood supply to meniscus — Discoid meniscus

Introduction

Although the intrauterine development of the human meniscus has been of interest to researchers and clinicians, three questions remain unresolved:

- Do menisci evolve through a discoid stage and does the discoid meniscus therefore indicate a lack of normal development? or is it a malformation? Despite the fact that many studies have failed to show a discoid meniscus in the fetal stages, a more detailed study may reveal some clues as to its development.
- The second question deals with the exact distribution of blood vessels in menisci and thus the mode of nutrition of these structures. Whereas certain studies describe the fetal meniscus as a well vascularized structure, in adults the lack of blood vessels inside the meniscus proper is well known [1]. If such a difference exists, when does the change occur?
- Another question, less often raised, deals with the kind of tissue. In children and adults, the menisci are composed of fibrocartilage. Is fibrocartilage already formed during the fetal period or does it develop after birth, in response to loading?

The present study was undertaken to clarify these questions.

Materials and Methods

Ninety-four spontaneously aborted embryos and fetuses aged 6 weeks to term, obtained from the Bone and Joint Research Laboratory, University of Ottawa, form the basis of this study. In accordance with Provincial laws, none of the specimens was processed before 3 months had elapsed after abortion. Having measured C-R (Crown-Rump) length and estimated the period of gestation and the stage of embryonic development according to Streeter [2], we fixed all embryos and fetuses in 10% neutral formalin. All embryos were sectioned in toto; in fetuses, the knees were removed and decalcified with EDTA (ethlenediaminetetraacetic acid), embedded in paraffin, then serially cut in either a sagittal or a frontal direction. The sections

[1] Bone and Joint Research Laboratory, Division of Orthopaedic Surgery, Ottawa General Hospital, University of Ottawa, Ottawa, Ontario, Canada K1H 8L6

were stained by Azan, Goldner's Trichrome, or HPS (hematoxyline phloxine safranine).

Results

The intrauterine development of the menisci will be divided into several stages:

1. Formation of a uniform interzone
2. Formation of a three layered interzone
3. Meniscal cell differentiation
4. Collagenous matrix formation inside menisci

Formation of a Uniform Interzone

An interzone of uniform cellular density between the cartilaginous anlages of femur and tibia can be observed at 6 weeks (stage 17 according to Streeter [2]) (Fig. 1).

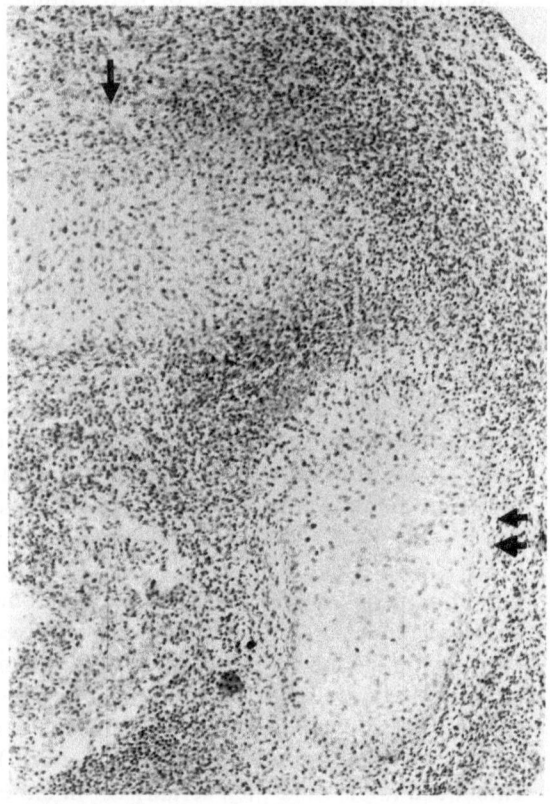

Fig. 1. Embryo 117N, 6 weeks. Sagittal section. The anlages of the femoral condyle (*arrow*) and tibia (*double arrow*) are separated by an interzone of uniform cell density. Goldner ×37.5

Formation of Three-Layered Interzone

In frontal sections of 6½ week old embryos, the triangular formation of increased cellular density indicates the developing menisci. Their presence can be observed with greater ease at 7 weeks (stage 19), (Fig. 2) when a layer of decreased cell density separates this structure from the femoral condyles leading to a three layered interzone. At the end of the embryonic period (8 weeks, stage 23), the cells of the menisci are round and randomly arranged. The superficial cells begin to exhibit an orientation parallel to the joint surface. Cavitation begins at about the same time. Cavitation denotes the presence of slits in the loose celled layer between the menisci and the anlages of the femur and tibia (Fig. 3). With time, they become confluent.

Meniscal Cell Differentiation

A layer of decreased cell density now separates the menisci from the tibial plateaus. Sagittal sections through the midline of the knee show a blastema of uniform density, whereas more medial or lateral sections permit menisci with plump cells in them to be distinguished. More superficially the meniscal cells start to become flatter.

By 10 weeks, the densely-celled menisci can be easily distinguished from a loose-celled tissue peripherally which contains blood vessels. The beginning of collagen formation inside both menisci is also noted (Fig. 4).

Collagenous Matrix Formation Inside Menisci

At 12 weeks, some blood vessels penetrate the peripheral third of both menisci. The collagen content has increased. A joint cavity is now formed (Fig. 5). The orientation of collagen fibers becomes obvious at 14 weeks; it is parallel to the joint surface on the inner part of the menisci. At that stage, the superficial cells of both menisci form a layer of cells which are flatter than the deeper cells (Fig. 6a,b).

At 18 weeks, in frontal serial section, blood vessels reach the tip of the lateral meniscus. The following serial sections, however, reveal that this has occurred at the anterior horn in proximity to the meniscal attachment. In none

Fig. 2. Embryo 150N, 7 weeks. Frontal section. The triangular formation of increased cell density indicates a developing meniscus. A layer of decreased cell density separates this structure from the femoral condyle (*arrow*), thus creating a three-layered interzone. Goldner ×150

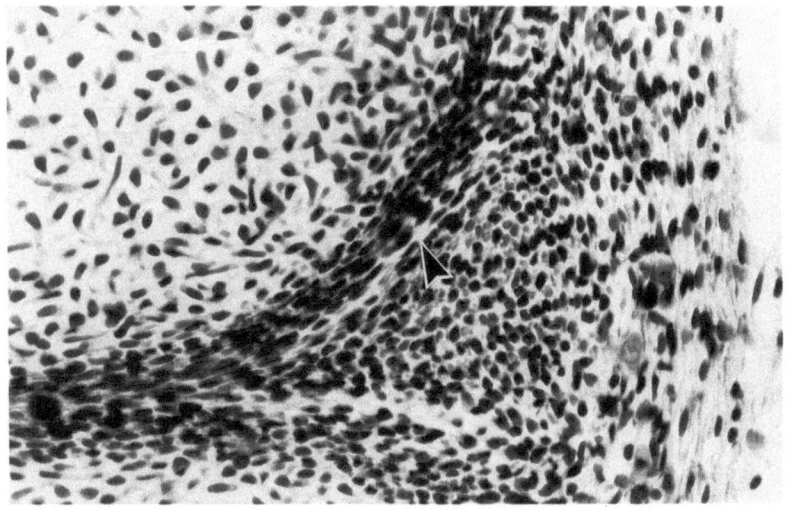

Fig. 3. Embryo 72, 8 weeks. Frontal section. The cells of the meniscus are round and randomly arranged. Multiple slits (cavitations) are also visible between femur and tibia (*arrows*). HPS ×150

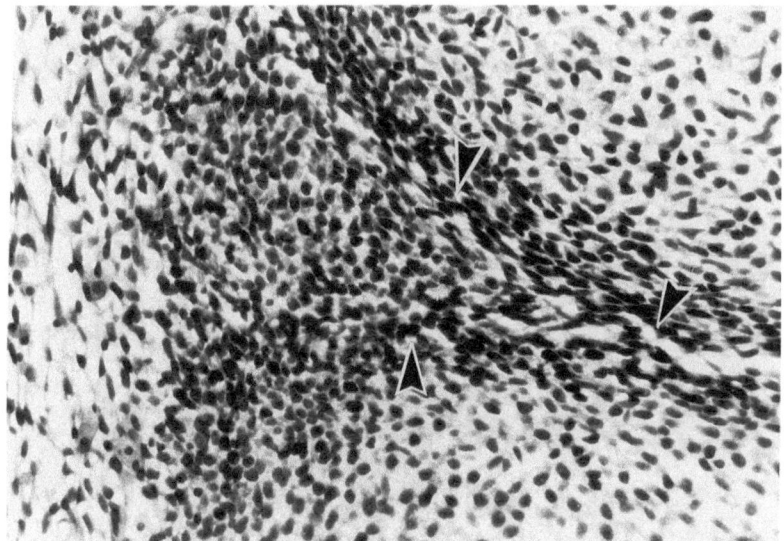

Fig. 4. Fetus 12, 10 weeks. Frontal section of the medial meniscus. The shape of the meniscus is now obvious. It can be clearly distinguished from the loose peripheral tissue. Note early blood vessel formation (*arrow*) at the periphery of the meniscus. HPS ×100

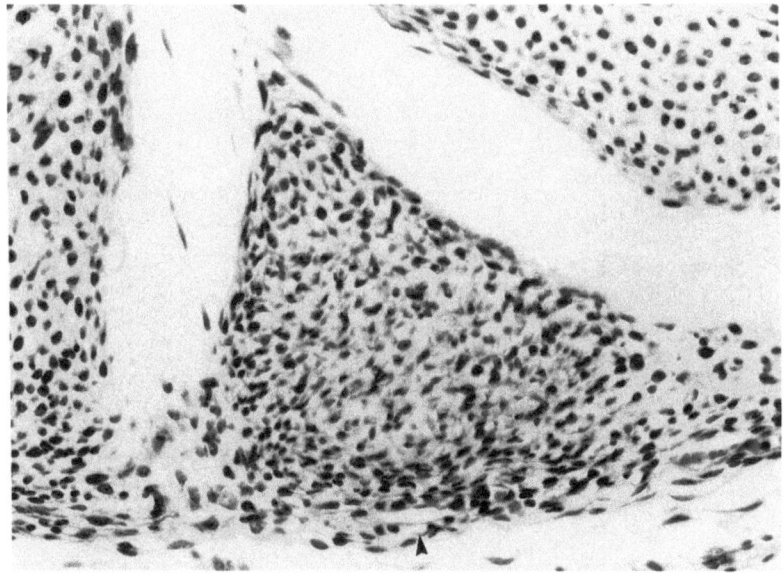

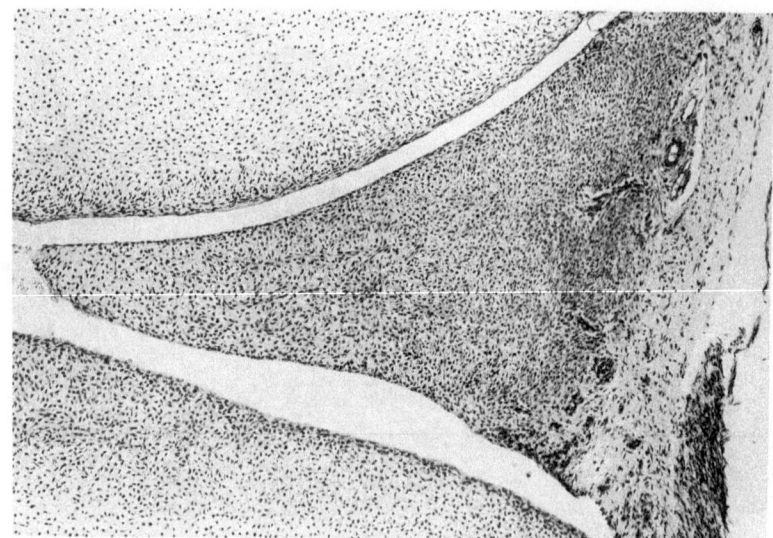

Fig. 5. Fetus 14N, 12 weeks. Frontal section of the lateral meniscus. Blood vessels penetrate the peripheral third of the meniscus. Goldner ×25

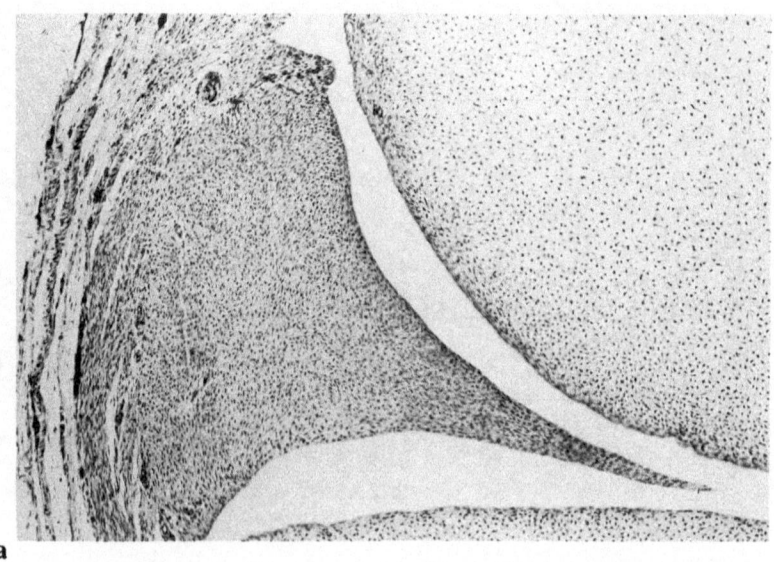

a

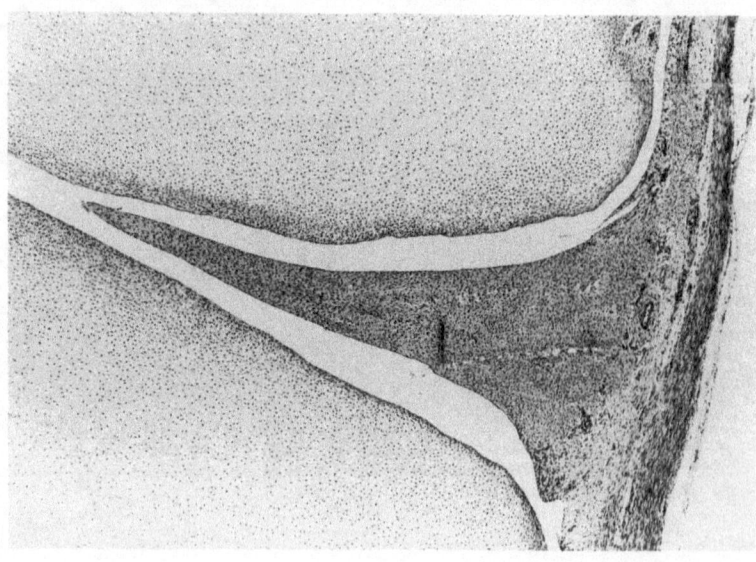

b

Fig. 6a,b. Fetus 41N, 14–14½ weeks. Frontal section of the middle segment of both menisci **a**, medial and **b**, lateral. The superficial cells are flatter than the more deeper cells. Their orientation is parallel to the joint surface. Vessels are located at the outer third of menisci. Goldner **a** ×25; **b** ×7.5

Fig. 7. Fetus 146, 20 weeks. Frontal section of lateral meniscus. The collagenous content of the matrix has increased. No fibrocartilage is seen. Goldner ×7.5

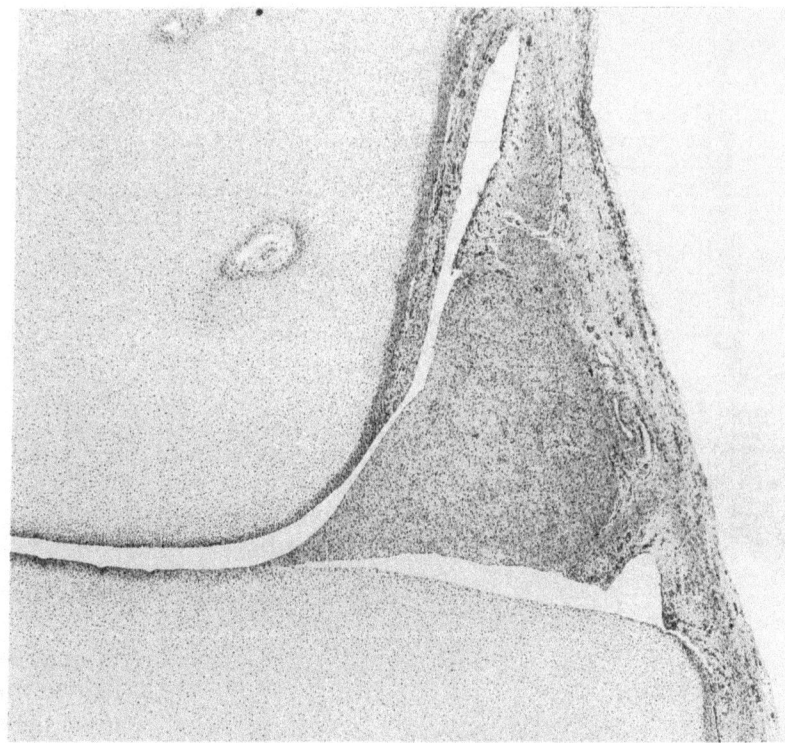

of the other sections could blood vessels be seen to penetrate deeper than the outer third of the menisci. A phenomenon similar to the anterior horn can be seen at the posterior horn.

At 20 weeks, the transition from menisci to peripheral tissues is still abrupt. The collagen content of menisci has further increased but there is no evidence of fibrocartilage (Fig. 7).

At term, there is essentially no change in the blood supply to both menisci. Also, there is no fibrocartilage (Fig. 8a,b).

In none of our specimens could we observe the presence of a completely discoid meniscus.

Discussion

Though the discoid meniscus was once considered a temporary feature during the embryonic period [3], Kaplan [4] and Levine and Blazina [5], among other authors, refuted such a view, based on examination of embryos and fetuses, and stated that this feature was not present during the embryonic or fetal periods. Later on, Smillie revised his assumption [6]. Our results also failed to show evidence of the so-called primitive or infantile type of meniscus. To find

evidence of discoid menisci in the fetal period, a detailed investigation of the posterior horn of the lateral meniscus seems of particular interest. However, even in frontal sections, which should demonstrate this part better than sagittal ones, we were unable to exactly reconstruct the posterior horn and its ligamentous attachment to the medial femoral condyle. We believe that horizontal sections of the knee joint are essential for that purpose.

From the point of view of meniscal repair, knowledge of the blood supply to the meniscus is of paramount importance. In adults, microvascular studies were established by Arnoczky and Warren [1], and similar studies were done in adults and in one fetus by Day et al. [7], showing a more extensive vascular pattern in the fetus which may allow greater reparative potential in the developing meniscus.

Gray and Gardner showed that more vessels are present in the anterior and posterior part of menisci at 19½ weeks, and that some of them reach the inner free margin between 30½ and 32 weeks [8]. McDermott documented the extension of blood vessels into the tips of menisci at 18 weeks [9]. He failed, however, to exactly localize the vessels. Our study seems to confirm Gray and Gardner's observation: the vessels

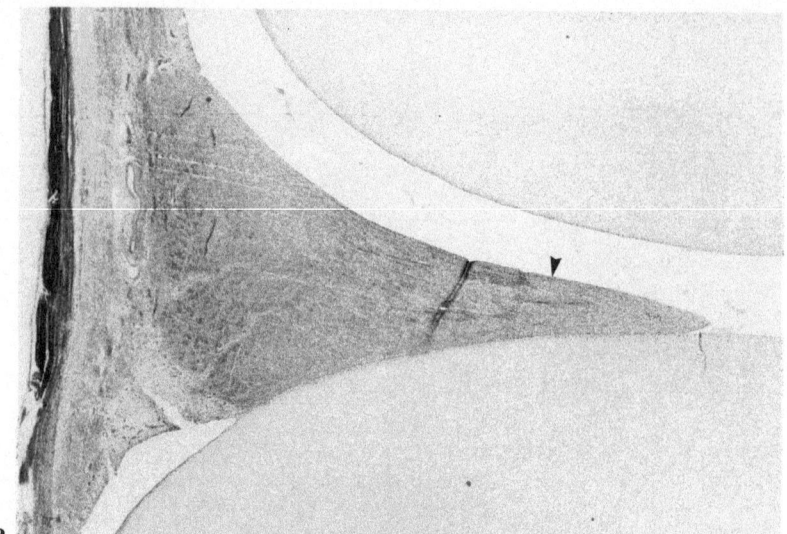

Fig. 8a,b. Fetus A 10917, at term. Frontal section, posterior horn of lateral meniscus. Note the presence of small vessels in the tip of the meniscus (*arrows*). Goldner **a** ×7.5; **b** ×37.5

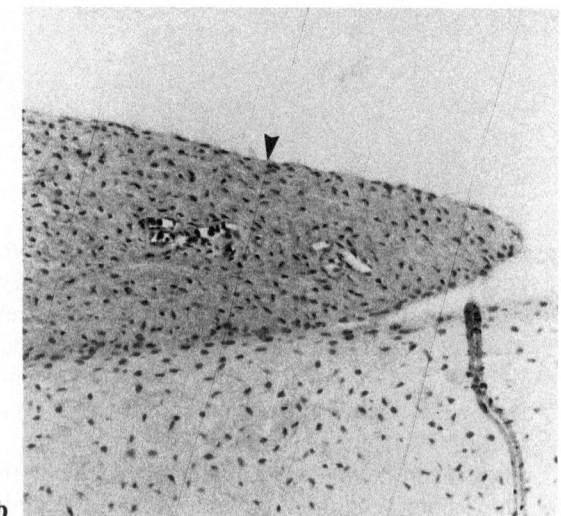

Conclusions

1. In none of the 94 knees from embryos and fetuses could a discoid meniscus be observed.
2. From the early fetal stage on, the inner two-thirds of both menisci are devoid of blood vessels. Their source of nutrition must be different from that of the outer third and that of the anterior and posterior horn.
3. During the entire fetal period, the menisci do not contain any fibrocartilage.

References

1. Arnoczky SP, Warren RF (1982) Microvasculature of the human meniscus. Am J Sports Med 10:90–5
2. Streeter GI (1951) Developmental horizons in human embryos. Carnegie Institution, Washington
3. Smillie IS (1948) The congenital discoid meniscus. J Bone Joint Surg [Br] 30:671–682
4. Kaplan EB (1955) The embryology of the menisci of the knee joint. Bull Hosp Jt Dis 16:111–124
5. Levine EF, Blazina ME (1966) Investigations of the lateral meniscus. Surg Forum 17:443–444
6. Smillie IS (1951) Injuries of the knee joint, 2nd edn. ES Livingstone, Edinburgh, pp 69–75
7. Day B, MacKenzie WG, Shim SS, Leung G (1985) The vascular and nerve supply of the human meniscus. J Arthroscopy, 1:58–62
8. Gray DJ, Gardner E (1950) Prenatal development of the human knee and superior tibiofibular joints. Am J Anat 86:235–287

reaching the tip of the meniscus are limited to the posterior and anterior horns, beginning at an age of 18–20 weeks of gestation. Thus the main part of the meniscus is devoid of blood vessels. The nutrition of this part must be assured through diffusion.

Formation of fibrocartilage was not found in any specimen during the embryonic and fetal periods, supporting Gardner and O'Rahilly [10] who questioned the finding of Andersen [11], who had reported the presence of fibrocartilage in fetal specimens. Detailed studies in infants and children are needed to determmine the moment of transformation into fibrocartilage and its possible relationship to weight bearing.

9. McDermott LJ (1943) Development of the human knee joint. Arch Surg 46:705–719

10. Gardner E, O'Rahilly R (1968) The early development of the knee joint in staged human embryos. J Anat 102:289–99

11. Andersen H (1961) Histochemical studies on the histogenesis of the knee joint and superior tibiofubular joint in human fetuses. Acta Anat (Basel) 46:279–303

Etiology of Congenital Dislocation of the Hip Joint

KAZUO HIROSHIMA[1]

Summary. Although many anatomical, biochemical, and hereditary factors have been proposed as causative factors for congenital dislocation of the hip joint (CDH), the pathomechanism of CDH can not be explained by these factors alone. In addition to these factors, it is necessary to consider the special forces which lead the femoral head to dislocate from the acetabulum. Activated muscle tone and contraction are primary intrinsic forces that are developed by postural neurophysiological reflexes in a limited number of muscle groups. These forces, plus the increased tension of muscles and tendons around the hip joint, produced by passive extension of the hip and knee joints in the presence of flexion contractures of these joints, are considered to be especially important in the establishment of CDH. Under some conditions, e.g., in the presence of neonatal structural instability of the hip joint, neonatal joint laxity, increased antetorsion of the femur, or primary acetabular dysplasia, passive or explosive active extension of the iliopsoas and hamstring muscles affected by contractures can produce dislocating forces that work against keeping the femoral head in its proper position in the acetabulum. Prevention of CDH has been partially accomplished by improving the method of applying diapers and by permitting free movement of the lower extremities in the neonatal period. The elimination of CDH, however, will be very difficult until new diagnostic measures for early detection and new approaches to treatment are developed for such causative factors as primary acetabular dysplasia, familial joint laxity, and so on.

Key words. Congenital dislocation of the hip joint — Joint instability — Joint laxity — Postural effect on the hip joint — Acetabular dysplasia

[1] The Division of Orthopedics, Osaka National Hospital, Osaka, 540 Japan

Introduction

Congenital dislocation of the hip joint (CDH) was formerly regarded as a classical representative pediatric orthopedic disease, along with congenital clubfoot. These two pathological conditions (deformities) are also observed in patients with diseases such as arthrogryposis multiplex congenita, Larsen syndrome, and many other neuromuscular conditions. In some respects both pathological conditions may be clinically similar, but there are some definite differences between them. Over the last 25 years, the number of operations for CDH (open reduction, femoral and/or pelvic osteotomy) has been markedly decreased due to early screening and early treatment, while the number of surgical cases of congenital clubfoot has remained unchanged (Fig. 1). In many cases of CDH, anatomical reduction and healing can be achieved by proper treatment, in contrast to the difficulty of achieving anatomical healing in even meticulously treated cases of congenital clubfoot.

In contrast to congenital clubfoot, the onset of CDH is considered to be much influenced by the perinatal environment. Moreover, the fact that the incidence of CDH has been about 1/100 live births over the past 40–50 years in Japan, suggests that all neonates have some common factors which might predispose them to CDH.

Though the gross pathology of the hip joint in CDH has been reported on by many authors, no specific changes which can definitely be considered to cause CDH have been identified. Most of the described changes (increased

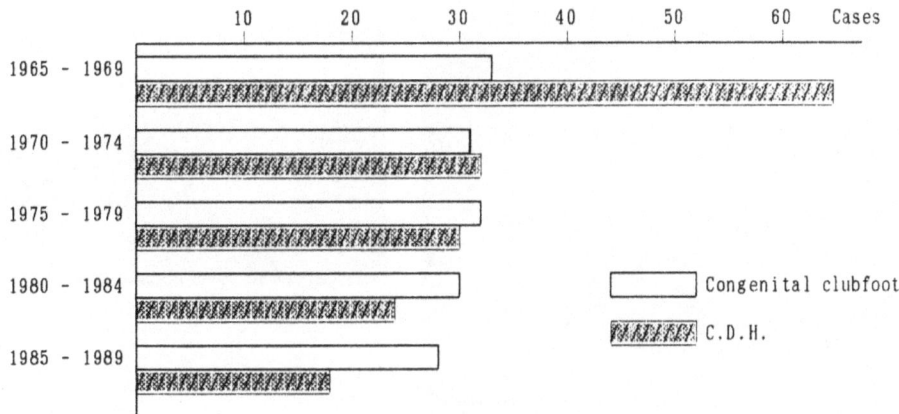

Fig. 1. Over 20 years, Comparison of the number of cases of open reduction for CDH and the number of surgical cases of congenital clubfoot over the last 20 years showing that the former has been markedly reduced, while the latter remained unchanged

antetorsion of the femur, shortened femoral neck, deformed femoral head, inverted limbus, hypertrophied and elongated ligamentum teres, fibrofatty mass, elongated joint capsule, impression on the acetabular rim, and ellipsoid deformity of the acetabular aperture) appear to be secondary changes that follow dislocation of the femoral head from the acetabulum.

The purpose of this paper is to describe several etiological factors that might cause CDH and to describe the possible pathomechanisms of CDH on the basis of recent studies.

Physiologically Unstable State of the Hip Joint During the Perinatal Period

The femoral head is deeply covered by the acetabular roof until the end of the second trimester, and after this period its size gradually increases disproportionately to the size of the acetabulum. During this period, the limbus plays an important role in stabilizing the femoral head in the acetabulum. This disproportion is marked in the 9th month of fetal life, and a steep and shallow cartilageous acetabulum with an overlarge femoral head is always observed in normally developed fetuses at autopsy [1]. According to Ralis, the ratio of the diameter of the acetabulum to that of the femoral head decreases to 70% by the time of birth [2]. This unstable state has also been confirmed clinically by ultrasonic examination [3]. When the hip joint in 90 degree

flexion is pushed posteriorily by axial compression, a certain amount of posterior instability of the femoral head is provoked, even in normally developed fetuses, but this instability normally disappears within 2 or 3 days after birth. Walker has reported that an abnormal impression on the acetabular rim or a deformed aperture of the acetabulum was observed at autopsy in 87% of 280 normal neonatal hip joints [4].

In conclusion, most neonatal hip joints are in an unstable condition that can lead to subluxation or dislocation if there are other factors that disturb hip stability.

Primary Acetabular Dysplasia and CDH

Almost all cases of CDH are associated with acetabular dysplasia, which is either of primary or secondary origin. Secondary acetabular dysplasia is defined as that which is caused by secondary growth disturbance following dislocation of the femoral head. In such an acetabulum, normal development would be expected if dislocation did not occur or if it were reduced anatomically at an early stage. Primary acetabular dysplasia, on the other hand, is a type of congenital hypoplasia of the pelvis and is considered to be a clinical entity distinct from CDH. Even though there have been no reports about the incidence of CDH in combination with primary acetabular dysplasia, such dysplasia is generally regarded as an important factor in

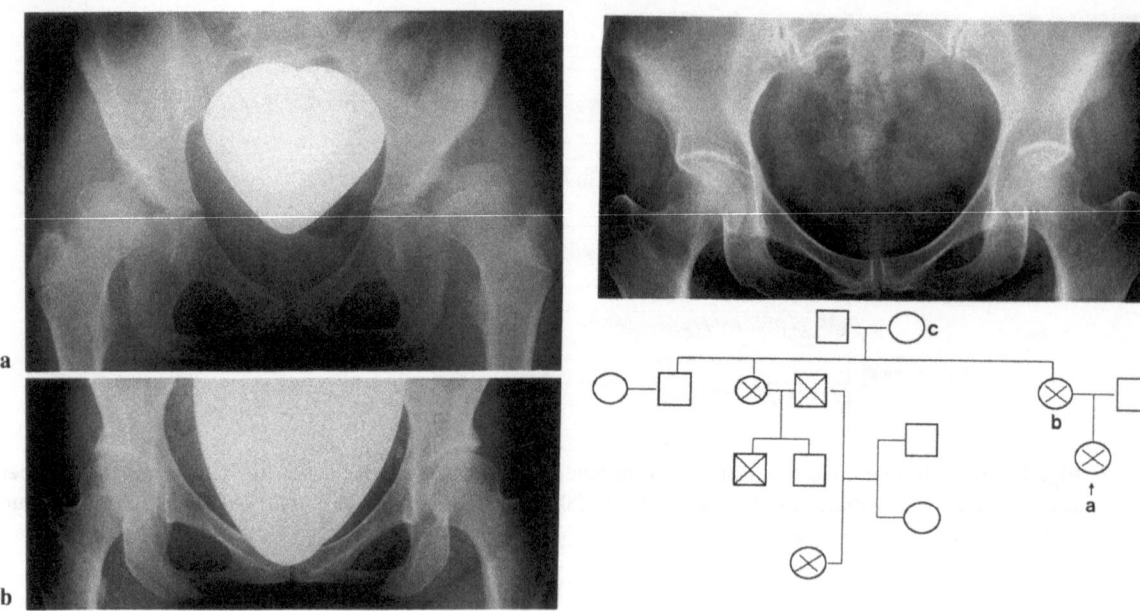

Fig. 2. a Family of the proband ([a]), who is a girl aged 8 years. She had closed manual reduction for bilateral CDH at the age of 1 year, after which she was not followed up by the orthopedic surgeon. She visited our department with coxalgia and low back pain when she was 8 years old. Marked bilateral acetabular dysplasia with subluxation was demonstrated on radiologic examination. **b** The child's mother ([b]) had also undergone closed reduction for left CDH during infancy. The mother is now 35 years old and she does not limp, nor does she have any coxalgia or dullness of the hip. Her X-ray picture shows mild acetabular dysplasia on the left side, without degenerative changes. **c** X-ray picture of the proband's grandmother ([c]), 65 years old, shows bilaterally normal hip joints. **d** Another four relatives were treated for CDH in infancy or early childhood

causing unstable hip joints, especially in the neonatal period. Figure 2 shows a CDH patient in whose family there were five members who suffered from CDH. The proband was treated conservatively in early infancy and the femoral heads have been concentrically kept in the acetabula, even though marked bilateral acetabular dysplasia has persisted. This is a typical case of primary acetabular dysplasia. Though the proband patient did not have generalized joint laxity at school age, the extent of joint instability at birth might have been more severe than at present, since normal neonatal joint laxity and structural instability of the hip (acetabulo-femoral disproportion) would have been present in addition to primary acetabular dysplasia.

Joint Laxity in the Neonatal Period

In normal neonates, temporary joint laxity, due to maternal hormones, is generally observed,

during the 2 or 3 days immediately after birth. This effect can be verified by urinary estriol measurements. Andren first reported the increased and prolonged urinary excretion of estriol in neonatal CDH [5]. By observation of vaginal smears in neonates, abnormal estrogen metabolism has also been pointed out in CDH patients [6]. The effect of estrogen on the laxity of ligamentocapsular tissue has been studied experimentally by several authors. It was found that estradiol had the strongest effect of all the estrogens in promoting joint laxity in the chicken [7], and that collagen production was inhibited by the combined administration of estrogen and progesterone [8]. Recently, a high ratio of type 3 to type 1 collagen was detected by the analysis of umbilical cord collagen in neonatal CDH [9]. The authors speculated that this increased ratio of type 3 to type 1 collagen indicated the immaturity of fetal collagen, and that such immaturity might be related to neonatal joint laxity in CDH.

Wynne-Davies reported on familial joint laxity in CDH patients and their families, and found that neonates with CDH had a higher frequency of joint laxity than patients with late-diagnosed CDH [10]. It was also reported that neonatal CDH tended to occur in families with joint laxity. The etiology of familial joint laxity might be some, as yet unknown, disturbance of collagen metabolism, rather than a disturbance of estrogen metabolism. Nevertheless, neonatal CDH patients with familial joint laxity would be more liable to be affected by the hyperfunction of estrogen metabolism that neonatal CDH patients without such a family history [11].

Fetal Presentation, Head Turning Predilection, Physiological Effects of Neural Reflexes on Motility of the Extremity, and CDH

Since the relationship of CDH and breech presentation was first reported by Vogel in 1905 [12], many authors have discussed this association, but no plausible explanation has yet been provided. Suzuki has reported differences between the incidence of CDH in cephalad and breech presentations [13]. Following single breech presentation, unstable hips in the neonatal period were present in 20% of infants, in contrast with a rate of 0.7% for cephalad presentation. Marked limitation of hip and knee extension, and hypertonicity of the hamstring muscles are co-existing problems that have been noted in neonates delivered by single breech presentation. The role of these prenatal postural deformities in the establishment of CDH will be discussed elsewhere.

Regarding postnatal postural deformities, it has been pointed out that the side of wryneck or the side of head turning predilection is related to the side on which CDH occurs [14,15]. In 92.0%−93.3% of neonates who have both CDH and wryneck/predilection for head turning, the side of head turning is related to the side on which occurs CDH, i.e., CDH occurs on the left side when the head turns towards the right and vice versa.

In the neonatal period, active flexion-extension movements of the upper and lower extremities are observed on the side of head turning, while the extremities on the opposite side are relatively inactive. Moreover, it has been confirmed by an electromyogram (EMG) study, using superficial electrodes, that the hip abductors on the side of head turning and the hip adductors on the other side were highly activated, even in neurologically normal cases [14]. Sakai observed gradual deterioration of the concentricity of the adducted hip joint when the direction of head turning was contralateral to the side of the adducted hip; this was considered to be related to the fetal position [16].

In conclusion, specific prenatal postural deformities related to breech presentation, specific postnatal effects of head turning on the muscular activity of the lower extremities, and a specific relationship between the side of CDH and the side of wryneck/direction of predilection for head turning are all considered to be important factors in the establishment of CDH.

Kinesiology and Pathomechanisms of CDH

Few reports have been written about the force required for the femoral head to dislocate from the acetabulum. This force can be divided into intrinsic and extrinsic components. Direct intrinsic force is produced by direct muscle contraction, e.g., the force produced by contraction of the iliopsoas and adductor muscles in paralytic hip dislocation corresponds to a direct intrinsic force. Indirect intrinsic force is produced by the stretching of contracted/shortened muscles and tendons. Direct extrinsic force acts on the femoral head as a dislocating force, rather than acting via the soft tissues, while indirect extrinsic force acts on contracted/shortened muscles and tendons to increase the tensile force. The indirect extrinsic force thus produces an indirect intrinsic force on the proximal femur, and this acts as a dislocating force. In this section several environmental factors related to indirect intrinsic force are discussed.

According to Wilkinson [17] and Michelson [18], dislocation of the hip joint was produced in young rabbits by rigid fixation of the knee in the extended position, while release of the hamstrings prevented dislocation. In 1974, Yamamuro reported that hypertonic hamstring muscles under the contracted/shortened iliopsoas muscle were an important factor in dislocation of the hip joint during rigid fixation of the rat knee joint in extension [19]. In 1975 Hinokida carried out a modified version of Michelson's experiment and showed a decreased incidence of dislocation and subluxation by release of the iliopsoas tendon [20]. In 1979 Hiroshima reported on the clinical pathology and surgical treatment of dislocation of the hip in cerebral palsy, the important findings being that dystonic contraction of the hamstring muscles caused dislocation of the femoral head from the acetabulum and that the femoral head was spontaneously reduced by fractional lengthening of the hamstring tendons [21].

Until 20 years ago, neonates in Japan were usually put in diapers by wrapping both hip joints in an extended and slightly adducted position. Until that time there was a very high incidence of CDH. However, since that time, a new method of putting on diapers with circumduction of the hips has been officially promoted and the incidence of CDH has been reduced surprisingly . In 1975 Ishida contributed greatly to this field work in Kyoto [22]. His opinion was that to prevent CDH the neonatal hip joint should not be extended passively but should be allowed to stay in the natural rest position, with natural movement of the lower extremities being permitted.

In considering the pathomechanism of CDH in flexion contracture of the hip joint, two situations should be taken into account. Passive extension of the hip and knee joints under flexion contracture of both joints (usually flexion contracture of the knee joint occurs when a hip flexion contracture already exists) acts on the femoral head with a force which will displace it upwards. This force is the increased tensile force produced by passive stretching of the iliopsoas and hamstring muscles. The other situation is single breech presentation, where marked hip flexion with extended knees results in hypertonicity of the hamstring muscles and tendons, even in utero. This hypertonicity produces a force that can displace the femoral head upwards. Moreover, the rectus femoris muscle is usually shortened because of the longstanding single breech posture. After birth, the hip joint will be in danger of dislocating when it is extended. Extension of both hip and knee joints will produce an increase of musculotendinous

tension in the rectus femoris and hamstring muscles, also providing an important force that shifts the femoral head cranially.

Even in infants without marked flexion contracture of the hip joint, displacing forces will act on the femoral head if the iliopsoas, hamstring, and rectus femoris muscles all contract together explosively and repeatedly, especially under passive extension of both hip and knee joints.

Late-diagnosed CDH, on the other hand, involves the action of another pathomechanism. Predilected head turning is associated with such accompanying pathology as primary acetabular dysplasia, marked neonatal hyperlaxity, marked neonatal joint instability, and/or increased antetorsion of the femur, so that the femoral head is at risk of subluxation or dislocation in this situation. The adductor muscles are considered to supply a direct intrinsic force. Hyperactivity of the hip flexors combined with hypoactivity of the hip extensors and abductors might also be considered an important intrinsic force. The exact pathomechanism of late-diagnosed CDH, however, is still uncertain.

Establishment of CDH

To explain the process of the establishment of CDH, many factors have been identified; however, none of them have been shown to be absolutely necessary or sufficient for the establishment of this condition. Figure 3 shows some important factors related to the onset of CDH that can be speculated on at present. Taking into consideration the numerous causative factors that have been proposed historically by many authors, and the possible pathomechanisms and varying clinical pathology of CDH, it would seem that this condition is a symptom-complex and not a single disease entity. No single decisive factor that is common to all CDH cases and that is absolutely necessary for the establishment of CDH has been identified. In addition to experimental studies, meticulous, well-organized, and prospective clinical studies involving primary acetabular dysplasia, familial joint laxity, late-diagnosed CDH, and neurophysiological analysis of neonatal movements of the lower extremities will be necessary to

Fig. 3. Possible pathomechanisms of CDH. Because the factors that can be excluded by our preventive efforts are very few and limited, the elimination of CDH will be very difficult

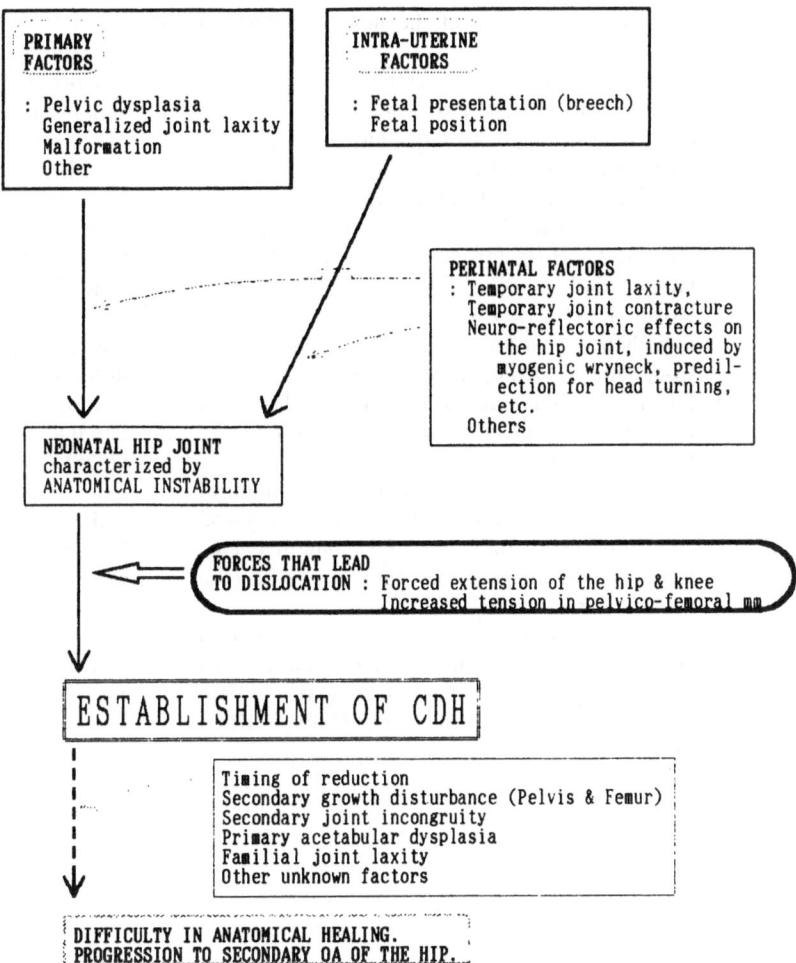

determine the pathomechanism of CDH and thus to allow for its prevention and cure.

References

1. Ito T, Marukawa T, Takco Y, Sakabe Y, Fujuwara S (1972) Arthrographical study of cartilageous acetabulum in immature naonates (in Japanese). Nippon Seikeigeka Gakkai Zashi 46:773–774
2. Ralis Z, McKibbin B (1973) Changes in shape of the human hip joint during its development and their relation to its stability. J Bone Joint Surg [Br] 55:780–785
3. Keller MS, Weltin GG, Ratner Z, Taylor KJW, Rosenfield NS (1988) Normal instability of the hip in the neonate: US standards 1. Radiology 169:733–736
4. Walker JM (1980) Morphological variants in the human fetal hip joint. J Bone Joint Surg [Am] 62:1073–1082
5. Andren L, Borglin NE (1960) A disorder of oestrogen metabolism as a factor of congenital dislocation of the hip. Acta Orthop Scand 30:169–171
6. Yu K, Takahashi M, Yanagida T, Kotani T, Shimazu A, Fukunishi O, Kadobayashi T (1969) Correlation of CDH in the neonate with changes in estrogen metabolism determined by vaginal smear (in Japanese). Nippen Seikeigeka Gakkai Zashi 43:820–821
7. Takeo Y (1965) Etiology of CDH — Especially from the hormonal aspect (in Japanese). Nippon Seikeigeka Gakkai Zashi 39:739–759
8. Hama H, Yamamuro T, Takeda T (1974) Experimental study of joint laxity (in Japanese). Nippon Seikeigeka Gakkai Zashi 48:688–689
9. Jensen BA, Reimann I, Fredensborg N (1986) Collagen type 3 predominance in newborns with

congenital dislocation of the hip. Acta Orthop Scand 57:362–365

10. Wynne-Davis R (1970) Acetabular dysplasia and familial joint laxity: Two etiological factors in congenital dislocation of the hip. J Bone Joint Surg [Br] 52:704–716

11. Funahashi K, Ikeda T, Shishime K, Abematsu N, Ueke T, Takai Y (1976) Significance of joint laxity in CDH (in Japanese). Nippon Seikeigeka Gakkai Zashi 50:868

12. Vogel K (1905) Zur Aetiologie und pathologischen Anatomie der Luxation Coxae Congenita. Z Orthop 14:132–159

13. Suzuki S, Yamamuro T (1986) Correlation of fetal posture and congenital dislocation of the hip. Acta Orthop Scand 57:81–84

14. Shimazu A, Nanbu K, Takemura E, Fukunishi O, Okajima M, Kadobayashi T (1968) Clinical study on cases combining CDH and myogenic wryneck (in Japanese). Nippon Seikeigeka Gakkai Zashi 42:786–787

15. Shionoya M (1969) A clinical study on lateral curvature of the infantile spinal column — In relation to congenital dislocation of the hip (in Japanese). Nippon Seikeigeka Gakkai Zashi 43:135–149

16. Sakai A (1989) A study on determinant factors of laterality in congenital dislocation of the hip (in Japanese). J Kurume Med Ass 52:29–39

17. Wilkinson JA (1963) Prime factors in the etiology of congenital dislocation of the hip. J Bone Joint Surg [Br] 45:268–283

18. Michelson JE, Langenskioeld A (1972) Dislocation or subluxation of the hip. J Bone Joint Surg [Am] 54:1177–1186

19. Yamamuro T, Hama H, Shikata J, Sanada H, Takeda T (1975) Influence of sex hormones on the development of experimental intracapsular dislocation of the hip (in Japanese). Centr Jpn J Orthop Traumat 18:738–740

20. Hinokida H, Adachi N, Murase M, Nakayama M (1975) Experimental study on CDH in rabbit — Role of iliopsoas muscle (in Japanese). Nippon Seikeigeka Gakkai Zashi 49:689–691

21. Hiroshima K, Ono K (1979) Correlation between muscle shortening and derangement of the hip joint in children with spastic cerebral palsy. Clin Orthop 144:186–193

22. Ishida K (1975) Prevention of CDH (in Japanese). Seikei Geka 26:467–474

Pathogenesis of Hallux Valgus

YOSHINORI TAKAKURA and YASUHITO TANAKA[1]

Summary. We analyzed the pathogenesis of hallux valgus, based on intrinsic factors, such as anatomical characteristics, and extrinsic factors, such as footwear. On radiological examination, anatomical characteristics of the hallux valgus foot included flatfoot, varus displacement and elongation of the first metatarsus, pronation of the sesamoid bone, and valgus displacement and pronation of the proximal phalanx. These anatomical factors influence one another to cause this deformity. However, the most important factors responsible for the pathogenesis of hallux valgus are instability between the first and second metatarsus and pronation of the plantar muscles, including the abductor hallucis muscle. An important extrinsic factor is the wearing shoes of for long periods, and we believe that the incidence of hallux valgus will thus increase more in future in Japan.

Key words. Hallux valgus — Pathogenesis — Flat foot — Metatarsus varus

Introduction

Hallux valgus was originally considered to be a rare disease in Japan, where people had traditionally worn geta (sandals), and tabi (special loose socks worn under the geta). However, as the lifestyle has changed in recent years and a vast majority of people wear shoes and socks all day long, the incidence of hallux valgus has increased rapidly. In the medical literature, hallux valgus was first reported in 1782 by Laforest [1], whereas, on the other hand, congenital clubfoot has been described since the era of Hippocrates. There is a considerable difference between the rate of occurrence of hallux valgus today and its occurrence in earlier times. We believe that changes in lifestyle, such as changes in footwear, have played an important role in the pathogenesis and etiology of this disease. In this report, we would like to discuss the etiology of hallux valgus based on intrinsic factors, such as the anatomical characteristics associated with hereditary and sexual factors, and on extrinsic factors, such as footwear.

Methods and Results

Intrinsic Factors

Hereditary and Sexual Factors

Hallux valgus is divided broadly into two categories, one occurring in teenagers and the other occurring in the middle-aged (those in their forties). The former is associated with a high familial incidence, suggesting the involvement of a hereditary factor in its etiology. Glynn has reported that 68% of patients who developed hallux valgus before the age of 20 had a family history of the condition [2]. These patients have certain anatomical characteristics of the foot, which are believed to be hereditary.

Ratios of male to female hallux valgus patients vary from 1:5 to 1:15 depending on reports, but it occurs predominantly in women. Extrinsic factors, such as wearing high-heeled

[1] Department of Orthopedic Surgery, Nara Medical College, Kashihara, Nara 634, Japan

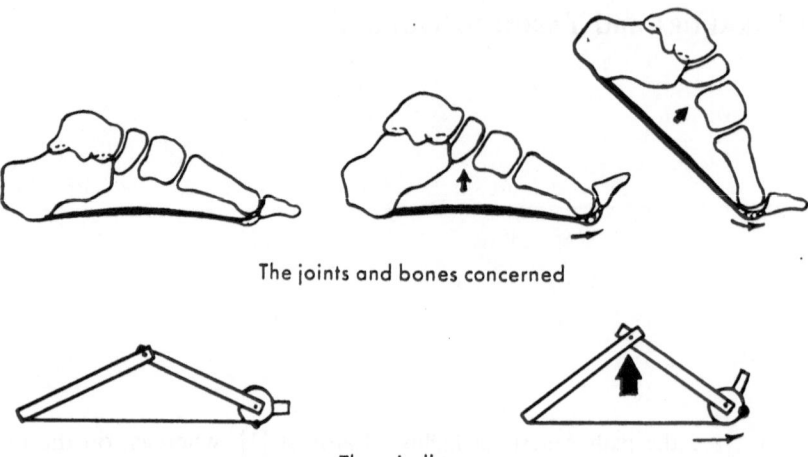

The joints and bones concerned

The windlass

Fig. 1. Windlass mechanism of the aponeurosis and the metatarsal head

shoes with pointed toes, are not the only reasons for the high prevalence of hallux valgus among women. Other factors, which have been of growing interest, are rapid weakness of the proprius muscles in the foot and an increase of body weight in middle-aged women.

Anatomical Factors

Various anatomical characteristics interact to produce hallux valgus.

Flatfoot

The foot consists of two arches, one longitudinal and one transverse. When both arches are flattened, hallux valgus occurs. If the longitudinal arch is flattened, the windlass mechanism of the plantar muscles and tendons collapses, causing subluxation of the proximal phalanx at the metatarsophalangeal joint of the great toe (Fig. 1) [3]. If the transverse arch is flattened, hypertonia of the adductor hallucis muscle holding this arch causes a valgus displacement of the proximal phalanx. To verify this, we measured the longitudinal arches of 100 normal feet and 106 hallux valgus feet in females. We found significant decreases in the longitudinal arch, the calcaneal pitch, and the first metatarsal gradient in the hallux valgus feet (Fig. 2). Thus, our study clearly indicates that the longitudinal arch in hallux valgus feet is significantly lowered (Table 1) [4].

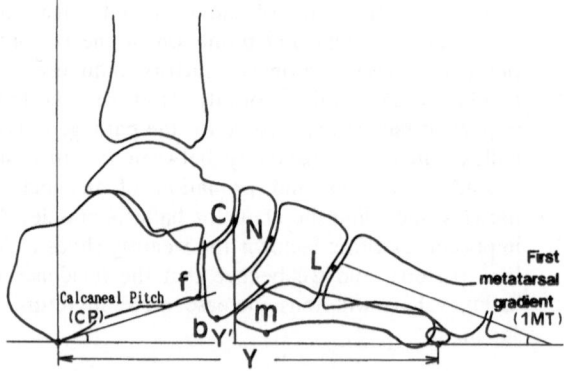

Fig. 2. Measurement of longitudinal arch by standing lateral radiograms:

$$\text{Cy (mm\%)} = \frac{\text{Cy}'}{\text{Y}} \times 100$$

Y (mm), Distance from the lowest point of calcaneus to the lowest point of sesamoid bone; f, b, m, The lowest point of tarsal bones; C, N, L, The middle point of tarsal joints Cy' (mm), The length of a perpendicular line from point C to y′

Metatarsus Varus

As the varus inclination of the joint surface between the first cuneiform and the metatarsus increases, a varus displacement of the metatarsus occurs (Fig. 3). In other words, in the varus joint surface, the distal portion of the metatarsus tends to drift to a varus position on weight-bearing. In some cases, metatarsus varus is not apparent on non-weight-bearing, but, on weight-bearing, marked metatarsus

Table 1. Radiological measurement of longitudinal arch in normal and hallux valgus feet

	Normal feet	Hallux valgus feet
Y	137.7 ± 8.4 mm	139.9 ± 8.4 mm
Ly	22.5 ± 1.8 mm%	20.6 ± 2.4 mm%
Ny	28.4 ± 2.6 mm%	25.6 ± 3.4 mm%
Cy	32.5 ± 2.9 mm%	29.2 ± 3.7 mm%
my	3.1 ± 2.0 mm%	3.6 ± 2.0 mm%
by	8.0 ± 2.2 mm%	7.1 ± 2.3 mm%
fy	12.7 ± 2.5 mm%	11.0 ± 2.6 mm%
CP	22.6 ± 4.2°	18.2 ± 4.5°
1MT	22.6 ± 2.4°	19.8 ± 3.0°

CP, Calcaneal pitch angle; 1MT, First metatarsal gradient angle; other symbols, refer to Fig. 2

varus, accompanied by instability between the first and second metatarsus, develops. On dorsoplantar radiographs of normal and hallux valgus feet, we measured the hallux valgus angle (HVA) and angles between the first and second metatarsus (M1M2), the second and fifth metatarsus (M2M5), and the first and fifth metatarsus (M1M5) (Fig. 4). We found that the HVA, and the M1M2 and M1M5 angles of

hallux valgus feet were significantly greater than those of normal feet (Table 2) [4].

However, there was no difference in the M2M5 angle between normal and hallux valgus feet. This means that the significant difference in the M1M5 angle between normal and hallux valgus feet can be attributed to the difference in the M1M2 angle. Our findings clearly indicate that the deformity of splayfoot results from a varus displacement of the first metatarsal and instability between the first and second metatarsals.

Round Shape Metatarsal Head

The greater the size and roundness of the metatarsal head, the more likely it is that the opposite articulating proximal phalanx is displaced to the medial or lateral direction. As a result, the proximal phalanx readily turns to a valgus position. However, in hallux rigidus, a deformity which is opposite in nature to hallux valgus, the metatarsal head is flat, and consequently the deformity of hallux valgus rarely occurs (Fig. 3) [5].

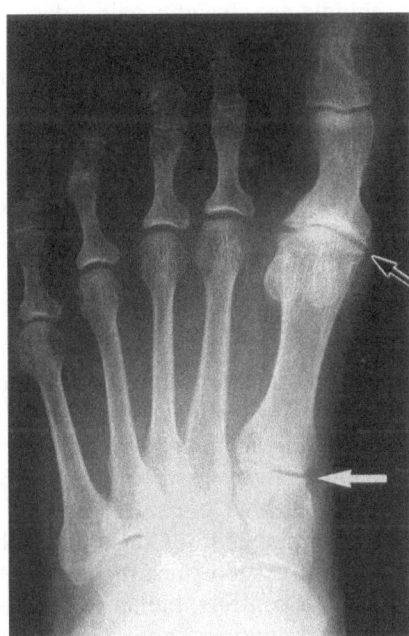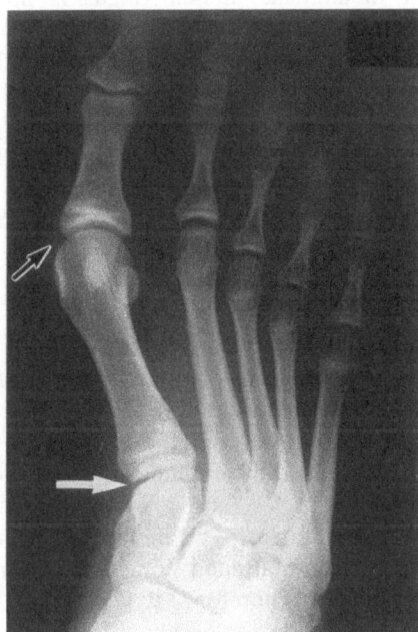

Fig. 3. A varus inclination of the joint surface between the first cuneiform and the metatarsus in hallux valgus is increased in comparison with hallux rigidus (*white arrows*). The metatarsal head is flat in hallux rigidus and round in hallux valgus (*black arrows*)

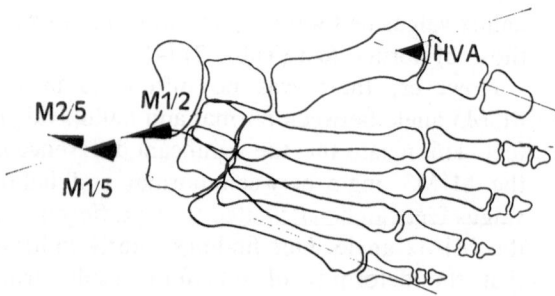

Fig. 4. Hallux valgus measurement by dorsoplantar radiograms

Table 2. Comparative results of dorsoplantar radiograms in normal and hallux valgus feet

	Normal feet	Hallux valgus feet
HVA	10.2 ± 5.3°	30.1 ± 8.4°
M1/2	10.0 ± 2.2°	15.1 ± 3.3°
M2/5	17.6 ± 3.1°	17.4 ± 4.0°
M1/5	27.6 ± 3.3°	32.5 ± 5.2°

HVA, hallux valgus angle; M1/2, first and second metatarsal; M2/5, second and fifth metatarsal; M1/5, first and fifth metatarsal

Naturally, if the first metatarsal is longer than the other metatarsals, hallux valgus is more likely to occur. In other words, the incidence of hallux valgus is statistically higher in the Egyptian-type foot (in which the great toe is longer than the other toes) than in Greek-type foot (in which the second toe is longer than the great toe). However, since this deformity is frequently observed in a foot with a short first metatarsal, the length of the metatarsal alone is not necessarily a predisposing factor.

Pronation of Medial Muscles
Pronation of the abductor hallucis muscle along with pronation of the sesamoid bone occurs in hallux valgus. This deformity is caused by a hypertonia of the adductor hallucis and flexor hallucis brevis muscles, and a varus displacement of the metatarsus. The metatarsus varus is caused by the flattened longitudinal and transverse arches. Therefore, it is difficult to conclude which deformity occurred first.

Proximal Phalanx Valgus
Metatarsus varus and a flattened transverse arch cause hypertonia of the adductor hallucis

muscle. Since this muscle is attached to the lateral side of the lateral sesamoid bone and to the proximal phalanx, this muscle tension causes a valgus displacement of the proximal phalanx and pronation of the sesamoid bone. This eventually leads to a valgus displacement and pronation of the proximal phalanx.

Hypertonia of the Plantar Muscles
A flattened longitudinal arch causes hypertonia of the plantar muscles, including the flexor hallucis brevis. This leads to a breakdown of the windlass mechanism (Fig. 1). On the other hand, a flattened transverse arch causes hypertonia of the adductor hallucis muscle. This results in hallux valgus.

The anatomical factors described above closely interact to produce hallux valgus. When simplified, their interaction can be expressed in the form of a hexagonal ring (Fig. 5). Patients who develop hallux valgus in their teens have congenital anatomical traits predisposing them to this deformity. As body weight gain and various extrinsic factors influence the anatomical factors during the growth process, hallux valgus sets in. In middle-aged or elderly patients, this deformity develops due to a combination of middle-age weight gain, decrease in muscle strength, and various extrinsic factors. However, close observation shows that they also frequently have the anatomical factors described above. Once the process of this deformity sets in, most muscles attached to the hallux work biomechanically to accelerate the process, and the disease therefore progresses rapidly.

Extrinsic Factors

The most important extrinsic factor associated with hallux valgus is footwear. For instance, according to some reports, the prevalence of hallux valgus was found to be 33% in people wearing shoes in contrast to only 1.9% in barefooted people [6]. Congenital clubfoot is known to have existed since the era of Hippocrates. In marked contrast, hallux valgus was not depicted in any sculptures in the Greek and Roman eras, and the first picture suggesting this deformity emerged in the Renaissance era. In medical history, hallux valgus was first recorded in the eighteenth century, which coincided with the

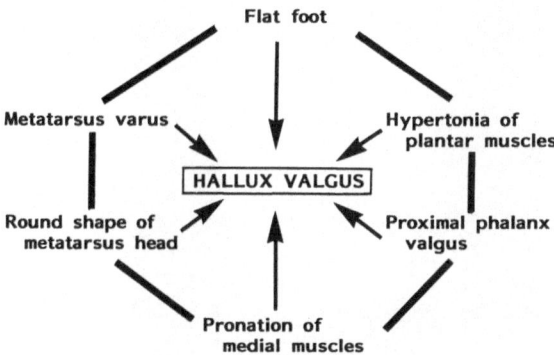

Fig. 5. Interaction of anatomical factors leading to the development of hallux valgus, expressed as a hexagonal ring

time when sandals with a thong were replaced by footwear with a closed front.

The history of footwear in Japan differs from that in the West. People in the Johmon period (about 10000–300 BC) wore footwear that covered the foot up to the instep, and later ordinary people wore sandals with a thong. Tabi became popular from the time of the Muromachi era (1333–1568 AD), and geta from the time of the Edo era (1600–1868 AD). Shoes have been worn widely by ordinary Japanese only since 1952, that is, after World War II. Reports on hallux valgus began to appear in the 1950s; the first report in Japan was presented by Mizuno in 1956 [7]. There has been a report, based on firm evidence, that showed a close correlation between the number of leather shoe manufacturers and the number of patients undergoing surgery for hallux valgus in Japan [8].

The above findings clearly indicate that wearing shoes and socks is a major etiological factor for hallux valgus. This deformity occurs with high frequency among women wearing high-heeled shoes. Even in women with normal feet, wearing high-heeled shoes with a pointed toe causes metatarsus varus and a valgus displacement of the phalanges, which are tightly squeezed into the pointed shoes (Fig. 6). Therefore, persons already having the anatomical characteristics predisposing to this deformity more readily develop hallux valgus when they wear such footwear (Fig. 7).

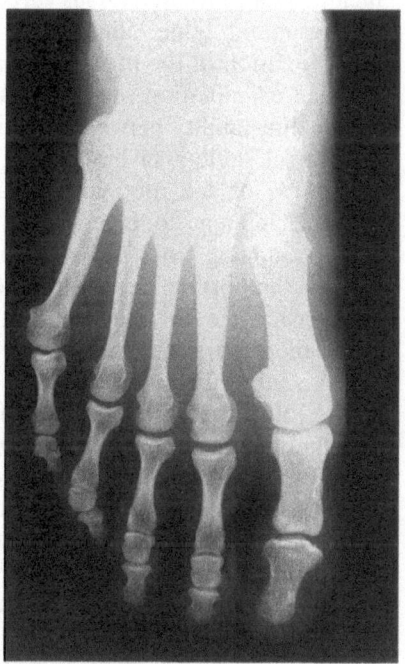
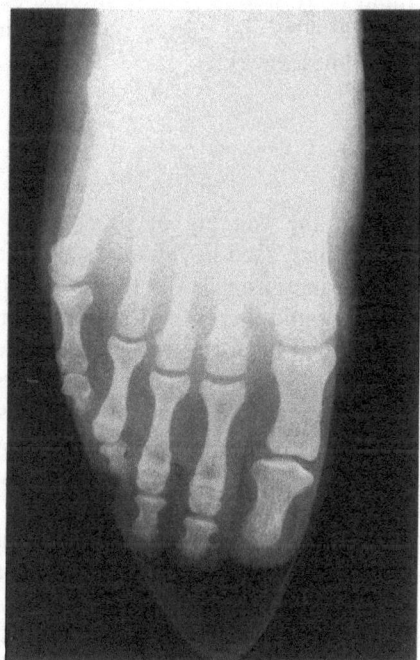

Normal foot   Wearing high heels

Fig. 6. Wearing high-heeled shoes caused metatarsus varus and valgus displacement of phalanges even in a woman with normal feet

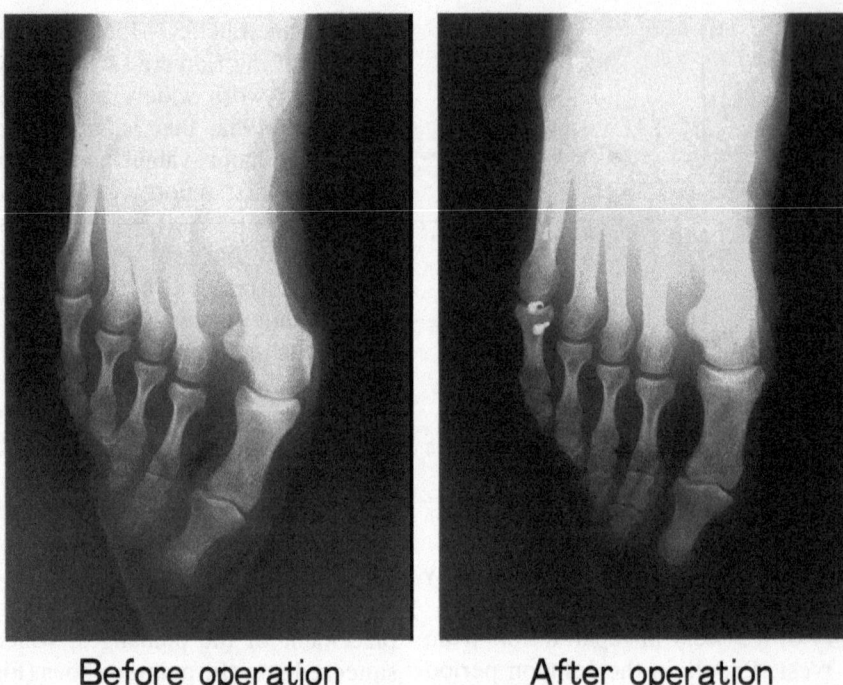

Before operation   After operation

Fig. 7. Wearing high-heeled shoes increased the development of hallux valgus deformity, while after correction the deformity did not appear even after wearing high-heel shoes

Another extrinsic etiological factor for hallux valgus is rapid body weight gain in middle age (primarily in the 40s) and during puberty (the latter half of adolescence).

Discussion

In recent years, the wearing of shoes with a closed front has increased in Japan, as the lifestyle has become increasingly Westernized. This has resulted in a rapid increase of patients with hallux valgus, which has been recognized as an important orthopedic disease. Therefore, investigation of the etiological factors of this disease is important not only from the point of view of treatment, but also in regard to preventive measures.

We analyzed the etiology of hallux valgus based on intrinsic factors, such as anatomical characteristics associated with hereditary and sexual factors, and extrinsic factors, such as footwear. A hereditary factor is thought to play a role in the occurrence of hallux valgus in teenagers, since many in this population have several congenital anatomical characteristics predisposing to this deformity. Anatomical characteristics of this deformity revealed by radiological examination of hallux valgus feet included flatfoot, metatarsus varus, pronation of the sesamoid bone, and valgus displacement and pronation of the proximal phalanx. Further detailed examination showed that hallux valgus feet had instability between the first and second metatarsal, metatarsal elongation, and increased roundness of the metatarsal head. These deformities influence one another in causing hallux valgus. Judging from our radiological findings, the most important factor ultimately influencing the occurrence of hallux valgus is instability between the first and second metatarsals (Fig. 8). This instability is produced by an inclination of the joint surface between the first cuneiform and the metatarsus. The deformity of splayfoot that accompanies hallux valgus gives an appearance of extension of the entire forefoot. However, our study clearly showed that the extension of the forefoot occurs mostly between the first and second metatarsals. Another important factor causing hallux valgus is pronation and hypertonia of the plantar muscles, such as the adductor hallucis, flexor hallucis brevis, and abductor hallucis muscle attached to the proximal phalanx.

In terms of extrinsic factors, shoes are an important influence on the pathogenesis of

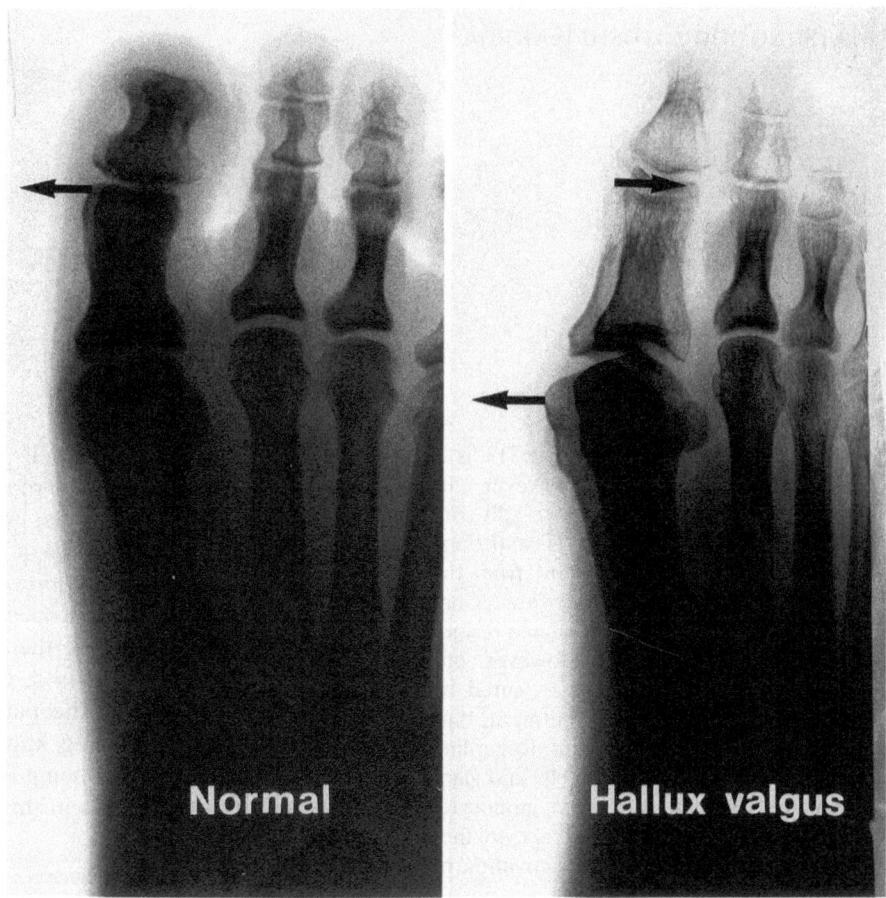

Fig. 8. Weight-bearing and non weight-bearing radiograms were underlapped in the center of the second metatarsus. The normal foot shows a stable position between the first and second metatarsals and varus displacement of the proximal phalanx. On the other hand, the hallux valgus foot shows instability of the first metatarsal and valgus displacement of the proximal phalanx. *Arrows* show the direction of displacement at the weight-bearing site

hallux valgus. Persons who have some anatomical predisposing factors readily develop this deformity by compressing the forefoot when wearing pointed-toe shoes. Therefore, it is important to wear shoes specifically designed for the hallux valgus foot. Ideal shoes provide a longitudinal arch support to correct the flattened longitudinal arch and a metatarsal arch support to correct the flattened transverse arch. They should also have adequate space to accommodate the phalanges.

References

1. Valentin B (1961) Geschichte der Orthopadie. Georg Thieme Verlag, Stuttgart, pp 187–190
2. Glynn MK, Dunlop JB, FitzPatrick D (1980) The Mitchell distal metatarsal osteotomy for hallux valgus. J Bone Joint Surg [Am] 62-A:188–191
3. Mann RA (1986) Surgery of the foot. CV Mosby, St Louis, pp 89–98
4. Tanaka Y, Takakura Y (1990) Anatomy and physiology of the forefoot. J Joint Surg (Japanese) 9:169–186
5. Mann RA, Coughlin MJ (1981) Hallux valgus: Etiology, anatomy, teatment and surgical conciderations. Clin Orthop 157:31–41
6. Lam SF, Hodgson AR (1958) A comparison of foot forms among the non-shoe and shoe-wearing Chinese population. J Bone Joint Surg [Am] 40-A:1058–1062
7. Mizuno S, Sima Y, Yamazaki K (1956) Detorsion osteotomy of the first metatarsal bone in hallux valgus. Nippon Seikeigeka Gakkai Zasshi 30:813–819
8. Kato T, Watanabe S (1981) The etiology of hallux valgus in Japan. Clin Orthop 157:78–81

Giant Cell Tumor of Bone: Current Controversies

Takeo Matsuno and Kiyoshi Kaneda[1]

Summary. Giant cell tumor of bone (GCT) is a distinct clinicopathological entity. However, its biological behavior and cells of origin are still controversial. Differential diagnosis of GCT and bone lesions with giant cells is most important from the radiological and histological points of view. Concerning its treatment, wide resection has been recommended by many previous workers. However, our results indicate that most GCT could be cured by curettage and bone grafting as initial treatment, thus preserving the function of the nearby joint. Regarding the histogenesis of GCT, both stroma cells and giant cells are speculated to be derived from monocyte-macrophage-osteoclast lineage, and several cytokines appear to have important roles in the activation of both stroma and giant cells.

Key words. Giant cell tumor of bone — Benign fibrous histiocytoma — Osteoclast

Introduction

Giant cell tumor of bone (GCT) was first described and named by Jaffe and Lichtenstein in 1940 [1]. Their name "giant cell tumor" has been the cause of confusion for some years, from diagnostic point of view, since pathologists who recognize giant cells in bone tumors tend to make a diagnosis of GCT, regardless of the fact that there are many bone tumors or tumorous conditions which exhibit giant cells histologically. (Table 1).

Histogenetically, GCT tumor cells are primitive mesenchymal bone marrow cells which can be divided into two types of cells, stroma cells and giant cells. Stroma cells are recognized to be representative GCT tumor cells; multinucleated giant cells result from the fusion of mononuclear stroma cells. Since its description by Jaffe and Lichtenstein, there has been no change in the concept of GCT, except for their histological grading, which is no longer used. GCT is still a controversial bone tumor, the pathogenesis of its tumor cells not yet being known, and the choice of treatment still being unclear. We intend to clarify these issues in this paper.

Clinical Features (Fig. 1)

According to a large series of reported GCT, GCT comprise about 5% of bone tumors [2–4]

Table 1. Bone tumors and tumorous conditions with giant cells

A. Malignant lesions
1. Fibrosarcoma (poorly differentiated type)
2. Osteosarcoma (telangiectatic type)
3. Malignant fibrous histiocytoma
4. Chondrosarcoma (clear cell type)

B. Benign lesions
1. Giant cell tumor of bone
2. Non-ossifying fibroma
3. Pigmented villo-nodular synovitis
4. Aneurysmal bone cyst
5. Solitary bone cyst
6. Chondroblastoma
7. Chondromyxoid fibroma
8. Brown tumor of hyperparathyroidysm
9. Giant cell reparative granuloma
10. Paget's disease
11. Metastasis

[1] Department of Orthopaedics, Hokkaido University School of Medicine, Sapporo, 060 Japan

and are categorized in the group of "unknown origin". Female patients have predominated in many series. However, in our series of 123 GCT, there were 67 male and 56 female patients. GCT tend to occur at the epiphyses of long tubular bones after the closure of the growth plate. More than 90% of the patients in our series were older than 15 years and 70% of them were aged 20–40 years. It is quite unusual to see GCT in patients under the age of 15 years, when the growth plate is open. In such instances this diagnosis would be doubtful and would probably be described as "giant cell lesions or a variant of GCT". Regarding the location of GCT, in more than 63% of the patients in our series these tumors were located about the knee. The distal end of the radius, the proximal humerus and the sacrum are also frequent locations. More than 99% of GCT in long tubular bones involve the epiphysis and in our series there were no cases in which the epiphysis was not involved. Lesions diagnosed as GCT when there is no involvement of the epiphysis should be further histologically reviewed; diagnosis should exclude the possibility of such variants of giant cell lesions as aneurysmal bone cyst (ABC), hyperparathyroidism, and giant cell-rich osteosarcoma (telangiectatic osteosarcoma).

To summarize the clinical features, more than 80% of GCT are located at the end (epiphysis) of long tubular bones after closure of the growth plate. Patients who are diagnosed histologically as having GCT before the growth plate is closed

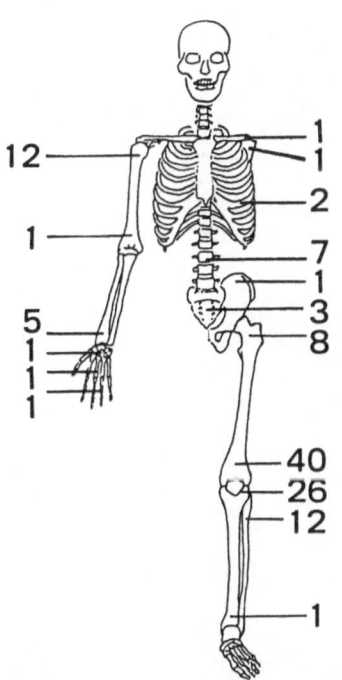

Fig. 1. Clinical features of GCT: Age and sex distribution and tumor locations in a series at the Deptartment of Orthopaedics Hokkaido University School of Medicine

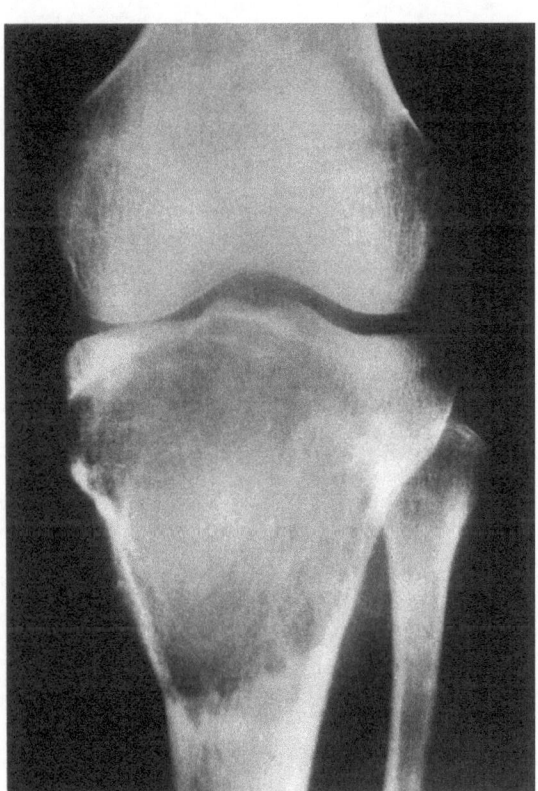

Fig. 2. Typical radiological features of GCT

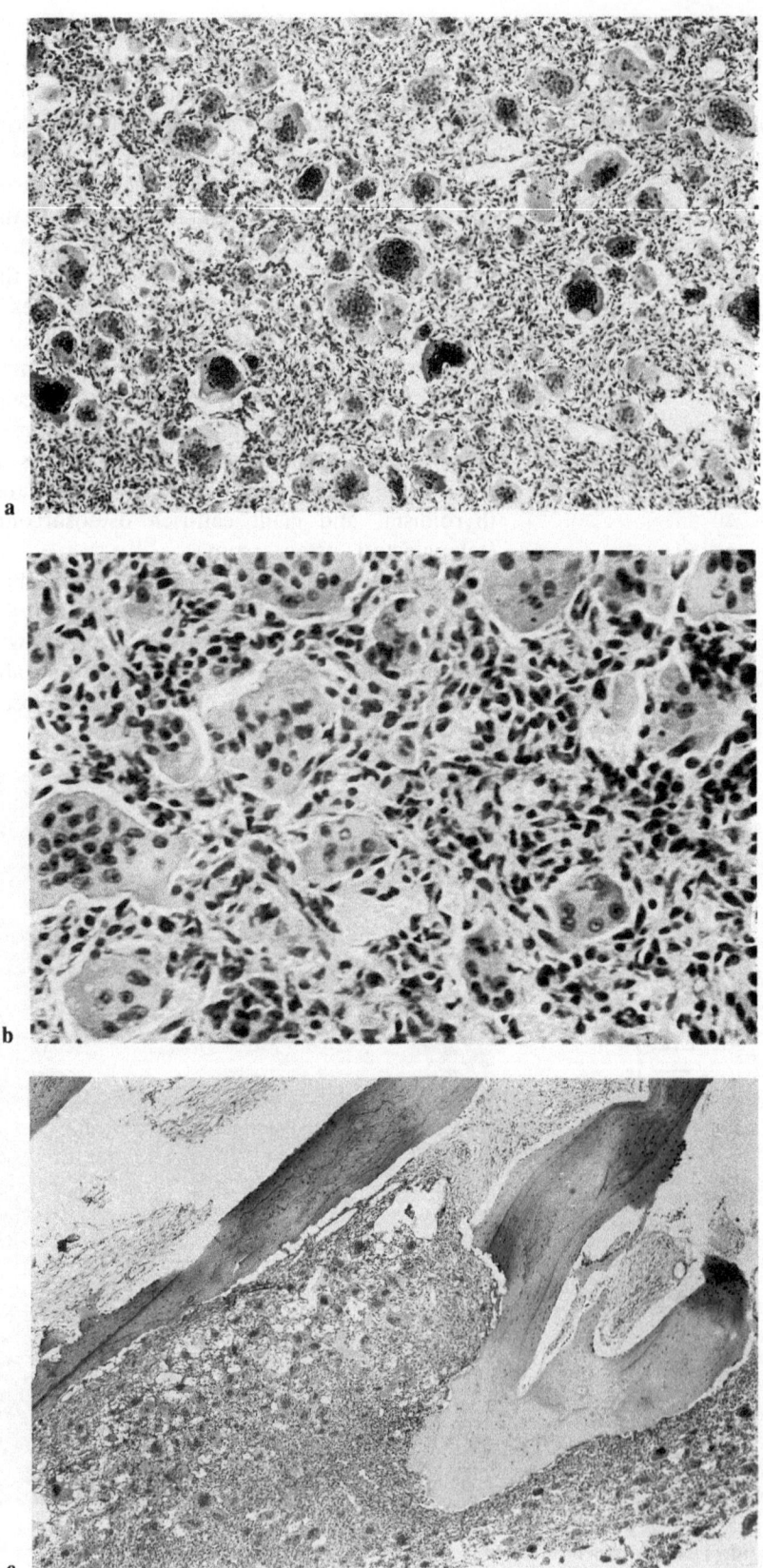

Fig. 3.

Fig. 3a Histological features of GCT (lower magnification); multinucleated giant cells are evenly distributed throughout the lesion. Stroma cells are spindle-shaped and intercellular production of collagen is not observed (×40, H and E stain). **b** Histological features of GCT (higher magnification; nuclei of stroma cells and giant cells are identical (×200, H and E stain). **c** Permeation of tumor cells between bony trabeculae. (×40, H and E stain). **d** Subchondral invasion of tumor cells (×40, H and E stain)

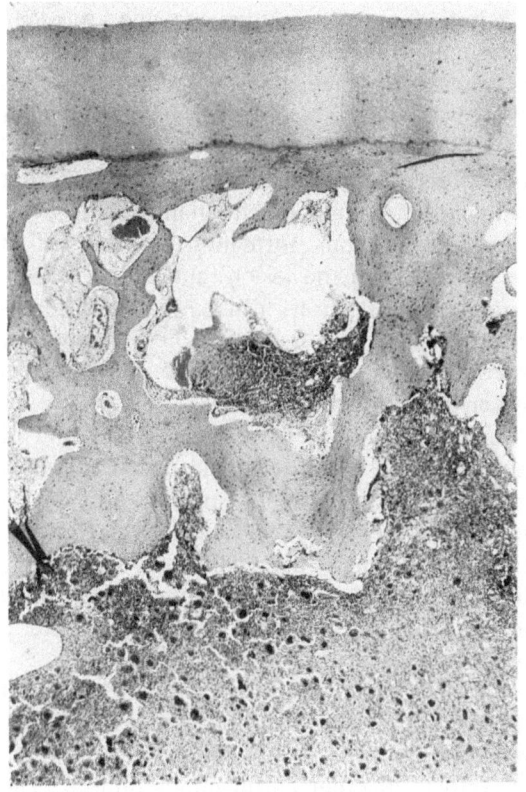

or when there is no epiphyseal involvement should be double-checked histologically to exclude giant cell lesions of bone tumors.

Radiological Features (Fig. 2)

The typical radiological features of GCT are expanding, lytic, and eccentrically located bone tumors at the ends of long tubular bones, with no abnormal ossification or calcification. The tumors tend to invade cortical bone without any bizzare periosteal reactions, which means that GCT can break down cortical bone but cannot break down periosteum as osteosarcoma does. The remaining destroyed cortical bone is radiologically observed as trabecular, with honeycomb-like patterns. The margins between surrounding normal cancellous bones show no sclerosis, and are characterized by gradually changing density. This has been categorized as IC growth rate by Lodwick's classification [5]. The tumors tend to invade subchondral bone and articular cartilage, sometimes directly invading the joint space. These phenomena are

never observed with osteosarcoma, in which tumor cells cannot extend into the joint space through the articular cartilage. Abnormal calcification and ossification are unusual radiological features in GCT.

Histological Features

The histological features of GCT can be divided into two patterns, typical (conventional) and atypical.

Typical Histological Features of GCT (Fig. 3a,b)

Typical GCT cells can be divided into two cell types, stroma cells and giant cells. Stroma cells are basic proliferating mononucuelear spindle cells with round to oval nuclei containing peppery chromatin and single small nucleoli. Intercellular collagen production is not a typical feature, except in the recurrent or so-called regressive form of GCT [6].

Mitotic figures are not unusual and are sometimes numerous, but do not relate to the aggressiveness or malignancy of the tumor. So-called abnormal mitosis and hyperchromatic or atypical cells are never be observed in GCT and this differentiates conventional GCT from other malignant bone tumors with giant cells.

Osteoid or bone formation is observed at the periphery of the lesion, and, in cases with pathological fractures, can easily be differentiated from tumor bone or osteoid formation by osteoblast rimming which is not observed in tumor osteoid tissue.

Another typical cell GCT pattern is that of multinucleated giant cells, the nuclei of which are identical to those of stroma cells, which proves that these giant cells are derived from the fusion of stroma cells. Giant cells are evenly distributed throughout the tumor and show no tendency of grouping together around a hemorrhage.

Cartilage and chondroid formation is not observed in GCT and its presence of is strongly indicative that the lesion is a chondroblastoma or consists of other cartilaginous tumors. The GCT tumor cells tended to permeate between surrounding bony trabeculae without sclerotic, reactive bone; this represents the radiological features of Lodwick's IC growth rate [5] (Fig. 3c). These tumor cells also invaded subchondral bone and articular cartilage, finally invading the joint space (Fig. 3d). Intravascular invasion of stroma cells or giant cells is also frequently observed. However, this GCT characteristic does not mean that these lesions tend to recur locally or to form lung metastases.

Histological grading of GCT has no value since it does not correlate with such indicators of tumor prognosis as recurrent and metastatic rates.

Atypical Histological Features

Aneurysmal Bone Cyst (ABC)-Like Pattern

Most ABC were secondary to certain bone lesions (so-called secondary ABC); primary ABC seems to be quite rare. When examining a lesion in which the histological features are those of ABC, although its clinical and radiological features are those of GCT, the physician should re-examine the histologial specimen; in most of cases the typical features of GCT can be found in a small part of the cystic wall. In such cases the diagnosis of GCT should be made, even if 99% of the histological features are those of ABC and only 1% are those of GCT.

Fibroxanthomatous Pattern

It is not unusual for GCT to show fibroxanthomatous patterns, which include storiform patterns and foam cells (macrophages). These features sometimes become prominent, especially in recurrent GCT and in the so-called regressive form of GCT. In such cases the histological differentiation between GCT, non-ossifying fibroma (NOF), and benign fibrous histiocytoma (BFH) becomes important. The differential diagnosis of NOF and GCT is usually easy to make on a clinical and histological basis. NOF is located on the metaphysis and its radiological features are quite distinct from those of GCT, even though its histological features are quite similar. The differential diagnosis of GCT and BFH causes many problems if BFH is located on the epiphysis. The authors believe that most bone tumors diagnosed as BFH are GCT of regressive form and suggest that, as these two types of bone tumors are closely related they could be categorized together in the histiocytic bone tumor group (Fig. 4).

Case Study — Case 1 (Fig. 5a–c)

The patient was a 30-year-old male with lytic destruction of his right proximal fibula. The initial histological diagnosis was BFH, even

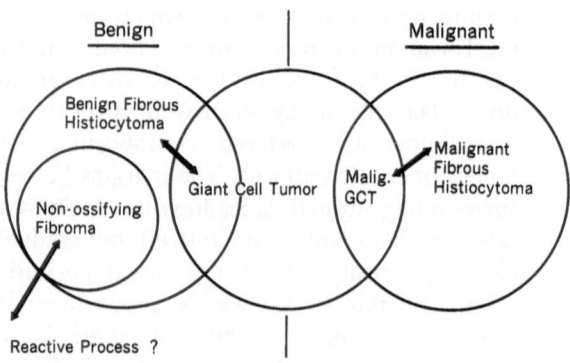

Fig. 4. Histiocytic tumor of bone

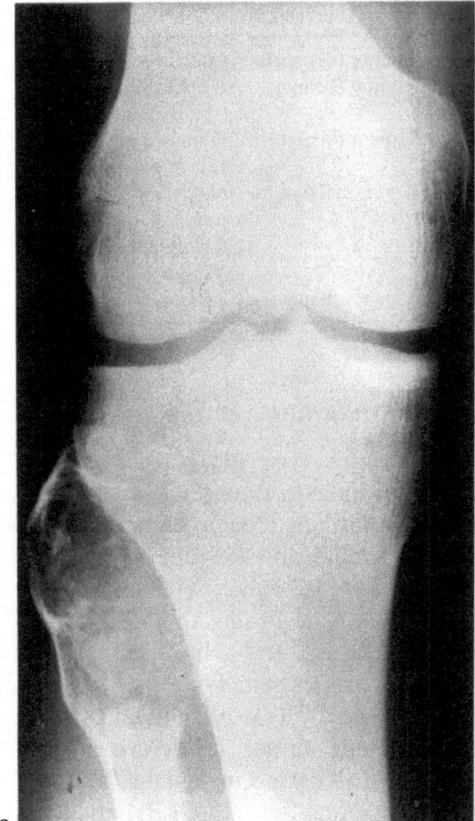

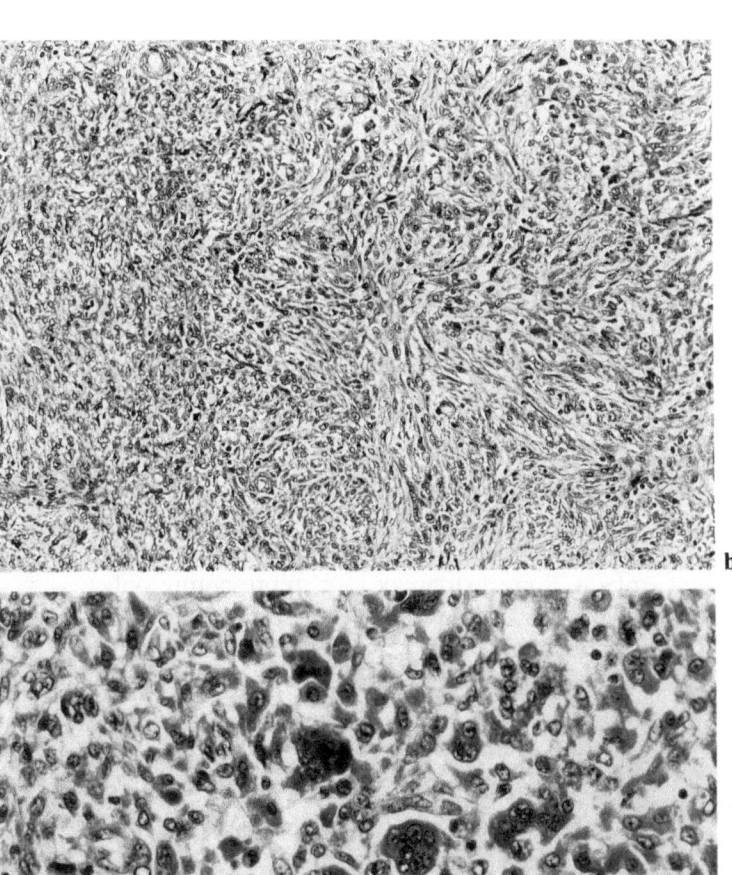

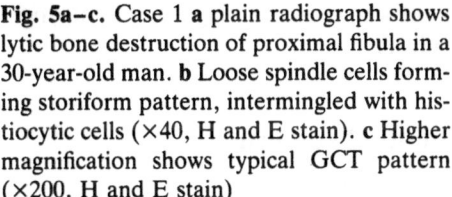

Fig. 5a–c. Case 1 **a** plain radiograph shows lytic bone destruction of proximal fibula in a 30-year-old man. **b** Loose spindle cells forming storiform pattern, intermingled with histiocytic cells (×40, H and E stain). **c** Higher magnification shows typical GCT pattern (×200, H and E stain)

though the radiological diagnosis was strongly suggested GCT. Thorough examination of histological sections revealed typical histological features of GCT, and the diagnosis was changed to GCT.

The diagnosis of BFH was critical; as indicated above, the authors believe that most BFH of epiphyseal origin could be the regressive form of GCT. So, in cases of radiologically typical GCT with a histological diagnosis of BFH, thorough histological re-examination of the specimen is necessary, and an effort should be made to identify any typical features of GCT. The authors believe that there are few, if any, BFH of epiphyseal orign.

Bone or Osteoid Formation

Bone or osteoid formation in GCT is not unusual. In our patients most bone formation was located on the boundary between the tumor and the surrounding bone or at the site of pathological fractures. The differentiation between GCT and osteosarcoma is important, but the lack of atypical tumor cells confirms the diagnosis of GCT.

Mitotic Figures

Mitotic figures are frequently observed in GCT. However, the mitosis observed in GCT is so-called normal mitosis; the abnormal mitosis that is frequently observed in malignant bone tumors is never observed in GCT. The grading of GCT according to the rate of mitosis or according to the atypical nature of the tumor cells is of no use at present. This grading system does not represent the aggressiveness, the recurrence rate or the malignancy of GCT. GCT grades 1 and 2 behave in a similar manner clinically and GCT grades 3 and 4 should be diagnosed as giant cell-rich osteosarcoma (telangiectatic osteosarcoma) or malignant fibrous histiocytoma, respectively.

Concepts of Malignant GCT

Malignant GCT and malignant transformations of GCT are extremely rare, representing only 0.7%–1.6% of GCT in large series [2–4]. We classified GCT into 5 types according to its clinical appearance (Table 2).

Type 1: Classical or Conventional Benign GCT

This is histologically benign and is completely cured by resection of the tumor; its recurrence rate was around 25%. On recurrence it was treated by curettage.

Type 2: GCT of Spinal Origin

This is histologically benign, but has a high recurrence rate because the location of the tumor makes resection impossible.

Type 3: GCT with Pulmonary Metastasis

Pulmonary metastasis of GCT does not necessarily mean that the tumor is malignant. Actually, rather than metastasis, this should be termed lung transplantation or embolization, because the metastasized, or transplanted, lung lesion never behaved in a malignant fasion, usually remaining in the lung tissue without causing any harm, even in cases when the lung lesion was multiple.

Type 4: Malignant Change of GCT After Radiation Therapy

We believe this should be termed radiation sarcoma and should not be called malignant GCT.

Table 2. Types of giant cell tumor

Type 1:	Giant cell tumor (benign):	Classic type
Type 2:	Giant cell tumor (benign):	Aggressive type (spine origin)
Type 3:	Giant cell tumor (benign):	Pulmonary metastasis (? transplantation)
Type 4:	Malignant giant cell tumor:	Malignant transformation after radiation therapy (radiation sarcoma)
Type 5:	Malignant giant cell tumor:	Extremely rare

Type 5: True Malignant GCT

We believe that this type of GCT is extremely rare and that most primary lesions of the type which have hitherto been diagnosed as malignant GCT should now be called MFH or giant cell-rich osteosarcoma (telangiectatic osteosarcoma). Also, according to the criteria established by Dahlin and Unni malignant changes of GCT are extremely rare [4]. The authors believe that GCT is a semimalignant, not malignant, bone tumor as described by Uehlinger [7], and that true malignant GCT is extremely rare. Among our 119 GCT patients, only 1 showed lung transplantation and there was no patient who could be diagnosed as having malignant GCT.

Treatment and Prognosis

Treatment of GCT is still controversial. Wide resection has been recommended as an initial treatment and more aggressive and radical treatments, including arthrodesis, osteochondral allograft, and total joint replacement have been performed. However, typical GCT always involves the epiphysis of long tubular bones, which makes wide resection of tumor and preservation of joint function difficult. The basic philosophy of treating GCT in our deaprtment has been, and still is, curettage and bone grafting (allografting) and good clinical results are obtained. Of our 123 GCT patients, 108 had GCT which arose in the epiphysis of long tubular bones; 96 of these patients were treated by curettage and bone grafting. Twenty-seven of these 96 patients (28%) had GCT recurrence. Twenty-two of these 27 patients were treated by curettage again and the remaining 5 patients

Fig. 6a–c. Case 2 **a** plain radiograph shows lytic, expansile destruction of distal femur. Diagnosis of GCT was made. **b** Plain radiograph 6 months after initial surgery (curettage and bone grafting). **c** Plain radiography 2 years and 6 months after initial surgery. Tumor recurrence is observed in the lateral condyle of the distal femur. **d** Plain radiograph 6 years after second surgery. Tumor was cured without any recurrence

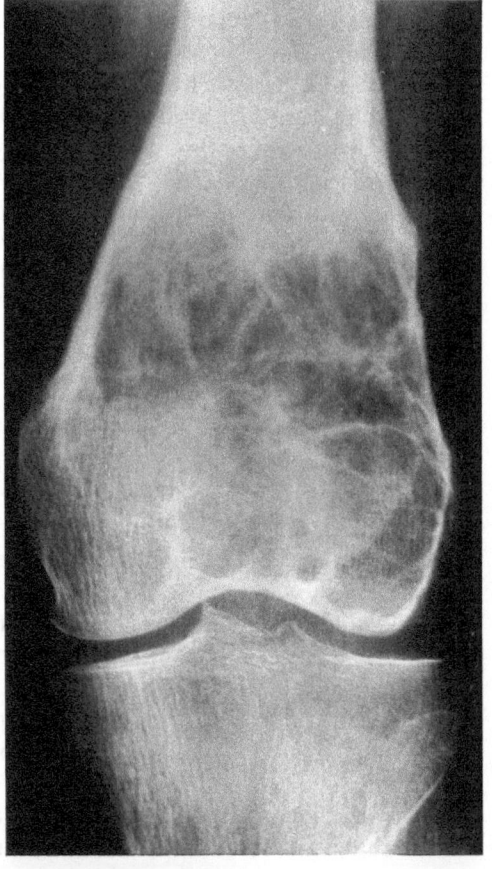

a

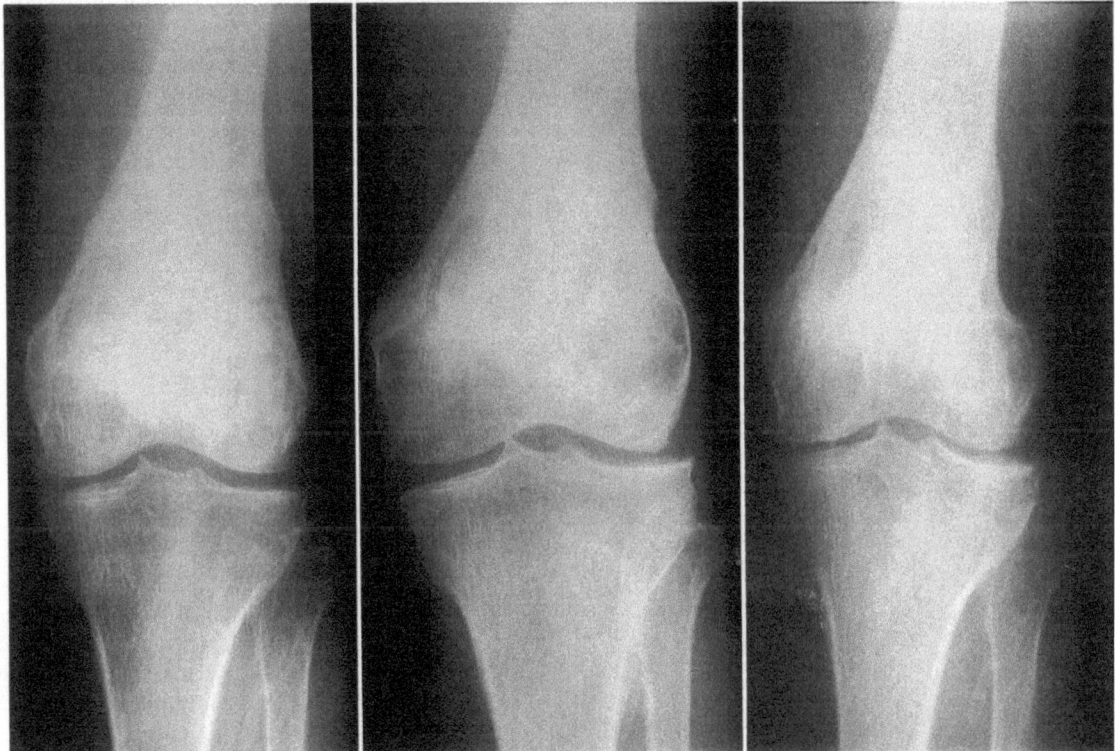

b
c
d

were treated by resection or amputation. Of the 22 patients 17 were cured and 5 again showed re-recurrence. These five patients were again treated by curettage, following which only one showed recurrence; this was treated by resection. In summary, 90 (94%) of our 96 GCT patients who were treated initially by curettage and bone grafting were cured, with nearby joint function being preserved, without the performance of arthrodesis or the need to use any prosthesis.

Case Study — Case 2 (Fig. 6)

The patient was a 57-year-old female with a lesion of her right distal femur. A diagnosis of GCT was made and she was subsequently treated by curettage and bone grafting. However, 2 years and 6 months after the initial treatment she showed a recurrence on the lateral condyle of the distal femur. Curettage and bone grafting were again performed on the recurrent lesion. Six years after the re-curettage she is doing well; she has no pain and does not limp. The range of motion of her right knee is now 110 degrees.

We believe that curettage and bone grafting is the treatment of choice for GCT, and that this treatment should be carried out even in recurrent GCT. The prognosis is good, even in recurrent GCT when these procedures are used. Radiation therapy should be reserved only for those cases not amenable to surgical excision.

Histogenesis of GCT Cells (Cells of Origin)

Since the histogenesis of adamantinoma has been determined (this tumor was found to be of epithelioid origin), GCT is the only bone tumor in which histogenesis remains unknown; indeed, its histogenesis is the subject of many controversies. Electron microscopic (EM) studies have confirmed that GCT giant cells showed some resemblance to osteoclasts, even though they have no ruffle border [8,9]. The authors of these studies speculated that as GCT giant cells usually do not participate in bone resorption they do not have a ruffle border. These workers further speculated that if these cells were needed in bone resorption they would be activated and the presence of a ruffle border would be discernible electron microscopically. Several studies have confirmed the EM resemblance of GCT stroma cells to macrophages [8,9]. In addition, research utilizing acid phosphatase has confirmed the resemblance between GCT giant cells and osteoclasts [9]. Precise histological examination of GCT, especially boundaries between the tumors and surrounding bony trabeculae, showed that there were no histo-

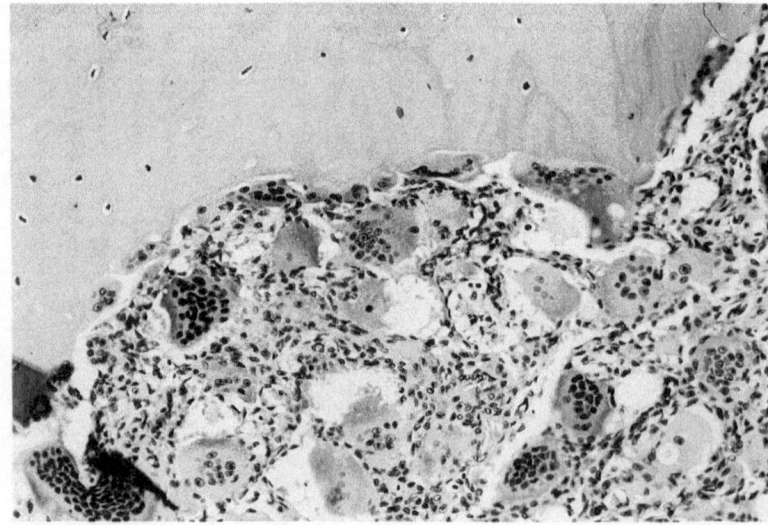

Fig. 7. Histological features of GCT. Boundary between GCT lesion and surrounding bony trabeculae. Osteoclastic activity is prominent. (×180, H and E stain)

logical differences between the appearance of GCT giant cells and osteoclasts which were actively participating in resorption of the surrounding bone (Fig. 7). Some parts of the lesion showed evidence that even the stroma cells participated in the resorption of bone. We therefore speculated that both stroma cells and GCT giant cells are closely related histogenetically to osteoclasts. Burmester [10] classified various GCT cells into four types, according to the differences found in an immunohistochemical study using monoclonal antibodies. These four different types of cells were all of mononuclear-phagocyte lineage and all the differences depended on differences of the stages from which osteoclasts are derived. Several immuno-histochemical studies have also confirmed that there is a close relationship between macrophages and osteoclasts [11-13].

We speculate that GCT stroma cells could be derived from monocyte-macrophage-osteoclast lineage and that GCT giant cells could originate from osteoclasts, and that these two different GCT cell types are closely related due to the actions of several cytokines, including prostaglandin-E, interleukin, and insulin-like growth factor.

References

1. Jaffe HL, Lichtenstein L, Portis RB (1940) Giant cell tumor of bone: Its pathologic appearance, grading, supposed variants and treatment. Arch Pathol 30:993-1031
2. Dahlin DC, Cupps RE, Johnson EW Jr (1970) Giant cell tumor: A study of 195 cases. Cancer 25:1061-1070
3. Campanacci M, Giunti A, Olmi R (1975) Giant-cell tumours of bone: A study of 209 cases with long-term follow-up in 130. Ital J Orthop Traumatol 1:249-277
4. Dahlin DC, Unni KK (1986) Bone tumors. General aspects and data on 8542 cases, 4th end. Charles C. Thomas, Springfield, Illinois pp 119-140
5. Lodwick GS (1971) The bones and joints, an atlas of tumor radiology. Year Book Medical, Chicago
6. Mirra JM (1989) Bone tumors. Clinical, radiologic, and pathologic correlations. Lea and Febiger, Philadelphia, pp 941-1020
7. Uehlinger E (1976) Primary malignancy, secondary malignancy and semimalignancy of bone tumors. In: Grundmann E (ed) Malignant bone tumors. Recent results in cancer research. Springer Berlin, pp 109-119
8. Aparisi T, Arborgh B, Ericsson LE (1977) Giant cell tumor of bone. Detailed fine structural analysis of different cell components. Virchows Archiv A Path Anat Histol 376:273-298
9. Aparisi T, Arborgh B, Ericsson LE (1977) Giant cell tumor of bone. Fine structural localization of acid phosphatase. Virchows Arch [A] 376:299-308
10. Burmester GR, Winchester RJ, Dimitriu-Bona A, Klein M, Steiner G, Sissons HA (1983) Delineation of four cell types comprising the giant cell tumor of bone. Expression of Ia and monocyte-macrophage lineage antigens. J Clin Invest 71:1633-1648
11. Brecher ME, Franklin WA, Simon MA (1986) Immunohistochemical study of mononuclear phagocyte antigens in giant cell tumor of bone. Am J Pathol 125:252-257
12. Goldring SR, Schiller AL, Mankin HJ, Dayer JM, Krane SM (1986) Characterization of cells from human giant cell tumors of bone. Clin Orthop 204:59-75
13. Athanasou NA, Bliss E, Gatter KC, Heryet A (1985) An immunohistological study of giant-cell tumour of bone: Evidence for an osteoclast origin of the giant cells. J Pathol 147:153-158

The Etiology of Osteoporosis

Kosaku Mizuno, Takayuki Takashima, and Kazushi Hirohata[1]

Abstract. The progress of diagnostic imaging and quantitative measurement of osteoporosis is significantly helping epidemiological studies to find the etiology of osteoporosis. Biochemical investigations have revealed that a deficiency in calcium absorption and imbalanced calcium regulating hormones are a cause of osteoporosis. Particularly, the decrease in estrogens at the time of menopause creates an imbalance in calcium regulating hormones. From electron microscopical studies, it can be seen that the decrease in the vasoconstrictive influence of estrogen at menopause influences the permeability of vessels in the Haversian canals which affects calcium homeostasis and influences the development of osteoporosis. It is likely that estrogen has both a direct and indirect effect on bone which can influence the development of osteoporosis.

Key words. Osteoporosis — Etiology — Calcium — Menopause

Introduction

In many societies throughout the world the number of individuals who achieve advanced age is steadily increasing. The presence of osteoporosis, and the frequency of fractures, in this elderly population is a significant problem. At this time, the etiology of osteoporosis in the elderly population is not completely understood; however, active research is being carried out into techniques and procedures that will lead to a better understanding of this important disorder. Epidemiological studies have shown that at the time of menopause there is an increase in fractures in women. The relationship between estrogen and the weakening of the skeletal system will be discussed.

Osteoporosis is encountered in both menopausal and aged individuals. In this chapter we discuss the etiology of osteoporosis and describe various clinical tests which can define and quantitate the extent and severity of this condition.

Definition of Osteoporosis

Albright defined osteoporosis as follows: "Osteoporosis is the condition in which there is no change in the ratio of the chemical components in bone, but there is decreased bone mass per volume" [1,2]. The pathological process of osteoporosis creates holes throughout bone. In 1885, Pommer observed the increase in holes throughout bone and recognized this as a condition in which bone porosity had significantly increased. He therefore named this condition "osteoporosis"; osteo, indicating bone, and porosis, indicating small holes [3].

The relationship between osteoporosis and post-menopausal women was not recognized until 1941. It had previously been believed to be a condition restricted to the aged skeleton. To distinguish the two presentations of osteoporosis they were called senile osteoporosis and post-menopausal osteoporosis. Although osteoporosis was present in these two different age groups the essential pathology of the two conditions was quite similar. In an effort to unify the two presentations of the same bone disorder Bauer in 1960 introduced the term osteopenia,

[1] Department of Orthopedic Surgery, Kobe University School of Medicine, 7-5-2 Kusunoki-cho, Chuo-ku, Kobe, 650 Japan

which indicated a syndrome of decreased bone mass [4].

Osteopenia is a term which can be applied to any skeletal disorder in which there has been a decrease of bone mass. Osteopenia is not a diagnosis; it is a specific word which can be used to describe a pathological decrease in bone mass.

Many pathological processes produce osteopenic bone. Discussion of all these conditions is beyond the scope of this chapter, which will focus on osteoporosis, which is a specific pathological disorder that produces osteopenic bone.

The rapid onset and extensive degree of osteoporosis in post-menopausal women was investigated by Riggs. Riggs called this condition involutional osteoporosis, to reflect the onset of the disorder with the decrease in estrogen in post-menopausal women [5]. He further classified involutional osteoporosis into Type I and Type II; Type I affecting menopausal women and predominantly involving trabecular bone and Type II being a senile condition affecting both male and female aged individuals and involving cortical bone.

The pathological process of osteoporosis, which creates weakened fragile bones that are easily fractured, is a condition in which bone absorption exceeds bone formation; the fundamental cause of this pathological imbalance is not well understood. One focus of this chapter will be the discussion of diagnostic imaging techniques which can aid physicians in determining the extent and etiology of osteoporosis.

Techniques for Diagnostic Imaging of Osteoporosis

Radiographic Examination

Effects of Osteoporosis on the Vertebral Spine

The morphology of bone can be objectively portrayed with standard radiographs. The standard radiograph was the first noninvasive diagnostic technique to be used for the identification of osteoporosis, and it has improved substantially since being introduced by Roentgen.

Osteoporosis is a systemic disease which effects the entire skeleton; pathological frac-

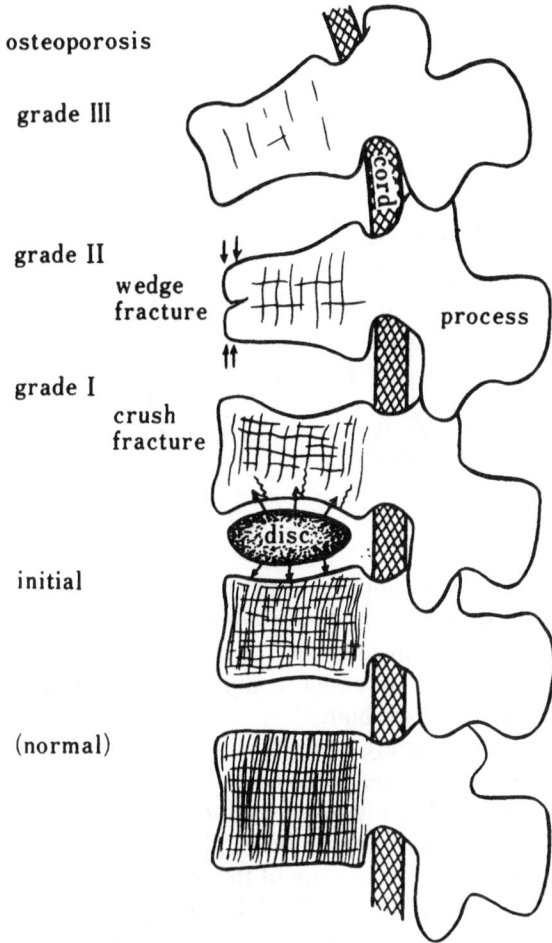

Fig. 1. Pathological changes of vertebral body in osteoporosis. Grade shows the density of the trabeculae within the vertebral body

tures are common throughout the axial and appendicular skeleton. Pathological compression fractures of the vertebral bodies are frequent, painful, and deforming.

X-ray of an osteoporotic vertebral body can reveal pathological changes in the bone (Fig. 1). The density of the bone is decreased due to the decrease in the trabeculae; this creates an obvious increase in the porosity of the vertebral body [6,7]. The osteoporotic vertebra has less bone mass and is therefore weakened and subject to pathological fracture [8].

The intervertebral disc and vertebral body endplates are also affected by osteoporosis. The intervertebral disc becomes sclerotic as it loses water. This unyielding sclerotic disc can exert force against the weakened osteoporotic

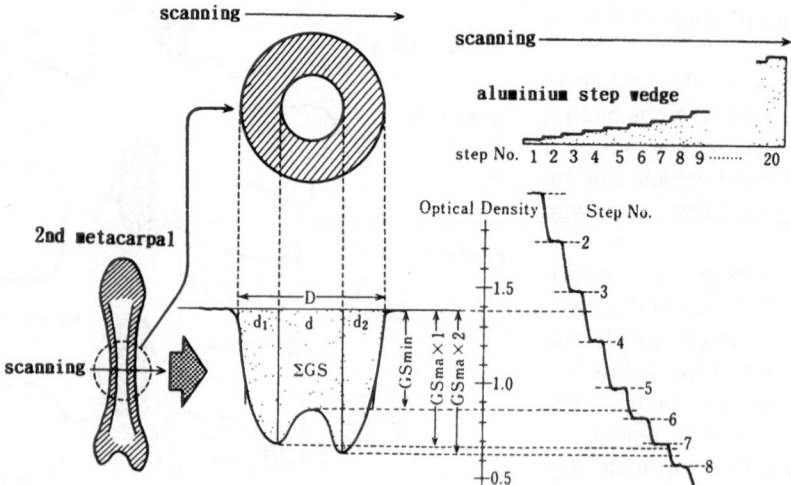

Fig. 2. Microdensitometry of the second metacarpal.

vertebral endplates and this process can result in pathological changes of the endplates. Such changes include a biconcave compression deformity or wedge compression deformity of the vertebral body.

The pattern and density of the trabeculae within the vertebral body can be revealed by standard x-ray examination. Radiographs of vertebral bodies can be helpful in estimating the approximate severity of the osteoporosis [9,10]. In Japan, this method is widely used and is known as the Jikei University System for stage classification of vertebral bone density in osteoporosis.

Effects of Osteoporosis on the Proximal Femur

Singh developed a radiographic classification of changes due to osteoporosis in the pattern of trabeculae in the proximal femur [11]. This classification system describes a progressive decrease in trabecular density in this region of the bone. There is a significant correlation between the decrease in trabecular density in the proximal femur and fracture of the femoral neck.

Effects of Osteoporosis on the Metacarpals

As osteoporosis is a systemic disease which weakens the entire skeleton, all bones will show decreased bone mass from osteoporosis. Useful measurements of the decrease in bone mass can be obtained from bones in the axial or appendicular skeleton. Measurement of the cortical bone width of the second metacarpal, the Nordin method, is frequently used to assess the extent of osteoporosis. In Japan this method is called Inoue's microdensitometry and it is used extensively (Fig. 2) [12].

Isotope Evaluation of Osteoporosis

Single photon absorptiometry is a quantitative technique which measures bone mass in the distal radius [13]. This technique is performed using ^{125}I. It is very sensitive and can detect minute changes in bone mass.

Quantitative Computerized Tomographic Evaluation of Osteoporosis

This is a technique in which bone mass within a designated area of trabecular bone can be measured accurately [14–16]. As trabecular bone is the most metabolically active bone component, the ability to selectively measure this tissue can provide valuable information on the metabolic activity of the skeletal system [17].

Dual Energy X-ray Analyzer (DEXA) Evaluation of Osteoporosis

This method is an advancement on both single and dual beam absorption techniques, this being the most precise instrument available to

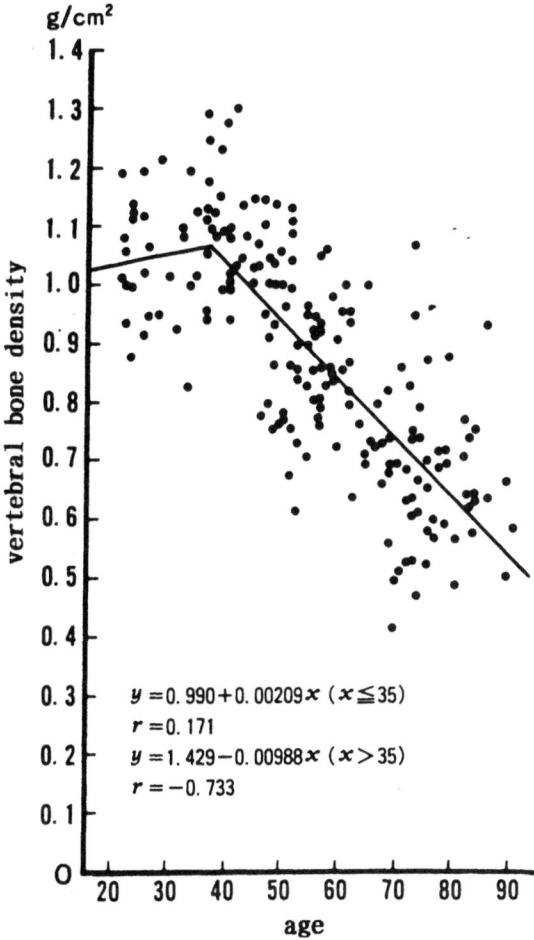

g/cm²

$$y = 0.990 + 0.00209x \quad (x \leqq 35)$$
$$r = 0.171$$
$$y = 1.429 - 0.00988x \quad (x > 35)$$
$$r = -0.733$$

Fig. 3. Regression of bone mineral density of the lumbar spine with age in normal women

measure bone mass; an additional benefit is its ability to neutralize the effects of measurement on surrounding soft tissues.

Epidemiological Evaluation of Osteoporosis

The technology required to accurately quantitate bone mass has steadily improved. Quantitative measurements resulting from advanced techniques have permitted epidemiologists to study osteoporosis in an effort to understand its etiology. Epidemiological evaluation has revealed that there is a negative correlation between aging and bone mass [8,18,19]. It has been shown that there is a dramatic decrease in bone mass in women toward the end of their fourth decade, prior to the onset of menopause (Fig. 3) [7].

The sensitivity of DEXA has provided objective quantitative measurements of decreases in bone mass in menopausal women (Fig. 4). Menopausal women who sustained vertebral compression fractures were evaluated with DEXA and were found to have a significant decrease in bone mass when compared to women who had not sustained this fracture.

These findings showed that the decreasing amount of estrogen in premenopausal women was related to their decreasing bone mass and also showed that there is a close relationship of estrogen to bone [20].

The Biochemical Approach to Osteoporosis

Human physiology requires blood calcium concentration to be maintained at a certain definite level [21]. Fluctuations in blood calcium concentration are associated with pathophysiological conditions. Normal blood calcium concentration is maintained by complex interaction between hormones, tissues and organs; the organs and tissues predominantly responsible for maintaining calcium homeostasis being the intestines, kidneys, and bones [22].

In elderly individuals, dysfunction of the kidneys and intestines can alter their ability to adequately regulate calcium concentration in the blood. The intestines will not adequately absorb calcium, and the kidneys will not adequately filter and conserve the calcium, thus blood calcium concentration is decreased. This hypocalcemia is corrected by the mobilization of stored calcium from the skeletal system and in this respect the skeletal system can be considered as a calcium reservoir. In elderly patients, the mobilization of stored calcium from the bones to maintain normal calcium homeostasis is one of the causes of osteoporosis.

Calcium regulating hormones respond to fluctuations in blood calcium concentration and can influence bone cells to either deposit or mobilize calcium. In the elderly population, regulation of these hormones may no longer be precise, and this can further influence the development of osteoporosis. Frequently, parathyroid hormone is increased, while calcitonin and active vitamin D are decreased [23-26].

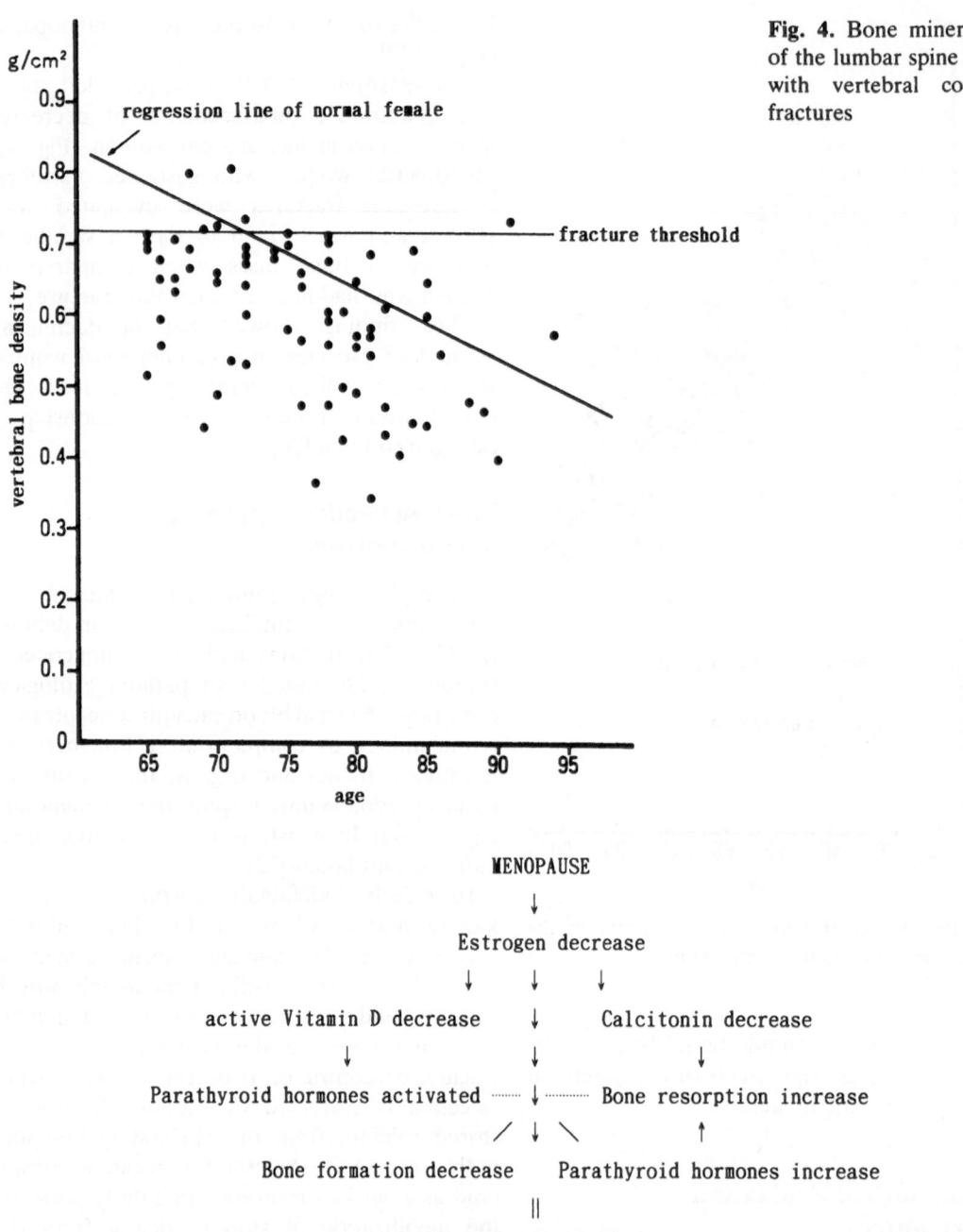

Fig. 4. Bone mineral density of the lumbar spine in women with vertebral compression fractures

Fig. 5. Relationship between estrogen deficit and calcium regulating hormones

It has been shown that there is a strong relationship between calcium regulating hormones and estrogens [27] and this relationship is one reason for the increased incidence of osteoporosis in women. Although it remains controversial whether parathyroid hormone is at the normal level or significantly elevated in patients with osteoporosis [25,28], it is generally believed that this hormone is slightly elevated in these patients [29]. Figure 5 shows that these biochemical changes are closely related to changes in the bones. The close relationship between hormones, bones, and calcium metabolism is well established; however, the precise mechanisms of their interaction and their relationship to the development of osteoporosis are being actively investigated by histological and other techniques.

Histological Approach to Osteoporosis

In many experimental studies rats have been maintained on a calcium restricted diet to assess the development of osteoporosis [30]; however, it has been found that dietary restriction of calcium alone does not produce this pathological bone condition. Female oophorectomized rats maintained on a calcium restricted diet have shown osteoporotic changes in their bones [31]. These rats have been used as an animal model to study osteoporosis.

Osteoporosis can arise from disuse of the skeletal system; experimental disuse of the extremities can result in the development of osteoporosis. The induction of disuse osteoporosis is also a useful technique for research on this condition [32,33].

Experiments involving the development of disuse osteoporosis and the use of calcium restricted oophorectomized rats have been helpful in clarifying the relationship between calcium regulating hormones and bone tissue [34,35].

We have investigated the imbalance between bone resorption and osteoporosis and the onset of fractures in osteoporosis patients. We have also created a reproducible animal model of osteoporosis with which we have investigated the influence of calcium regulating hormones on the prevention and treatment of fractures [36].

Parathyroid Hormone and Bone Tissues

To investigate the relationship of parathyroid hormone and bone tissue I carried out various experiments in rats. The femur of a rat was fractured and excessive parathyroid hormone was then administered. Following this treatment, radiographs of the rat skeleton showed thinned trabeculae and the skeleton appeared to be weak and fragile. Histological evaluation of the bone revealed increased osteoclastic activity.

Osteogenesis at the fracture site was altered and delayed by the administration of parathyroid hormone. In this model of osteoporosis,

fracture occurred repeatedly with a diminished healing response. This model is analogous to the clinical presentation of human patients with advaced osteoporosis.

In contrast to rats which received excessive parathyroid hormone a rat was developed which had no parathyroid hormone. This research rodent was called a "PTX" rat. These rats were treated using the same research protocol. The femur was broken and the healing response was observed both radiologically and histologically. In these rats osteoclast activity was restrained, and bone resorption was decreased, i.e., in the absence of parathyroid hormone osteoclastic activity was diminished. However, osteoblastic activity was also diminished and osteogenesis was delayed (Fig. 6). These findings suggested that parathyroid hormone, while predominantly stimulating osteoclast activity, can also stimulate osteoblastic activity. Adequate parathyroid hormone is required for normal bone physiology [37].

Calcitonin and Bone Tissue

Creation of a calcitonin deficient animal model was unsuccessfully investigated by the authors. Therefore, in contrast, I created an animal model in which excessive calcitonin was administered. Histological examination of bone from these animals revealed decreased populations of osteoclasts and chondroclasts in response to the calcitonin. Metabolic activity within these cells was also suppressed and decreased bone absorption was observed. Electron microscopic examination revealed shortening of the ruffled border of the osteoclasts, which provided additional evidence of their suppressed metabolic activity. Thus, it can be seen that although calcitonin is effective in suppressing bone absorption, it does not appear to influence bone reformation [36,38].

Vitamin D and Bone Tissue

Administration of vitamin D activated both osteoclast and osteoblast cell populations (Fig. 7). Vitamin D increased the remodelling and metabolic activity in all bones [38].

The metabolic activity of bone is regulated by many hormones and although vitamin D can

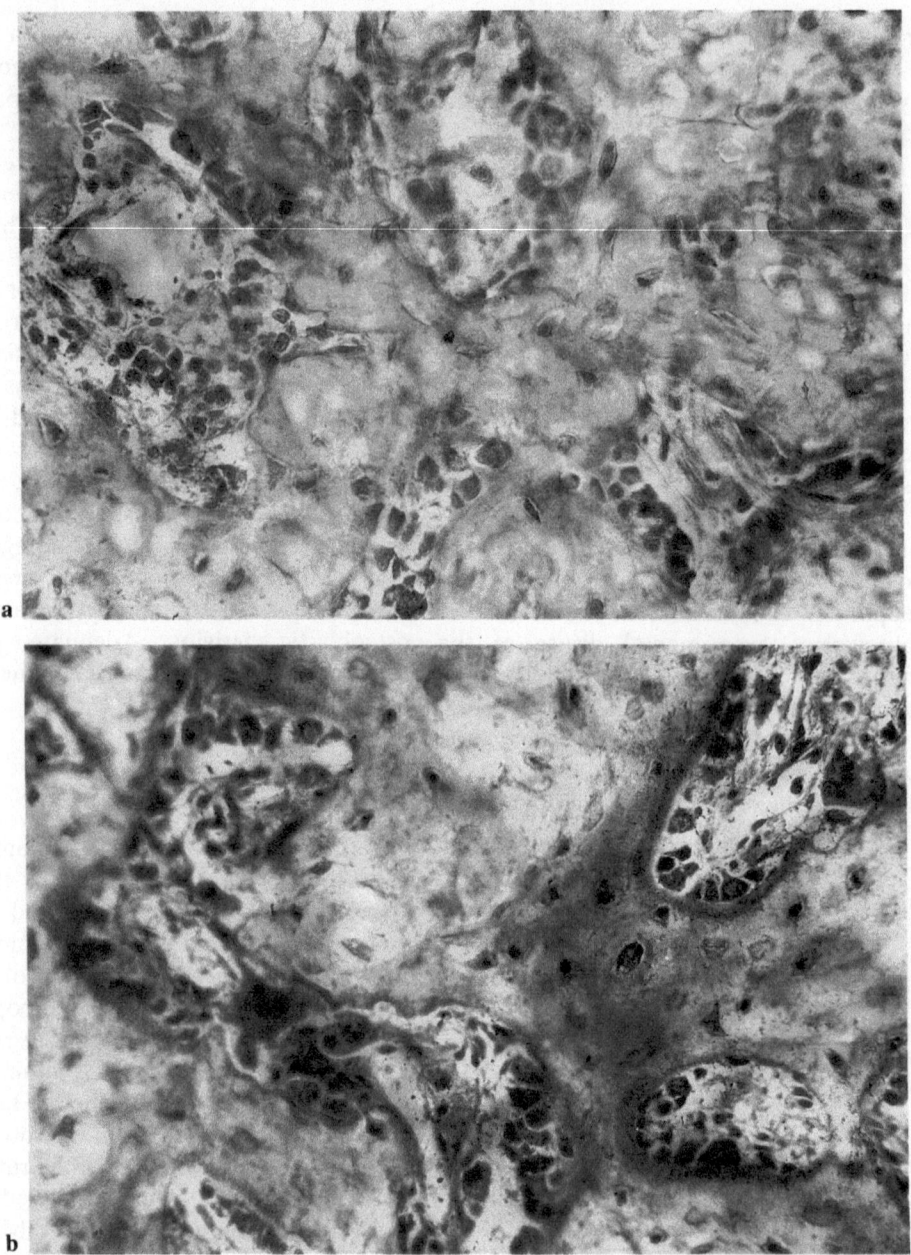

Fig. 6a,b. Bone cell activity in rats, showing less activity of osteoclasts and osteoblasts in the PTX rat (**a**) than in the control (**b**)

increase the rate of remodelling of bone, this alone will not strengthen the bone. The only hormone which can provide a strengthening effect on bone is calcitonin. Proper maintenance of bone metabolism requires that all the calcium regulating hormones function in harmony; disruption of this proper balance can result in osteoporosis.

Electron Microscopy and Osteoporosis

The diameter of the Haversian canals in osteoporotic bone was found to be significantly enlarged. Electron microscopy was used to define their detailed architecture.

Fig. 7a-c. Bone cell activity at fracture site in rats given vitamin D. **a** Osteocytic osteolysis and enlarged lacunae due to osteocyte activity. **b** Osteoclastic osteolysis due to osteoclast activity is seen along the inner surface of the uniting enlarged lacunae. **c** A bone multicellular unit consisting of osteoclasts causing bone resorption (*arrow*) and osteoblasts with osteoid seams in bone formation (*double arrow*)

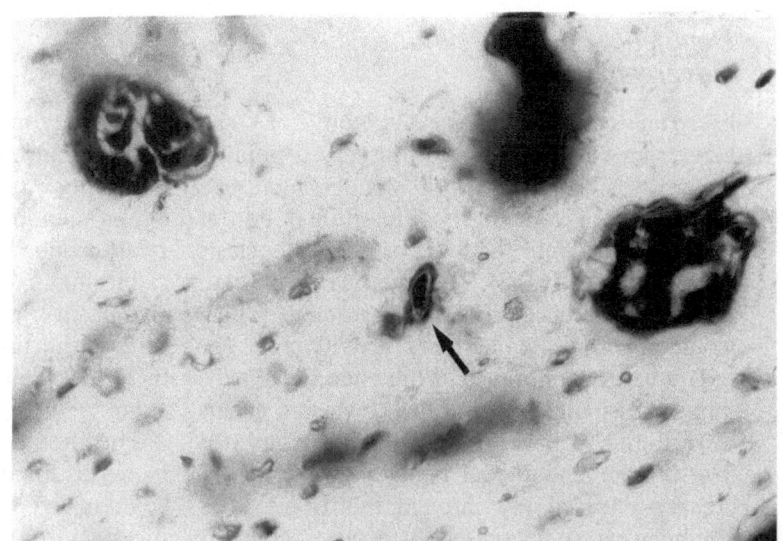

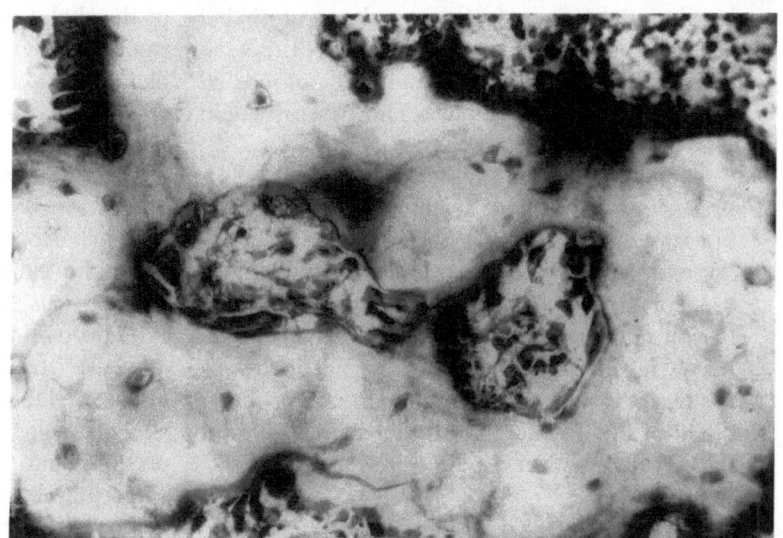

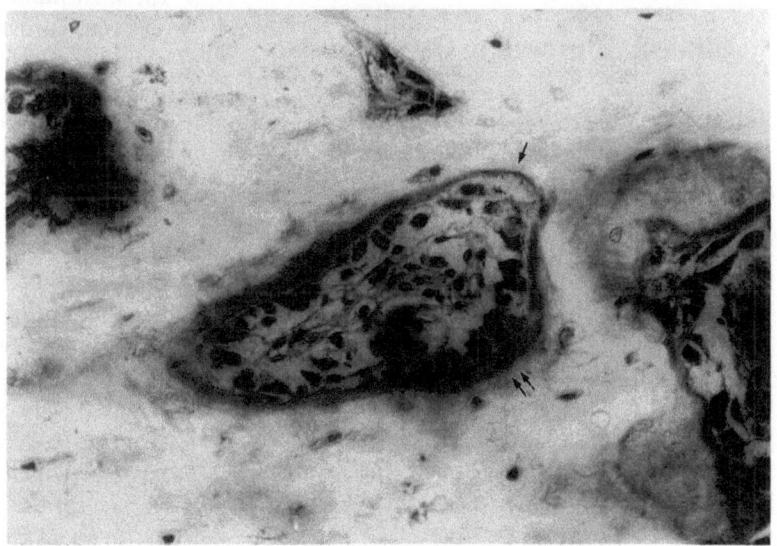

Detailed Architecture of the Haversian Canal

Electron microscopic evaluation of the Haversian canal revealed an increased population of osteoclasts and a slightly increased population of osteoblasts. The ruffled border and the metabolic activity of the osteoclasts was decreased (Fig. 8). The osteoblasts revealed decreased mitochondria and ribosomes which would also indicate decreased activity (Fig. 9).

The basal membranes of the endothelial cells lining the small vessels of the Haversian canals were found to have become thinner (Fig. 10). The thinner endothelial lining may permit increased permeability through this tissue. The combination of increased osteoclasts, thinner basal membranes of the vascular endothelial cells, and the increased permeability of this tissue could enable stored calcium to be mobilized and pumped from the bones. This process would produce osteoporosis.

The thinning of endothelial cell basal membranes may also have an impact on the development of osteoporosis through the influence of estrogens. Since estrogens can produce vasoconstriction, the absence of estrogens could permit increased vessel dilation which would result in increased permeability through this tissue. This increased permeability, as a direct effect of the absence of estrogens, could permit the development of osteoporosis.

Clinical Approach to Osteoporosis

Osteoporosis weakens the skeletal system, making it more susceptible to fractures. As the skeletal system ages, different patterns are found, in the frequency of fractures in men and women [39–41].

The significantly increased frequency of fractures in women at the time of menopause strongly suggests that the decreasing amounts of estrogen adversely affect the strength of bone. However, when both sex and age are analyzed with respect to the incidence of fractures in patients over 45 years of age, the results reveal that fractures do not arise exclusively from osteoporotic bone.

Riggs provided data which showed relationships between specific fracture patterns, sex, and age [5] (Fig. 11). He showed that the frequency of spinal compression fracture deformity was very rare in men, whereas the frequency of this deformity was sharply increased in women at the age of menopause. In men there was no special relationship between fractures of the distal radius and age, whereas in women, there was a significant transient increase in this type of fracture at the time of menopause. However, this increased frequency was not sustained with aging.

The frequency of femoral neck fractures increases for both men and women at about 60 years of age. The increase in the frequency of this fracture occurs as a direct response to aging of the skeleton and does not appear to have the same etiology as menopausal fractures of the distal radius. Menopause and aging both have an impact on decreasing the strength of the skeleton but these two factors appear to affect the frequency of fractures in different bones.

Riggs described two forms of osteoporosis which he called Type I and Type II. Type I osteoporosis has been called post-menopausal osteoporosis [42]. In this condition there is a decrease in estrogen which directly impacts upon metabolically active trabecular bone. As the distal radius and vertebral bodies are predominantly supported by their internal trabecular bone, they are therefore the bones most susceptible to weakening and fracturing in the post-menopausal period.

Type II osteoporosis, which has also been called senile osteoporosis, is directly influenced by aging and calcium metabolism. Type II osteoporosis affects both men and women and occurs as a result of prolonged calcium imbalance and calcium deficiency. It has an impact predominantly upon cortical bone. The fractures in Type II osteoporosis generally include those of the femoral neck, pelvis, proximal humerus, and proximal tibia.

It can be very difficult to distinguish the origin of osteoporosis, as this bone condition arises from alterations in normal calcium homeostasis, from estrogen deficit, and/or due to aging, each of which, alone or together, can have an impact on the strength of bones. The changes in estrogen at menopause appear to be the most

Fig. 8. Electron micrograph of an osteoclast in the inner surface of a Haversian canal in an osteoporotic patient, showing the decreased ruffled border N, nucleus; Mx, matrix. (×5400)

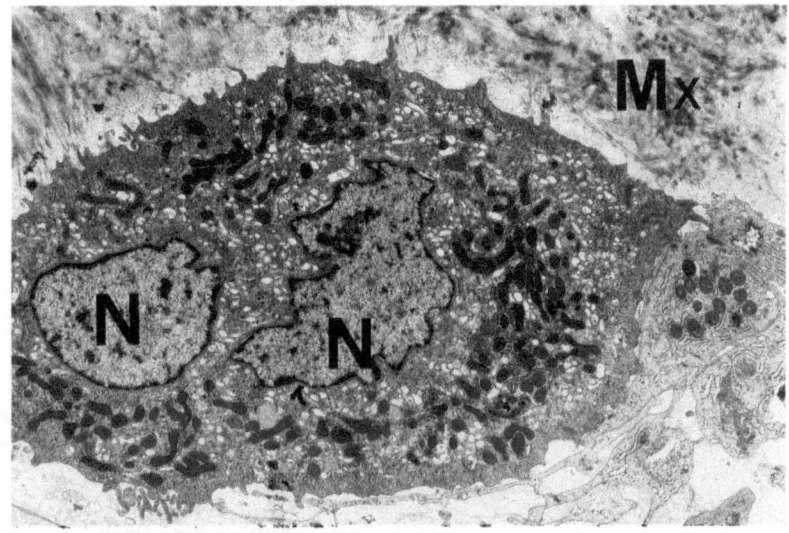

Fig. 9. Electron micrograph of an osteoblast lining the inner surface of a Haversian canal in an osteoporotic patient, showing decreased ribosomes and mitochondria on the endoplasmic reticulum N, nucleus: Mx, matrix. (×2600)

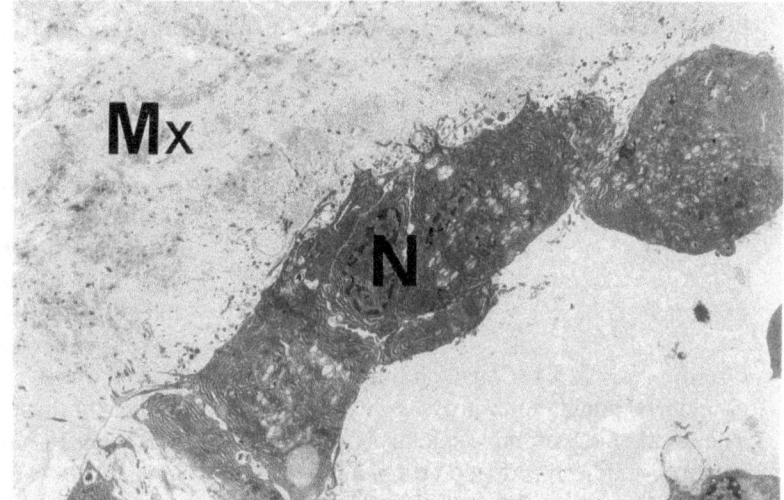

Fig. 10. Electron micrograph of a Haversian vessel in an osteoporotic patient, showing the thinner basal lacunae V, blood vessel; EC, endothelial cell; PC, pericyte; BL, basal laminae. (×10700)

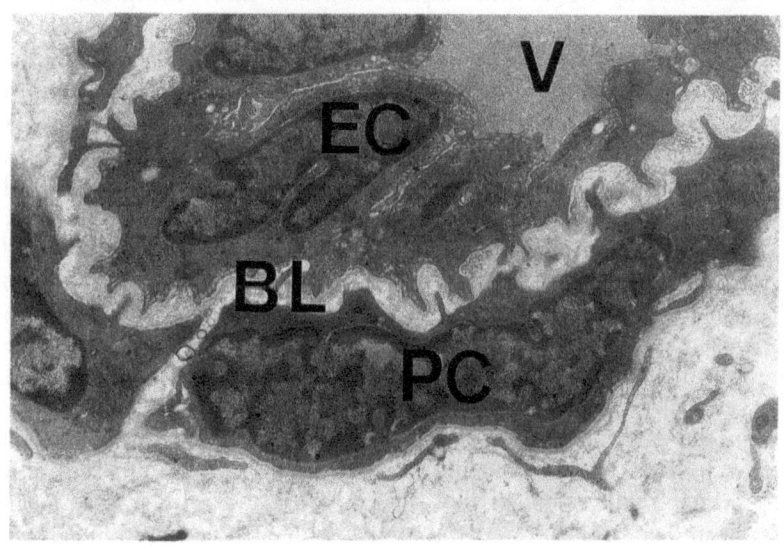

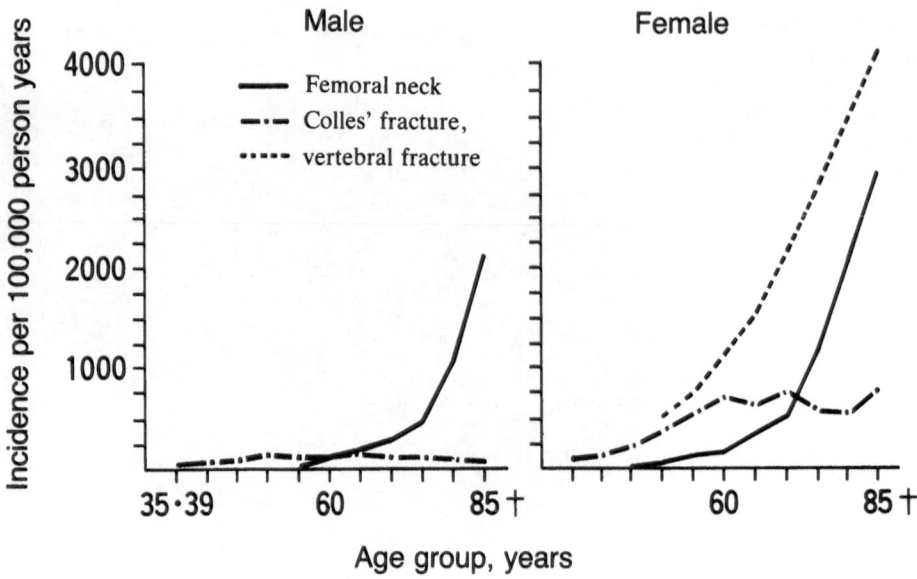

Fig. 11. Incidence rates of common fractures in osteoporosis (from [5], with permission). —— Femoral neck fractures, – · – Colles' fracture, ----- vertebral fracture.

significant in creating sudden fragility of the skeleton [43].

Discussion

Osteoporosis is a serious condition worldwide, as elderly populations are steadily increasing. The weakening of the skeletal system due to osteoporosis has produced an epidemic of fractures in this population and this phenomenon is thus making a significant impact on health care systems all over the world.

In this chapter have indicated the pathological conditions causing osteoporosis, while considering the many possible factors which can influence its etiology. The sharp decrease of estrogen at menopause, the imbalances in calcium regulating hormones, and the increased bone resorption and associated decrease in bone mass, are the primary pathological conditions which produce osteoporosis [44].

The frequency of fractures increases significantly at the age of menopause. This suggests that there is an age-related alteration in the physiology governing bone metabolism [45]. This alteration could be considered as an age-related collapse of the bone metabolism "control tower"; this collapse and the

menopausal decrease in estrogen are certainly related.

Neither the biological influence of estrogen on bone nor its relationship with or influence on the other calcium regulating hormones is completely understood. It is thought, however, that estrogen may act directly on the bone tissue, or indirectly through calcitonin.

Recent research has shown that estrogen can have a direct effect on bone [46–48], since it was reported that osteoblast cells had estrogen receptors and that estrogen influenced the production of TGF-β and worked with interleukin 1 [49,50]. Additional research is necessary to reveal the complex relationship between estrogen, bone metabolism, menopause, and the development of osteoporosis [51,52].

Estrogen and menopause are related to the development of Type I osteoporosis. However, there are other factors which must be influential in the etiology of osteoporosis. The incidence of this condition varies among different races and habitats [53], which suggest that genetic and environmental factors can influence its occurrence [54]. Osteoporosis has a very strong heterogenetic character, and therefore, in determining the etiology of this skeletal condition, we must examine many interrelated factors which can influence bone metabolism [55].

Conclusions

1. Improvements in diagnostic imaging and the quantitative measurement of osteoporosis have been of significantly help in the conduct of epidemiological investigations into the etiology of osteoporosis.
2. Deficiencies in calcium absorption and imbalanced calcium regulating hormones are causes of osteoporosis.
3. The decrease in estrogens at the time of menopause creates an imbalance in calcium regulating hormones.
4. The decrease in the vasoconstrictive influence of estrogen at menopause influences the permeability of vessels in the Haversian canals which, in turn, affects calcium homeostasis and influences the development of osteoporosis.
5. Estrogen has both direct and indirect effects on bone; these can influence the development of osteoporosis.

References

1. Albright F, Smith PH, Richardson AM (1941) Postmenopausal osteoporosis, its clinical features. JAMA 116:2465–2477
2. Albright F (1943) Cushing's syndrome: Its pathological physiology; its relationship to the adreno-genital syndrome and its connection with the problem of the reaction of the body to injurious agent. Harvey Lect 38:123–186
3. Pommer GA (1977) Osteomalazie und Rachitis. Leipzig 1885. In: Avioli LV, Krane SM (eds) Metabolic bone disease. Academic, New York, pp 307–310
4. Bauer GCH (1960) Osteopenia In: Rodahl K Nicholson JT, Brown EM Jr (eds) Bone as a tissue. McGraw-Hill, New York, pp 118–127
5. Riggs BL, Melton LJ III (1986) Involutional osteoporosis. N Engl J Med 314:1676–1686
6. Boukhris, Becker KL (1973) The interrelationship between vertebral fractures and osteoporosis. Clin Orthop 90:209–213
7. Riggs BL, Wahner HW, Dunn WL, et al. (1981) Differential changes in bone mineral density of the appendicular and axial skeleton with aging: Relationship to spinal osteoporosis. J Clin Invest 67:328–335
8. Smith DM, Khairi MRA, Johnston DD Jr, et al. (1975). The loss of bone mineral with aging and its relationship to risk of fracture. J Clin Invest 56:311–318
9. Pogrund H, Makin M, Robin G, et al. (1977) Osteoporosis in patients with fractured femoral neck in Jerusalem. Clin Orthop 124:165–172
10. Saville PD, Kharmosh O. (1967) Osteoporosis of rheumatoid arthritis: Influence of age, sex, and corticosteroids. Arthritis Rheum 10:423–430
11. Singh M, Nagrath AR, Maini PS, et al. (1970) Change in trabecular pattern of the upper end of the femur as an index of osteoporosis. J Bone Joint Surg [Am] 52:457–467
12. Inoue T, Kusida K, Miyamoto S, et al. (1983) Quantitative assessment of bone density. Nippon Seikeigeka Gakkai Zasshi 57:1923–1930
13. Wasnich RD, Ross PD, Heilbrun LK, et al. (1985) Prediction of post-menopausal fracture risk with use of bone mineral measurements. Am J Obstet Gynecol 153:745–751
14. Can CE (1988) Quantitative CT for determination of bone mineral density: A review. Radiology 166:509–522
15. Fujii Y, Tsunenari T, Tsutsumi M, et al. (1988) Quantitative computed tomography. Comparison of two calibration phantoms. J Bone Mineral Metab 6:71–74
16. Kalender WA, Bresowsky H, Felsenberg D (1988) Bone mineral measurement. Automated determination of midvertebral CT section. Radiology 168:219–221
17. Ruegsegger P, Dambacher MA, Ruegsegger E, et al. (1984) Bone loss in premenopausal and postmenopausal women: A crossectional and longitudinal study using quantitative computed tomography. J Bone Joint Surg [Am] 66: 1015–1023
18. Geusens P, Dequeker J, Verstraeten A, et al. (1986) Age-, sex-, and menopause-related changes of vertebral and peripheral bone; population study using dual and single photon absorptiometry and radiogrammetry. J Nucl Med 27:1540–1549
19. Mazess RB (1982) On aging bone loss. Clin Orthop 165:239–252
20. Riggs BL, Jowsey J, Goldsmith RS, et al. (1972) Short and long term effects of estrogen and synthetic anabolic hormonc in postmenopausal osteoporosis. J Clin Invest 51:1659–1663
21. Nordin BEC (1964) Osteoporosis. Advances in metabolic disease. Academic, London, p 125
22. Nordin BEC, Smith DA, McFadyen I, Johnston S (1965) The relation between urinary hydroxyproline and calcium balance in osteoporosis. In: Richelle LJ (ed) Calcified tissues. L Université de Liège, pp 431–435
23. Deftos LJ, Weisman MH, Williams GW, et al. (1980) Influence of age and sex on plasma calcitonin in human beings. N Engl J Med 302: 1351–1353

24. Gallagher JC, Riggs BL, Eisman J, et al. (1979) Intestinal calcium absorption and serum vitamin D metabolites in normal subjects and osteoporotic patients: Effect of age and dietary calcium. J Clin Invest 64:729–736

25. Hurley DL, Tiegs RD, Wahner HW, et al. (1987) Axial and appendicular bone mineral density in patients with longterm deficiency or excess of calcitonin. N Engl J Med 317:537–541

26. Tiegs RD, Body JJ, Wahner HW, et al. (1985) Calcitonin secretion in post-menopausal osteoporosis. N Engl J Med 312:1097–1100

27. Falch JA, Oftebro H, Haug E (1987) Early postmenopausal bone loss is not associated with a decrease in circulating levels of 25-hydroxyvitamin D, 1,25-dihydroxyvitamin D, or vitamin D-binding protein. J Clin Endocrinol Metab 64:836–841

28. Gallagher JC, Riggs BL, Jerpbak CM, et al. (1980) The effect of age on serum immunoreactive parathyroid hormone in normal and osteoporotic women. J Lab Clin Med 95:373–385

29. Fujita T, Orimo H, Okano K, et al. (1972) Radioimmunoassay of serum parathyroid hormone in postmenopausal osteoporosis. Endocrinol Jpn 19:571–577

30. Larsson S (1969) Studies on the development of experimental osteoporosis. I. The effect of prolonged calcium restriction on the skeletal tissue of adult male rats. Acta Orthop Scand [Suppl] 120

31. Orimo H, Fujita T, Yoshikawa M, et al. (1972) Increased sensitivity of bone to parathyroid hormone in ovariectomized rats. Endocrinology 90:760–763

32. Burkhart JM, Jowsey J (1967) Parathyroid and thyroid hormones in the development of immobilization osteoporosis. Endocrinology 81:1053–1062

33. Okumura H, Yamamuro T, Kasai R, et al. (1987) Effect of 1α-hydroxyvitamin D$_3$ on osteoporosis induced by immobilization combined with ovariectomy in rats. Bone 8:351–355

34. Hock JM, Gera J, Fonseca J, et al. (1988) Human parathyroid hormone increases bone mass in ovariectomized and orchidectomized rats. Endocrinology 122:2899–2904

35. Hori M, Uzawa T, Morita K, et al. (1988) Effect of human parathyroid hormone on experimental osteopenia of rats induced by ovariectomy. Bone and Mineral 3:193–199

36. Mizuno K, Tanaka J, Sumi M, Hirohata K (1981) Bone cell activities and calcium regulating hormones. Kobe J Med Sci 27:251–261

37. Mizuno K, Fukuhara H, Sumi M, Kawai K, Hirohata K (1986) Effect of parathyroid hormone on the process of fracture healing. Orthop Trans 10:315–316

38. Mizuno K, Kawai K, Tanaka J, Sumi M, Hirohata K (1985) Effect of calcitonin and vitamin D on the process of fracture healing. Orthop Trans 9:268

39. Kreiger N, Kelsey JL, Holford TR, et al. (1982) An epidemiologic study of hip fracture in postmenopausal women. Am J Epidemiol 116:141–148

40. Jensen GF, Christiansen C, Boesen J, et al. (1982) Epidemiology of postmenopausal spinal and long bone fractures. A unifying approach to postmenopausal osteoporosis. Clin Orthop 166:75–81

41. Jensen GF, Christiansen C, Boesen J, et al. (1983) Relationship between bone mineral content and frequency of postmenopausal fractures. Acta Med Scand 213:61–63

42. Riggs BL, Melton LJ III (1983) Evidence for two distinct syndromes of involutional osteoporosis. Am J Med 75:899–901

43. Judd HL, Meldrum DR, Deftos LJ, et al. (1983) Estrogen replacement therapy: Indications and complications. Ann Intern Med 98:195–205

44. Lafferty FW, Spencer GE, Pearson OH, et al. (1964) Effects of androgens, estrogens, and high calcium intakes on bone formation and resorption in osteoporosis. Am J Med 36:514

45. Meema S, Bunker ML, Meema HE, et al. (1975) Preventive effect of estrogen on postmenopausal bone loss. JAMA 135:1436–1440

46. Eriksen EG, Colvard DS, Berg NJ, et al. (1988) Evidence of estrogen receptors in normal human osteoblast-like cells. Science 241:84–86

47. Ernst M, Schmid C, Froesch ER (1988) Enhanced osteoblast proliferation and collagen gene expression by estradiol. Proc Natl Acad Sci USA 85:2307–2310

48. Komm BS, Terpening CM, Benz DJ, et al. (1988) Estrogen binding, receptor mRNA, and biologic response in osteoblast-like osteosarcoma cells. Science 241:81–84

49. Pacifici R, Rifas L, Teitelbaum S, et al. (1987) Spontaneous release of interleukin 1 from human blood monocytes reflects bone formation in idiopathic osteoporosis. Proc Natl Acad Sci USA 84:4616–4620

50. Pacifici R, Rifas L, McCracken R, et al. (1989) Ovarian steroid treatment blocks a postmenopausal increase in blood monocyte interleukin 1 release. Proc Natl Acad Sci USA 86:2398–2402

51. Ettinger B, Genant HK, Cann CE (1985) Longterm estrogen replacement therapy prevents bone loss and fractures. Ann Intern Med 102:319–324

52. Massague J (1987) The TGF-β family of growth and differentiation factors. Cell 49:437–438

53. Mizuno K (1979) Treatment of osteoporosis with special reference to the coexistence of osteoporosis and osteomalacia. Endocrinologia Jpn 26:43–56

54. Tylavsky FA, Bortz AD, Hancock RL (1989) Familial resemblance of radial bone mass between premenopausal mothers and their college-age daughters. Calcif Tissue Int 45: 265–272

55. Centrella M, Canalis E (1985) Transforming and nontransforming growth factors are present in medium conditioned by fetal rat calvariae. Proc Natl Acad Sci USA 82:7335–7337

Index